||Shree||

JAIKRISHNADAS AYURVEDA SERIES

114

DRAVYAGUNA VIJÑĀNA

(Fundamental Principles of Pharmacotherapeutics in Ayurveda)

Vol. I

Dr. J. L. N. Sastry

M.D (Ayu.)

CHAUKHAMBHA ORIENTALIA

A House of Oriental and Antiquarian Books

VARANASI

Publishers :
CHAUKHAMBHA ORIENTALIA
Post Box No. 1032
Gokul Bhawan, K. 37/109, Gopal Mandir Lane
Golghar, Maidagin
VARANASI - 221001 (U.P.)
(India)

Telephone: 0542-2333476, 2334356 Fax No. : 0542-2334356
E-mail : covns@sify.com

Edition : Reprint 2007
Price : Rs. 400-00

ISBN : 978-81-7637-056-1

Type setting and Printed by: Charu Printers, Gopal Mandir Lane, Varanasi-1

FOREWORD

I am indeed happy to write a foreword to the book entitled Dravyaguna vijnana– "principles of pharamcotherapeutics in Ayurveda" written by Dr. J.L.N. Sastry. Dr. Sastry has taken a Herculean task to compile this book in English after referring voluminous literature of past and present in Ayurveda. He has meticulously prepared the text siting the original references from the textbooks of ayurveda and contemporary writers. In the introduction he has mentioned the objective of this book is to provide a comprehensive knowledge about the subject "Dravyaguna" prepared in accordance with the CCIM syllabus for undergraduates in Ayurveda. This compendium of dravyaguna vijnana is not totally a substitute for the most refered "Materia medica" of Indian medicinal plants. But this book will be very useful for the students, practitioners and researchers on medicinal plants, both in its contents and structure. The distribution of core subjects into different chapters viz. Dravyaguna sasthra, Concept of Drug, Classification of drugs, concept of Karma, Botanical classification of plants, their collection, preservation, parts used in the preparation of medicines, various dispensing forms medicines, administration of drugs, the role of anupanas, brief history of dravyaguna in Vedas and Samhithas, glossary of Nighantus and their authors and an index to references makes this book more informative and easy to use.

The pharmacological, toxicological and clinical efficacy of a drug are attributed to the five qualities of the drug broadly classified as Rasa, Guna, Veerya, Vipaka and Prabhava. The Physical, Chemical and Physiological properties of dravyas are different to each other so as their Rasa, Guna, Veerya, Vipaka and Prabhava. The pharmacodynamic and pharmacokinetic actions of Ayurvedic single and compound medicinal preparations are difficult to explain in terms of modern Pharmacology. It is not the single chemical entity as in the case of allopathic drugs, acts on a receptor and elicits a response. Moreover, the drug therapy is individualized taking into account of Prakruthi of the individual and not generalized as in the case of allopathic drugs. The drug selectivity for a particular disease is further determined by the predominance of Doshas. There is also said to have compatibility of Panchbowthik principles of dravya with that of the individual.

The sources of dravyas, occurrence in the nature and their broad classification into Ahara and Oushadha dravyas have been elaborately discussed. The classification of dravyas according to their potency viz. Tikshna, Madhyama and Laghu is an eye opener to modern therapeutics on the rationale of selection of drugs for the treatment of various diseases in the appropriate dispensing and dosage forms.

The term veerya, is a confusing terminology with its equivalent term potency in modern pharmacology. The author has made an attempt to classify the 120 main drugs in the CCIM syllabus to the ushna veerya and seethveerya groups. This is an open challenge to the readers to accept it or modify it according to their experience with the drug.

Ayurvedic system of medicine has been practiced in the country and elsewhere from time immemorial and has stood the test of many adversities. In this book the auther deals with the pharmacotherapy of Ayurvedic drugs in lucid fashion and it can be seen how some of the new drug regimen have their genesis in the herbarium of ancient Science of life.

This book on Dravyaguna vijnana will be a welcome and timely contribution to students, practitoners and researchers of ayurvedic medicines. The purpose of this book will be served only by the progressive suggestions and criticism by the readers and I am sure the readers will be benefited immensely by this book. I wish Dr. Sastry to get more opportunities to write books of this type in English to popularize Ayurveda globally.

5th Sept. 2001 **Prof. Dr. S. Venkataraman**

INTRODUCTION

Ayurveda, the Knownledge of life sciences bestowed health and longivity in the form of preventive and curative measures. 'Swastha Vritta' and 'Sad Vritta' will cover the preventive aspects of 'body' and 'mind' respectively while 'Sodhana' and 'Samana' (curative & palliative measures) drugs are used in the management of different diseases. Except few exceptions the preventive aspects are covered by 'Adravya Chikitsa' (treatment without medicaments) and the curative aspects are mainly covered by 'Dravya Chikitsa' (Treatment using drugs).

We often come across references about Dravya under Shat padarthas while learning Padartha Vijnana. Similarly dravya is an integral part of Dravyaguna Vijnana also. But the former branch deals with the Kāraṇa dravya (causal material) and the later branch deals with the Kārya dravya (Effectual material). Therefore first branch may be called as 'materiology' and second branch as 'materia medica'. The author is of the opinion that even today Materia Medica is the fittest term to denote Dravyaguna Vijnana.

'Materia medica' (medical matter) is defined as "that branch of science which deals with all drugs used in the treatment of diseases, their source, preparation, dosage and use". Where as 'Pharmacology' is "a treatise on the properties of drugs'. Pharmakon = a drug or an active principle and logos = a study. Therefore pharmacology is defined as "the study of drugs, their origin, nature, properties and their effects upon living organisms".

Dravya guna deals with the Karya dravyas like Haritaki, Aswagandha, Guggulu, Vacha etc. There are seven basic aspects considered in this branch viz., Dravya, Rasa, Guna, Virya, Vipaka, Prabhava & Karma.

Initially Dravyaguna Sastra was not mentioned as a seperate branch of Ayurveda. But all the treatises contain elaborate descriptions about the herbs, their properties and indications. It is Raja Nighantu (17 AD) which recognized Dravyaguna as the first branch of Ayurveda.

Though Kāraṇa dravyas (nine basic factors of creation) do not have a direct role to play in Dravyaguna, they are indirectly showing their importance in the form of chemical constituents of Kārya dravyas. Therefore panchabhuta theory is as important as medicinal chemistry.

Charaka identified the necessity of complete knowledge on herbs and their utility in therapeutics. H : made a simile between poison, weapon, fire and thunderbolts on a par with indiscriminately used drug. On the other hand drug used with perfect knowledge is compared to elixer (Amrita). He also indicated that a deadly poison may be used as medicine if used with logic. Similarly a very good drug may act as deadly poison if used indiscriminately.

Further, Charaka documented that the mis-use or abuse of drugs may adversely effect the society by causing Janpadoddhwamsa (mass affect on society). He claimed that using a drug without proper knowledge is a social crime and moral defeat of the conduct of a physician. Such physicians deserve expulsion from the society.

It is concluded that chikitsa ultimately depends upon scientific approach. A physician who will utilize the Yukti (logic) and the knowledge of drugs together in practice will become the ultimate authority in the management of diseases.

With this background, one should realize the value of the fundamental principles of Ayurveda in genreral as those of dravyaguna vijnana in specific. Among the students we find a common expression that dravyaguna is a very dry subject and is not of practical importance. To aquire perfect knowledge on Rasa, Guna, Virya, Vipaka etc., one should know about the Panchabhuta theory. After wards its practical applicability is to be studied. It will be surprising for many to know that still there are some practitioners who practice Ayurveda on the basis of Panchabhutas. A foundation for Panchabhutas is functioning from Sangli town of Maharashtra. Vaidya Datar Sashtri was the founder who followed Panchabuta theory in practice and today many of his students are following the same concepts.

Exquisite knowledge on fundamentals of dravyaguna is always advised because of their utility in practice. For example, 'Pandu' which occurs as Rasa Pradoshaja Vikara as well as Rakta kshayaja vikara requires 'Soumya' & 'Agneya' dravyas respectively. Similarly the Rasayana group of drugs have both Seeta and Ushna Virya dravyas. Therefore one should know which dravya is to be prescribed in a given condition. Hence the necessity of fundamental principles of dravyaguna are more emphasized.

As a student the author did experience difficulties in compiling these aspects from different texts. There are good texts on dravyaguna written by scholars like: Yadavji Trikamji, P.V Sharmaji, S.C. Dhyaniji, Viswantha Dwivediji and K. Nisteswar etc in different languages. But there is no complete text in English on dravyaguna in accordance with CCIM syllabus. Earlier some attempts were made by H.V. Savnur and Moss in English. Still a comprehensive English text is in demand.

With this background, the author has decided to prepare a unique text on fundamental concepts of dravyaguna as well as on drugs in English. This will be useful to the under graduate as well as the post-graduate students of Ayurveda. At the same time practitioners and teachers will also appreciate the references and subject matter.

This book mainly covers the first paper of Dravyaguna for B.A.M.S. students as per the CCIM syllabus. There are sixteen (16) topics in the syllabus which are divided into two parts (A&B). Each part will cover eight topics. After careful examination of the syllabus, several repetitions were found by the author.

Karma chapter is discussed more elaborately with modern pharmocological actions. Several herbs screened for biological and pharmacological activities are mentioned with relavent references.

Research works related to Rasa, Virya etc., are also quoted wherever relavent or necessary. The panchabhoutik aspects of Rasa, Guna, Virya etc., are duscussed in respective chapters with scientific background.

The history of Dravyaguna and the chapter on Nighantu will be helpful to many. Different Nighantus, their authors along with time and inner matter are discussed elaborately.

Overall, the text is meant for every one who is interested to learn about fundamental principles of dravyaguna in Ayurveda. One can not forget the dictum– "a good physician is a good pharmacologist too". It clearly indicates that a thorough knowledge in the science of drugs engenders excellent success in clinical practice to the physician.

The author welcome suggestions and corrections from the readers if any notice.

Publishers sri Chaukhambha Orientalia, Varanasi are really appreciated for their relentless efforts on Ayurvedic literature publication.

31-07-2000

Dr. J.L.N. Sastry
(Author)

This work is dedicated
to
my grand parents (paternal)

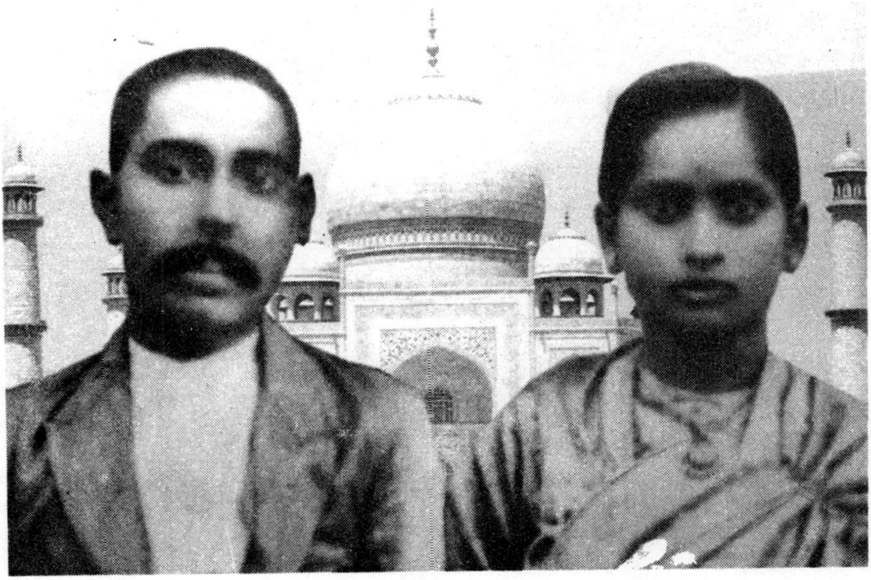

Late. Jatavallabhula Lakshmi Narayana Sastry
(Ayurveda Visarada– Ayurvedacharya)
&
Late. Smt. Jatavallabhula Seeta Maha Lakshmi

Dravya Guṇa-Vijyāna

In this subject, there will be two question papers of 100 marks each. Practical and viva voce examination will be of 200 marks. There will be total 180 lectures and 90 practical demonstrations

First Paper of 100 marks

(Part A : 50 marks)

1. **Characteristics of Dravyaguṇa Śastra :** Sapta Padārtha. General information regarding Rasa, Guṇa, Vīrya, Vipāka, Prabhāva and karma of Dravya.
2. **Characteristics of Dravya :** Panca bhautikatva, Auṣa-dhatva, reasons for the superiority of Dravya.
3. **Classification of Dravya :** According to Cetana - acetana (living-nonliving); Kārya-Kārana (effect-cause); utpatti (evolution), Yoni (Source) and Prayoga (use); rasaskandha classification-Candanādi varga, Agurvādi. The duality of Dravya on the basis of doṣa karma. Samśodhana dravya. Classification of medicines on the basis of evolution, class, shape, age. Comparative knowledge of the properties of the dravyas quoted by caraka-suśruta and vāgbhaṭa. The classification methods of other Nighantus.
4. **Etymology of Guṇa :** Characteristics, types, detailed knowledge with examples of Gurvādi, Parādi Guṇas. Reasons for the superiority of Guṇa.
5. **The Etymology, meaning, characteristics, and number of Rasa :** Analytical determination of the general principle and the various opinions of differents Acaryas regarding the number of Rasa. Pancabhautikata of Rasa. Its evolution. Special order. difference between rasa and anurasa. The speciality of Rasa and Bhautika composition. Effect of seasons, determination of bhautika evolution. Causes of the sense of Rasa (taste). Transformation of rasa. General classification. Characteristics, functions and properties of six rasas. The arrangement of Guṇas of rasa as best, medium and worst. Directions along with exceptions. Knowledge of Śamana and kopana of Doṣa and Duṣya along with rasa. The order in the usage of rasa in context of Auṣadha and Āhāra.
6. **Etymology and characteristics of Vipāka :** Analysis and determination of various opinions followed by the general principle

in context of vipāka. The properties and functions of vipāka; discussion on vipāka, causes which help to percieve vipāka. Difference between rasa and vipāka Reasons for the superiority of vipāka.

7. **Etymology, characteristics and nature of virya :** Analytical determination of the general principle and the various opinions of different acaryas in context of vīrya. Thoughts regarding the number of vīrya; Bhūtotkarṣa in vīrya. Fuctions of vīrya; Causes which help to percieve vīrya. Derivation of the general principle along with exceptions in context of determination of vīrya. Discussion of the superiority of vīrya with examples.

8. **Etymology of Prabhāva :** Characteristics, functions, vicitra pratyārabdhata and discussion on the superiority of prabhāva.

(Part B : 50 marks)

9. Discussion on the mutual relationship between Rasādi Guṇas present in Dravya.

10. Etymology of karma, characteristics, nature, types and discussion on the modality of karma from ancient and modern perspective. Classification of karma, Different tests of the Kārmukata (effect) of dravyas (drugs). Detailed discussion with examples of the following words denoting karma : Dīpana, Pācana, Saṁśodhana, Saṁśamana, Anulo-mana, Bhedana, Recana, lekhana, Grāhī, Stambhana, Madakāri, Pramāthi, Vyavāyi, Vikāsi.

11. Determination of the botanical classification according to shape, properties, actions, class, famous effects, similarities etc. such as – Daśamūla, various panca mūla, panca valkala, panca pallava, Triphala, Trikatu, Trimada, Caturūṣana, Panca kola, Ṣadūṣana caturbīja, Jīvanīya gana, Aṣta varga, Trijātaka, catur jātaka, panca tikta, pancamla, mahapanca viṣa and upaviṣādi. In drugs of animal origin -kṣirāṣṭaka, Mūtrāṣṭaka, Pittapancaka.

    In drugs of mineral origin - lavanapancaka, kṣāra dravya and kṣārāṣṭaka.

12. **The basis of the Nomenclature and synonyms of Drugs :** Country-soil-divisions. The collection of drugs and the characteristics of the collected drugs. Knowledge of the method of collection. Knowledge of drugs of plant origin according to different parts. Knowledge of the time for collection. Collection of the dravya according to vīrya. Collection of food articles and drugs of animal origin. Preservation

methods of the collected drugs. Drug storage area. The preservation of collected drugs by dry and wet methods. Definition of māna (measurements)– 1. Pautava 2. Druvaya 3. Pāyya mānās and discussion according to ancient and modern view.

13. Various impurities of drugs. Purification of drugs, methods of purification of drugs, and knowledge of synthetic drugs.

14. Good medicinal drug, usage of medicinal drug. The part used as medicine, combinations of drugs and incompatible drugs. Yogās of auṣadhis (medicinal formulae); discussion on the quantity and posology of drugs. Role of age, Bala (Immunity), sex, Agni, Doṣa, Dūṣya, Vyādhi, Koṣṭha, Nature of the drug, Habit, Sattva (mental condition), Place, time and formulation in determining the dose. Anupāna, Times of medication. Routes of medication. Knowledge of writing Prescriptions.

15. A Brief history of the science of Dravya-Guṇa. The seed of Dravya guṇa śaṣtra in ancient times and in the vedas. The doctrine of Dravya guṇa in Āyurvediya Saṁhitās and the list of drugs.

16. **During medieval times :** Aṣṭāñgā Nighantu, Paryaya ratnamāla, Dhanvantari nighanṭu, Soḍhala nighanṭu, Hṛdaya dīpaka, Siddhamantra prakāra, Mādhava kṛta dravyaguṇa, Cakrapānidatta kṛta dravya guṇa Samgraha. Madana pāla nighanṭu, Rājanighanṭu, Kaiyadeva nighanṭu etc. Discussion regarding the period and authors of these works. Knowledge of the subject and arrangement. Knowledge of the Books of Dravyaguna Śastra written by modern scholars.

CONTANTS

Foreword III to IV

Introduction V to VIII

1. *Chapter-I* 1-3
Introduction to Dravya guna Sastra

2. *Chapter-II* 4-18
Concept of Dravya

3. *Chapter-III* 19-44
Classification of Dravya

4. *Chapter-IV* 45-88
Concept of Guna

5. *Chapter-V* 89-129
Concept of Rasa

6. *Chapter-VI* 130-153
Concept of Vipaka

7. *Chapter-VII* 154-171
Concept of Virya

8. *Chapter-VIII* 172-182
Concept of Prabhava

9. *Chapter-IX* 183-184
Relation between Rasidi gunas

10. *Chapter-X* 185-267
Concept of Karma

11. *Chapter-XI* 268-291
Botanical Classification and Different Groups of Drugs used in Ayurveda

12. *Chapter-XII* 292-318
Nomenclature; Soil-types; Collection of Drugs; Preservation Methods and Measurements

13. *Chapter-XIII* 319-336
Impurities in Drugs and their Purification Methods

14. *Chapter-XIV* 337-380
Ideal Drug; Parts used; Drug Combinations; Incompatible Drugs; Posology; Anupana (Vehicle); Times of Drug administration; Routs of Drug Administration and Prescription writing

15. *Chapter-XV* 381-401
Brief History of Dravya Guna in Vedas and Samhitas

16. *Chapter-XVI* 402-435
Knowledge about Various Nighantus and their Authors, Dravya Guna Books by Modern Scholars

17. *Index* 436-441

✸

Chapter -I

Introduction to Dravyaguna Sastra

1. Characteristics of Dravyaguna Sastra

The first mentioning of Dravyaguna is traceable from the descriptions of Charaka who defined Ayurveda as the science which deals with the Dravyas-Gunas & Karmas of helpful and harmful materials[1].

Dravyaguna Sastra has been identified as a seperate speciality by Narahari; the author of Raja Nighantu (17.AD)[2]. Actually Ayurveda advocates the concept of pharmacotherapeutics and clinical pharmacology but not pharmacology and therapeutics seperately.

Acharya Priyavrata Sharma defined Dravyaguna Sastra as the branch which deals with the properties, action and therapeutic effects of various dravyas (drugs).[3]

2. Seven Constituents of Dravya

Bhavamishra (16-17 AD) quoted about the five constituents of a dravya viz.; Rasa (taste). Virya (potency), Vipaka (metabolite), Guna (property) and Prabhava (non-specific activity)[4]. Adding Dravya and Karma (action) to the above five Acharya Yadavji Trikamji mentioned about Sapta Padarthas' (seven constituents of Dravya). Dravyaguna Sastra mainly deals with these seven aspects under the fundamental principles.

(1) Dravya *(Drug)*

A substance which possess Guna (properties) and Karma (action) with inhernt relation in it is known as Dravya[5].

---

१. यतश्चायुष्याणि अनायुष्याणि च द्रव्यगुणकर्माणि वेदयत्यतोऽप्यायुर्वेदः। (च.सू. ३०)

२. द्रव्याभिधानगदनिश्चयकायसौख्यं । (रा.नि.)

३. द्रव्याणां गुणकर्माणि प्रयोगाः विविधास्तथा ।
सर्वशो यत्र वर्ण्यन्ते शास्त्रं द्रव्यगुणं हि तत् ।। (द्र. गु. वि.)

४. द्रव्ये रसो गुणो वीर्यं विपाकः शक्तिरेवच ।
पदार्थाः पञ्च तिष्ठन्ति स्वं स्वं कुर्वन्ति कर्म च।। (भा. प्र.)

५. यत्राश्रिताः कर्मगुणाः कारणं समवायि यत् तद्रव्यं । (च.सू.१)

It is further clarified that a karya dravya (drags etc.) which is used in the health management as well as the disease management will definitely possess some or the other pharmacological properties e.g. dravyas like Haritaki, shatavari, Godhuma, Brahmi etc.

(2) Rasa *(Taste)*

The property which is percieved through the taste-buds i.e.Rasanendriya) is known as Rasa[1].

The taste of a substance will be detected only when it is exposed to the tongue and when the taste buds are functioning corre-ctly. Ayurveda accepted six tastes viz., Madhura (sweet), Amla (Sour), Lavana (Salt), Katu (Spice), Tikta (bitter) & Kashaya (astringent).

(3) Guna *(Physical Property)*

It is the property which will have inherent relation with the dravya but remain inactive. That means it can not perform any activity of its own without the help of other ingredients. It also acts as non-inherent reason (Asamavaya Karana) for a given therapeutic effect[2] e.g., Snigdha (unctuous) Seeta (cold), Tikshna (stimulant) etc.

Though all the physical and chemical properties are considered as Gunas, specifically physical properties are acceptable under Guna in this context. Chemical properties at various stages will fall under rasa, virya & vipaka.

(4) Virya *(Potency)*

It is the property by which the drug produces the therapeutic effect. It is also mentioned that every action of a drug is under the control of virya. e.g., Seeta virya (endothermic) and Ushna virya (exothermic)[3].

This may be considered as the unmetabolized pharmacologically active ingredient of a drug which performs the pharmacological activity e.g. morphines toxicity of 1st and 2nd stages

१. रसनार्थो रसः........................। चक्रपाणिः रस्यते आस्वाद्यते इति रसः । (च. सू.१)
२. समवायी तु निश्चेष्टः कारणं गुणः । (च. सू. १)
३. वीर्यं तु क्रियते येन या क्रिया।
ना वीर्यं कुरुते किञ्चित् सर्वा वीर्यकृताः क्रियाः ॥ (च. सू. २६)

occur before metabolization and after conjugation the 3rd state of toxicity occurs (i.e., after metabolized).

(5) Vipaka *(Drug Metabolism)*

It is the property of a durg which is responsible for the change in the original taste etc., on exposure to GIT enzymes and which is responsible for the final form of the drug in side the body[1] e.g., Madhura, Amla, Katu vipaka.

(6) Prabhava *(non-specific activity)*

When a drug produces a result which is not in accordance with the constituents viz.; Rasa, Guna, Virya, Vipaka, then it is denoted as Prabhava or Shakti[2]; e.g., Sirisha acting as Vishaghna, Pushkara-mula acting as Hridya etc.

(7) Karma *(pharmacological action)*

The inseperable reason for the association (Samyoga) and dissociation (Vibhaga) of a drug in exhibiting its pharmacological action is known as 'Karma' and it is independent[3], e.g., Deepana (appetizer), Pachana (digestive) etc.

---

१. जाठरेणाग्निना योगाद्यदुदेति रसान्तरम् ।
रसानां परणियान्ते स विपाक इति स्मृतः ॥ (अ. हृ. सू. १)

२. रसवीर्यविपाकानां सामान्यं यत्र लक्ष्यते ।
विशिष्टः कर्मणां चैव प्रभावस्तस्य स स्मृतः ॥ (च. सू. २६)

३. संयोगे च विभागेच कारणं द्रव्यमाश्रितम् ।
कर्तव्यस्य क्रिया कर्म, कर्म नान्यदपेक्षते ॥ (च. सू. १)

Chapter -II

Concept of Dravya

1. Definition of Dravya

A drug (dravya) is defined as a substance which will possess properties (guna) and actions (karma) together with an inherent relation[1,2] .In this context chakrapani explained that Guna term includes rasa, virya, vipaka also[3].

Vaiseshika Philosophy and Sushrita Samhita have accepted similar definition for dravya i.e., kriya and guna will have an inherent relation with the drug[4,5].

To understand the relation between Kārana (cause) and Karya (effect), certain principles were mentioned.

(i) Samavāyi or Upādāna Kārana (Inherent or material Cause) e.g: threads in the fabric.

(ii) Asamavāyi Kārana (Non-inherent cause) e.g.: urnion of threads to make a piece of cloth.

(iii) Nimitta Kārana (Efficient or auxillary cause) e.g.: means for weaving the fabric e.g.: weaver, machinery etc.

Charaka quotes an example that "a drug is like a fabric material and its properties and action are like the yarn of the fabric". Though the definition of dravya given by charaka is intended for kārana dravyas, the same is applicable to kārya dravyas like Shatavari, Guduchi etc. These drugs will exert different Guna-Karmas when used in therapeutis.

---

१. द्रव्यं = द्रोरिव । द्रु + द्रव्यश्च भव्ये । (वाचस्पत्यम्)
२. यत्राश्रिताः कर्मगुणाः कारणं समवायि यत् । तद्द्रव्यम् ....। (च. सू. १)
३. गुणशब्देनचेह धर्मवाचिना रसवीर्यविपाकप्रभावाः सर्व एव गृह्यन्ते । (चक्रपाणि - च. सू. १)
४. क्रियागुणवत् समवायिकारणं द्रव्यम् । (वै. द. १ अ. १५ सू.)
५. द्रव्यलक्षणं तु क्रियागुणवत् समवायिकारणम् इति । (सु. सू. ४०/३)

Badhanta Nagarjuna defined dravya as the site of operation for the activities of rasa, guna, virya, vipaka and karma[1].

2. Concept of Panchabhutas in Dravyaguna

For Ayurveda, Panchabhuta theory is as important as medicinal chemistry is for modern medicine. There are evidences about five element theory (ether, air, fire, water and earth) in the western medicine during ancient times.

'Bhuta' is defined as the minutest matter which will prove its existance through certain characteristic features or it is the factor which produces all the inorganic and organic materials[2].

Charaka concluded that all the dravyas in the universe (i.e; Kārya dravyas) are composed of pancha bhutas (five elements)[3]. Here chakrapani clarified that the Kārya dravyas are only Panchabhoutik but not the Kārana dravyas[4].

Suśruta mentioned about the process of conversion of food (which is panchabhoutik) into body constituents through the action of Agni[5]. The human body which is made up of Panchabhutas will need diet (Ahara) which in turn is composed of Panchabhutas. Therefore these dravyas will undergo Vipaka (digestion & metabolism) and improve their respective biochemical equivalents. Dr. C. Dwarakanath consider that the Bhutagni paka occures in the Yakrit (Liver).

With this back ground Suśruta correctly claimed that the treatment ultimately depends upon Panchabhutas[6].

---

१. द्रव्यमाश्रयलक्षणं पञ्चानाम् । (र.वै.)
भाष्यं:- रसादीनां पञ्चानां भूतानां यदाश्रभूतं तद् द्रव्यम् ।

२. भू सत्तायां इति धातोः निष्पन्नः। (वाचस्पत्यम्)
भवन्ति निन्यं सत्तामनुभवन्तीति भूतानि अथवा
भवन्ति उत्पद्यन्ते येभ्यः द्रव्याणि इति भूतानि । (द्र. गु. वि.)

३. सर्वं द्रव्यं पाञ्चभौतिकमस्मिन्नर्थे । (च. सू. २६/१०)

४. सर्वंद्रव्यमिति कार्यद्रव्यं । अस्मिन्नर्थे अस्मिन् प्रकरणे (आत्रेयभद्रकाप्यीये)।
(चक्रपाणि- च. सू. २६/१०)

५. पञ्चभूतात्मकेदेहे आहारः पाञ्चभौतिकः ।
विपक्कः पञ्चधासम्यक गुणांस्तानभिवर्धयेत् । (सु. सू. ४६ /८०)

६. भूतेभ्यों हि परं यस्मान्नास्ति चिन्ता चिकित्सिते । (सु. शा. १/९)

Before discussing about the Panchabhuta theory it is important to note that Ayurveda accepted Vaiseshika philosophy for Shat Padarthas (six basic materials). Regarding Pancha Vimshati Tattwas (25 elementary factors), Acharyas of Ayurveda followed the Sankhya philosophy mainly. Therefore it is important to demarcate that Panchabhutas discussed in Padartha vijrnana are mainly Karana dravyas and those discussed under Dravyaguna are Karya dravyas mainly. In other words, the former subject deals with Materiology while the later deals with Materia Medica.

The main difference is that Vaiseshikas explain their concept on the basis of Paramanus and Trasarenus, where as Sankhyas denote them as Tanmatras and Mahabhutas which is widely accepted in Ayurveda. Vaiseshika texts mention that two Paramanus become 'Dwyanuka' and three dwyanukas will make a Tryanuka or Trasa renu. The matter is claimed to be invisible upto dwayanuka state. Even Sarangdhara explained the measurements on the basis of Paramanu and Trasa renu. Sankhya texts mention that Tanmatra (Sukshma bhuta) becomes 'Maha bhuta' and 'Drisya bhuta'. However it is commonly accepted by both the philosophies that their physical and chemical characters increase one by one in a chronological order.

The order of creation is mentioned in the following manner in the Ayurvedic texts[1,2].

---

१. सर्वभूतानां कारणमकारणं सत्त्वरजस्तमोलक्षणमष्टरूपमखिलस्य जगतः संभवहेतुरव्यक्तं नाम । तदेकं बहूनां क्षेत्रज्ञानामधिष्ठानं समुद्र इवौदकानां भावानाम् ॥ (सु. शा. १/३)

२. तस्मादव्यक्तान्महानुत्पद्यते तल्लिङ्ग डाव। तल्लिङ्गाच्चमहतस्तल्लक्षण एवाहंकार उत्पद्यते; सत्रिविधो वैकारिकस्तैजसो भूतादिरिति । तत्र वैकारिकादहंकारात् तैजससहायात्तल्लक्षणान्येवैकादशेन्द्रियाण्युत्पद्यन्ते, तद्यथा- श्रोत्रत्वक्चक्षुर्जिह्वाघ्राणवाक्हस्तोपस्थापायुपादमनांसीति; तत्र पूर्वाणि पञ्च बुद्धीन्द्रियाणि, इतराणि पञ्चकर्मेन्द्रियाणि, उभयात्मकं मनः; भूतादेरपि तैजससहायात्तल्लक्षणान्येव पञ्चतन्मात्राण्युत्पद्यन्ते- शब्दतन्मात्रं, स्पर्शतन्मात्रं,रूपतन्मात्रं, रसतन्मात्रं, गन्धतन्मात्रमिति; तेषां विशेषाः- शब्दस्पर्शरूपरसगन्धाः; तेभ्यो भूतानि- व्योमानिलअनलजलोर्व्यः; एवमेषा तत्त्वचतुर्विंशतिर्व्याख्याता ॥ (सु. शा. १/४)

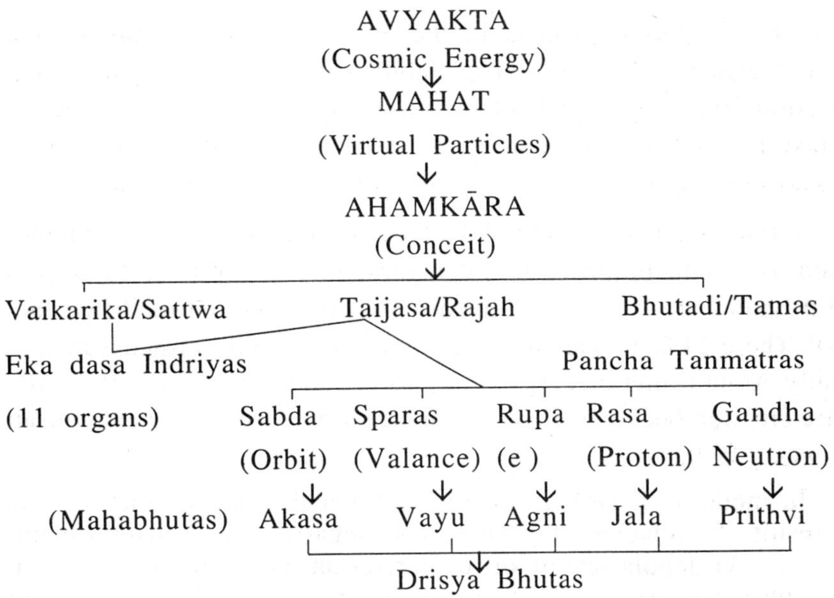

It is stated that the creation begins with 'Avyakta' or 'Prakriti' which is impercievable in nature. In biochemistry it is denoted as unknown cosmic energy or radiation coming from the galaxy. Entire energy in the universe is as a result of it only. The next phase 'Mahat' is comparable to 'virtual particles' or highly charged energy particles like meson, positron, neutrino etc. But these are highly unstable and can not have active part or direct part in formation of Karya dravyas. After Mahat we have Ahamkara (self-sufficient conceit) with three fragments viz., Vaikarika (sattwa), Taijasa (Rajah) Bhutadi (Tamas). These three will represent the more stable energy particles which take part in atom i.e., Sattwa is proton, Rajah is electron and Tamas is neutron. These three are together known as Trividha Ahamkaras (three conceits) since- Sattwa considers ifself as the only source of positive charge, Rajah considers itself as the only source of negative charge and Tamas considers itself as the only neutrally charged particle.

Actually, from these stable particles only the material world begins to form. Eka dasa Indriyas (11 functional aspects of sensory, motor and senso-motor organs) will emerge from sattwa and Rajah (with the support of Tamas in the end). Pancha Tanmatras (five phyical aspects of atom) viz., Sabda (orbit/sound), Sparsa (valence/touch), Rupa (electron activity/shape), Rasa (proton activity/taste) and Gandha (neutron activity/smell) will emerge from Tamas and Rajah (with the support of sattwa in the end)[1].

Trividha Ahamkaras and Pancha Tanmatras will be together called as 'Ashta Prakritis' (eight natural factors). While, 11 organs and 5 bhutas are known as 'Shodasa Vikritis' (Sixteen modified factors)[2]. These 24 factors are together known as 'Chaturvimshati Tattwa's. Finally Atma (kinetic energy of atom) is added to this and therefore entire creation becomes alive and thence are called as 'Panchavimsati Tattwas' (25 factors).

In modern physiology all the motor and sensory functions are the result of exchange of positive and negative ions across a membrane. Either depolarization or repolarization across the resting membrane by means exchange of positively charged ca^+, K^+, Na^+ etc., or negatively charged Cl^-, O^- etc., result in bodily activities. The same is the basis for considering Sattwa and Rajah for Ekadasa Indriyas.

Pancha Tanmatras mainly indicate the physical properties of matter or atom while Pancha Maha bhutas mainly indicate the chemical properties of atom along with physical properties. Therfore Pancha tanmatras have horizontal expansion in evolution like periods in the modern periodic table. Pancha Maha bhutas have linear or vertical expansion like groups in the periodic table.

The pancha tanmatras and panchabhutas are represented in the following way scientifically:

Pancha Tanmatras	**Sabda**	**Sparsa**	**Rupa**	**Rasa**	**Gandha**
Physical	Orbit	Valance	Electron	Proton	Neutron
Chemical		H^+	O^-	P^+	N^- C^+
Pancha Mahabutas	**Akasa**	**Vayu**	**Agni**	**Jala**	**Prithvi**
Physical	Vacuum	Gases	Plasma	Liquids	Solids

१. खादीनि बुद्धिरव्यक्तमहानहंकारस्तथाऽष्टमः । भूतप्रकृतिरूद्दिष्टा विकाराश्चैव षोडश ॥
बुद्धीन्द्रियाणि पञ्चैव पञ्च कर्मेन्द्रियाणि च ।
समनस्काश्च पश्चार्था विकारा इति संज्ञिताः ॥ (च. शा. १/६३-६४)

२. अव्यक्तं महानहंकारः पञ्चतन्मात्राणि चेन्यष्टौ प्रकृतयः ; शेषाः षोडश विकाराः ॥ (सु. शा. १/६)

Chemical Hydrogen Oxygen Phosphorus Nitrogen Carbon

Sabda, Sparsa, Rupa, Rasa and Gandha are the five Tanmatras as well as the inherent properties of Panchamahabhutas.

Sabda is compared to orbit size because by beating gases audible sound is not produced. But by beating a solid metal sound is produced. From gases to metallic elements the orbit size increased and the property of sound increased. Sparsa is considered as valance since vayu is known for movement. The electrons are revolving in orbits because of this force only. Rupa i.e., colour and luminiscence differ from each element and hence calorimetry. The change of one element to the other is decided by the number of electrons in the outer shell. Therefore rupa is simile to electron activity. Rasa is compared to proton activity since it is the base of Jala. Hydrogen acts as water forming element because of its proton peculiarity. On the other hand liquid medium is a must for the perception of taste i.e., for transportation of ions accross the taste buds. Gandha is related similar to neutron because solid particles (i.e., heaviest fundamental particles) are essential for olfactory function and neutron provides the weight to the atom.

Chemically panchamahabhutas may be related to elements like hydrogen, oxygen, nitrogen, phosphorus (or sulphur) and carbon respectively. These five are the constituents of protoplasm and proteins. These five elements in the form of five compounds are major constituents of the body. They are: CO_2, CH_3, PO_3, H_2O and NH_3.

It is mentioned in the classics that the bhutas at the minutest level have their individual characteristics like sabda, sparsa etc. These features add one to another as the evolution of bhutas complete. This process of quantiplication is denoted as Anyonyana pravesa or Panchapanchikarana in Ayurveda and Vendanta respectively[1].

---

१. महाभूतानि खं वायुरग्निरापः क्षितिस्तथा। शब्दः स्पर्शश्चरूपं च रसोगन्धश्च तद्गुणः ॥
तेषामेकगुणः पूर्वो गुणवृद्धिः परे परे ।
पूर्वः पूर्वगुणश्चैव क्रमशो गुणिषु स्मृतः ॥ (च. शा. १/२७-२८)
अन्योन्यानुप्रविष्टानि सर्वाण्येतानि निर्दिशेत् ।
स्वे स्वे द्रव्येतु सर्वेषां व्यक्तं लक्षणमिव्यते ॥ (सु. शा. १/२१)

As Avyakta is inactive, activity is provided by Atma or Purusha. This may be compared to kinetic energy of atom. There are three types of activities or three kinds of Atma described in the ancient texts.

(i) Bhutatma - activity in the inorganic matter
(ii) Jeevatma - activity in the organic matter
(iii) Paramatma - activity in the galaxy (which is imperceivable).

Acharyas of Ayurveda have described the dravya on the basis of bhuta predominance in it. The structure related activity of a drug is quite similar to the pharmacological action of dravya resulting from its panchabhoutik configuration.[1,2,3,4] According to Vedentik view bhuta predominane in a dravya is assessed by this formula: "the main bhuta will be 1/2 part and the remaining bhutas will be 1/8th part each[5]."

(1) Akasiya dravya- Ak 1/2 + Va 1/8 + Ag 1/8 +Ap 1/8 + Pr 1/8
(2) Vayaviya dravya-Ak 1/8 + Va 1/2 + Ag 1/8 + Ap 1/8 + Pr 1/8
(3) Agneya dravya -Ak 1/8 + Va 1/8 + Ag 1/2 + Ap 1/8 + Pr 1/8
(4) Apya dravya - Ak 1/8 + Va 1/8 + Ag 1/8 + Ap 1/2 + Pr 1/8
(5) Parthiva dravya - Ak 1/8 + Va 1/8 + Ag 1/8 + Ap1/8 + Pr 1/2

The panchabhoutik configuration of rasa-virya-vipaka are explained in the respective chapters.

3. Medicinal Properties of Dravya

It is discussed earlier that all the Kārya dravyas are composed of five elements (Panchabhoutik). These dravyas may be

१. आकाशादीनि भूतानि सर्वाण्येकगुणान्यथ । महाभूतेषु जन्येषु गुणवृद्धिः प्रजायते ॥ डाकद्विद्विचतुःपञ्चगुणत्वं खादिषु स्मृतम् । गुणस्तत्रैक आस्मीयः शेषः संसर्गजः स्मृतः॥ अन्योन्यानुप्रविष्टानि दृश्यभूतानि निर्दिशेत तस्मात् पञ्चगुणान्येव सर्वाणीति विनिश्चयः॥ (पं. भू.)

२. तत्र पृथिव्यप्तेजोवाय्वाकाशानां समुदायाद् द्रव्याभिनिवृत्तिः, उत्कर्षस्त्वथिव्यञ्जको भवति- इदं पाथिवम् इदमाप्यं,इदं तैजसम् , इदं वायव्यम् , इदमाकाशीयमिति । (सु. सू. ४१)

३. खर द्रव चल उण्णत्वं भूजलानिलतेजसाम् ।
आकाशस्याप्रतीघ्रातो दृष्टं लिङ्गं यथाक्रमम् ॥ (च. शा.१/२९)

४. तत्र सत्त्वबहुलमाकाशं, रजो बहुलो वायुः, सत्त्वरजोबहुलोऽग्निः, सत्त्वतमोबहुला आपः, तमोबहुला पृथिवीति॥ (सु. शा. १/२०)

५. व्यपदेशस्तु भूयसा । (सु.सू. ४१)

either the drugs or the constituents of human body. Therefore, the sthana (balance or homoeostasis), vriddhi (increase) and kshaya (decrease) of Tridoshas (three humors) i.e., physiology and pathophysiology are under the control of dravyas (either Ahara or oushadha)[1].

It is further claimed that the constituents of dravya viz., rasa,guna, virya & vipaka are responsible for the kshaya or vriddhi or samya of dosha-dhatu-malas[2].

Basically, Ayurveda elaborate the disease and health on the account of vitiation or balance of Tridoshas[3]. Thence, treatment is also two folded[4]:

(i) Swastha Urjaskara (preventive aspects)
(ii) Ātura roganut (curative aspects)

Among the quartet of medical management (Chikitsa chatushpāda), drug is placed next to physician in chronology[5]. An ideal dravya must possess the following four characteristics[6].

(1) Bahuta		should be abundently available.
(2) Yogyatwa	-	should be of maximum utility.
(3) Aneka vidha kalpana	-	should be made into defferent forms.
(4) Sampath	-	should possess the best qualities.

After having this back ground it is very essential to identify which material is medicinally valuable. In reply to this quiry we find references from the samhitas that no material in this universe is devoid of medicinal properties[7]. Charaka mentioned that even a

---

१. गुणा य उक्ता द्रव्येषु शरीरेष्वपि ते तथा ।
स्थानवृद्धिक्षयास्तस्माद् देहिनो द्रव्यहेतुका: ॥ (सु. सू. २)

२. द्रव्यरसगुणवीर्यविपाकनिमित्ते च क्षयवृद्धी दोषाणां साम्यञ्च। (सु. सू. ४६)

३. रोगास्तु दोषवैषम्यं दोषसाम्यमरोगता । (अ. हृ. सू. १)

४. स्वस्थस्योर्जस्करं किञ्चित् किञ्चिदार्तस्यरोगनुत् । (च. चि.। अ.। या.)

५. भिषग्द्रव्याण्युस्थाता रोगी पादचतुष्टयम् । (च. सू. ९)

६. बहुतातत्रयोग्यत्वमेनेकविधकल्पना ।
संपच्चेति चतुष्कोऽयं द्रव्याणां गुण उच्यते ॥ (अ. सं. सू. २)

७. (क) जगत्येवमनौषधम् । न किञ्चिद्विद्यते द्रव्यं वशान्नानार्थयोगयो: ॥ (अ.स.सू. ९)

क्रमश: पृष्ठ १२ में ....

deadly medicine may be used as an effective medicine or vice versa[1].

It is generally proposed that similar properties enhance the respective qualities inside the body while the opposite properties reduce[2].

However Chakrapani highlights the importance of logic (yukti) in utilizing the drugs. Parthivadi dravyas may enhance their related qualities usually but it is not a hard and fast rule. Similarly opposite qualities may become useful in management when used with certain modification (samskara etc)[3]. Dalhana also concluded that all Sthavara and Jangama dravyas act as good medicines because of their panchabhoutik nature[4].

4. Importance of Dravya

Charaka samhita accepted dravya as the supreme matter among Dravya, Rasa, Guna etc. At later times, Sushrita and Vagbhata have specifically mentioned about the superiority of Dravya. According to Suśruta dravya is important than the quartet (rasa, guna,virya

---

पृष्ठ ११ से क्रमशः........

(ख) अनेनोपदेशेन नानौषधिभूतं जगति किञ्चिद्द्रव्यमुपलभ्यते तां तां युक्तिमर्थं च तं तमभिप्रेत्य। (च.सू. २६/)

(ग) अनेन निदर्शनेन नानौषधिभूतं जगति किञ्चिद्द्रव्यमस्तिः । (सु. सू. ४१/५)

(घ) रसादि भेदैरिति भेषजानां दिङ्मात्रमुक्तं न यतोऽस्ति किञ्चित् ।
अनौषधं द्रव्यमिहावबोधो .... ॥ (अ. सं. सू. १२)

(ङ) इत्थं च नानौषधिभूतं जगति किञ्चिद् द्रव्यमस्ति विविधार्थप्रयोगवशात् ॥ (अ. सं. सू. १७)

१. योगादपि विषं तीक्ष्णं उत्तमं भेषजं भवेत् । भेषजं चाणि दुर्युक्तं तीक्ष्णं संपद्यते विषम् ॥ (च.सू. १)

२. सर्वदा सर्वभावानां सामान्यं वृद्धिकारणं । ह्रासहेतुर्विशेषश्च .... ॥ (च. सू. १)

३. ....यत् पार्थिवादि द्रव्य यद्गणं तद्गणे देहे संपद्यते तद् भेषजं भवतीत्यर्थः ।
तच्च पार्थिवादि द्रव्यं न सर्वथा न च सर्वस्मिन् व्याधौ भेषजमित्याह- तां तां युक्तिमित्यादि। युक्तिमिति उपायं, अर्थमिति प्रयोजनम् अभिप्रेत्येति अधिकृत्य,तेन केनचिदुपायेन क्वचित् प्रयोजने किञ्चिद्द्रव्यमौषधं भवति न सर्वत्र। तेन यदुच्यते- वैरोधिकानां सर्वदाऽपथ्यत्वेन 'नानौषधं द्रव्यम्' इति वयो विरोधिः; तत्र भवति, वैरोधिकानि हि संयोगसंस्कारदेशकालाद्यपेक्षाणि भवन्ति, वैरोधिकसंयोगाद्यभावे तु पथ्यापथ्यानि कूचित् स्युः । (चक्रपाणि- च.सू. २६/)

४. .....सर्वस्यैव जगतः स्थावरङ्गमाख्यस्य पाञ्चभौतिकत्वेन सर्वमौषधं क्रियागुण-योगादिभिर्दर्शयन्नाह- अनेनेत्यादि । नानौषधिभूतमिति अनौषधिभूतं द्रव्यं नास्तीति संबन्धः । युक्तिविशेषमिति युक्तिविशेषो योजनाविशेषस्तीयाग्नि - संस्कारभावनामात्राकालाद्यपेक्षः । अर्थः प्रयोजनं नानाव्याधिनिर्घातनं ....॥ (डल्हण - सु.सू. ४१/५)

and vipaka) since dravya is the seat for the later[1]. Vagbhata also expressed similar view[2].

It is observed that vipaka is depended upon virya; virya can not exist without rasa and rasa can not exist without dravya. In this manner there is a continuous linkage between the constituents of a dravya. Hence dravya is claimed to be the ultimate or superior thing[3].

In this context Chakrapani further clarify that- "a Seeta virya drug which is composed of Prithi and Jala will give rise to Madhura/ Guru vipaka. Similarly, a Ushna virya dravya which is made up of Agni and Akasa will under-go Katu/Laghu vipaka. Thus dravya is acting as a medium for the existance of virya, vipaka etc. Hence dravya is of primary importance."

The origin of dravya and rasa is simile to Agni (fire) and Dhuma (smoke) respectively. The former can yield the later but vice versa is not possible. Rasa, guna etc., will have their genesis simultaneously with dravya but not seperately. Their relation is compared with Deha/Sareera (body) and Dehina (Atma (soul). Even the eight types of viryas are depended upon the dravya. On broad out look Guravadi gunas and rasa etc., are also considered as gunas only. Usually gunas are deviod of any activity indepedently (Nirguna). That is why it is not possible to obtain guna from rasa. However one dravya may possess several rasas and several gunas. Similarly vipaka also depends upon dravya but not on rasas alone. Hence dravya is explained with primary importance in dravyaguna sastra[4].

Suśruta and Badhanta Nagarjuna have given the following explanations and examples for the importance of dravya:

---

१. पृथक्त्वदर्शिनामेष वादिनं वादसंग्रहः । चतुर्णामणि सामग्र्यमिच्छन्त्यत्र विपश्चितः ॥ (सु.सू. ४०)

२. द्रव्यमेव रसादीनां श्रेष्ठं, तेहि तदाश्रयाः । (अ.हृ.सू.१/१)

३. पाको नास्ति विना वीर्यात् वीर्यं नास्ति विना रसात् ।
रसो नास्ति विना द्रव्यात् द्रव्यं श्रेष्ठतमं स्मृतम् ॥ (सु.सू.४०/१५)

४. जन्म तु द्रव्यरसयोरन्योपेक्षिकं स्मृतम् । अन्योन्यापेक्षिकं जन्म यथा स्थाद्देहदेहिनोः ॥
वीर्यसंज्ञा गुणायेऽष्टौ तेऽपि द्रव्याश्रयाः स्मृताः । रसेषु न भवन्त्येते निर्गुणास्तु गुणाः स्मृताः ॥
द्रव्ये द्रव्याणि यस्माद्धि विपच्यन्ते न षड्रसाः । श्रेष्ठं द्रव्यमतो ज्ञेयं, शेषा भावास्तदाश्रयाः ॥
(सु.सू. ४०/१६-१८)

(1) Vyavasthitatwa: ***(Stability)***

The dravya is only stable in nature but not the constituents like rasa, guna etc[1]. For example : taste of unripen mango will keep on changing till it ripens. But the fruit is known as mango fruit till the end. In between the taste etc, will change from astringent to sour and sour to sweet. Similarly, the green colour of black Jamoon fruit when it is very tender will turn into Brinjal colour after some time and finally becomes black like collyrium (Anjana) when fully ripen. Accordingly taste, smell etc, will also change whereas dravya do not[2].

(2) Nityatwa: ***(Eternity)***

Certain qualities/properties of a dravya may be lost after some time. But the original dravya will remain as it is e.g., kalka, swarsa etc., may loose taste and smell. Still they will be called as kalka or swarasa of the given material. There-fore dravya is considered to be of primary importance[3].

---

१. व्यवस्थिततत्वात् , इह खलु द्रव्यं व्यवस्थितं न रसादयः, यथा- आमेफले ये रसादयस्ते पक्के न सन्ति।
(सु.सू. ४०/३)

* चक्रपाणि:- व्यवस्थिततत्वदिति अवस्थाभेदेन रसादिभेदेऽपि द्रव्यस्यव्यवस्थिततत्वात्; यथा-आम्रफलं प्रथमं कषायाम्लं, मध्येऽम्लं,एवं रसाव्यवस्थानेऽपि द्रव्यमात्ररूपतया व्यवस्थिततत्वम् ।

** डल्हन:- व्यवस्थिततत्वादिति द्रव्यं हि व्यवतिष्ठति न रसादयः, यथा- आम्रफलसे- कमेव प्रथमं कषायाम्लं पश्चादम्लं ततो मधुरमपि भवति, न तु तदेवाम्रफल- यथातकं कोशाम्रं वा भवति ।

२. व्यवस्थानात् ......। (र. वै. १/१०२)

* भाष्यं:- व्यवस्थानादिति द्रव्यं व्यवस्थितं, गुणाः अनवस्थिताः ।

उक्तं च- 'दूर्वाङ्कुरनिभं भूत्वा फलं जम्ब्वास्ततः पुनः। मेचकं भजते वर्णं पुनरञ्जनसन्निभम् । इति एवं तद्गताश्च स्पर्शरसगन्धाश्चानवस्थिताः । जम्बूफलमिति द्रव्यम् सामान्यम् ।

३. नित्यत्वाच्च, नित्यं हि द्रव्यमनित्या गुणाः, यथा कल्कादिप्रविभागः व्यवस्थिसंपन्नरसगन्धो व्यापन्नरस-गन्धो वा भवति ॥
(सु.सू. ४०/३)

* चक्रपाणि:- नित्यत्वाच्चेति नित्यत्वं रसादिनाशेऽप्यवस्थिततत्वमिह ज्ञेयं, व्यवस्थिततत्वं तु रसान्यथात्वे तद्रूपतया व्यवस्थिततत्वमिति भेदः। कालादीत्यत्रादिशब्देन जलवातादयो गृह्यन्ते ।

** डल्हण:- नित्यत्वात् क्रियाकालावस्थिततत्वादित्यर्थः। अनित्या गुणा इति विनाशन इत्यर्थः। कल्केत्यादि आदिग्रहणात् स्वरस श्रृतशीतफाण्टानामपि ग्रहणम। सएव कल्कादिप्रविभाग एव। संपन्नरसगन्धा वा भवतीति संयुक्तरसः संयुक्तगन्धो वा भवतीन्यर्थः। एतैनेतदुक्तं भवति,- कल्काद्यवस्थाष्वपि द्रव्यं तदेव नान्यतरद्द्रव्यं, रसगन्धौ त्वन्यो संयुक्तौ भवत इति, गुणादनियतात् द्रव्यं नित्यम् । अन्ये कल्कादि-

क्रमशः पृष्ठ १५ में.........

(3) Swajatyavasthanatwa: ***(Geno-specificity)***

No substance belonging to one genus/group will change into another. e.g. a prithvi dravya remains to be so till the end. Similarly milk will become curd but not salt or honey. During the process only certain characters/properties will change. Hence dravya is important[1].

(4) Panchendriya grahyatwa: ***(Perceptible through all the senses)***

Only dravya is perceptible through all the five senses (viz., sabda, sparsa, rupa, rasa and gandha). Rasa, Guna etc. are not so e.g., rasa is perceivable through rasanendriya, virya is identified through adhivasa[2,3].

पृष्ठ १४ से क्रमशः.........

स्थाने 'कालादिप्रविभांगात्' इति पठन्ति । तेषां मले आदिग्रहणाज्जलवातदेशसोमसूर्या गृहान्ते । तद्यथा- 'ता एवौषधयो ग्रीष्मे निः सारा रूक्षा (सू. अ. ६) इत्यादि।

*** हारणचन्द्रः- अनियतावस्थायिनो गुणा अनित्या उच्चन्ते, द्रव्यं च तदपेक्षथा नियतावस्थायि नित्यामाख्यायते। नित्यत्वं च द्रव्याणां कालपरिणामेनान्यथाथावेऽपि तदेवेदमिति प्रत्यभिज्ञायमानत्वाद-वगन्तव्यम् ॥

१. स्वजात्यवस्यानाच्च, यथा हि पार्थिवं द्रव्यमन्यथाभावं न गच्छत्येवं शेषाणि। (सु.सू. ४०/३)

* चक्रपाणिः- स्वजात्यवस्थानादिति परणिामेऽपि द्रव्यं स्वजातावतिष्ठते न जात्यन्तरं भवति, पार्थिवं तु पार्थिवमेव यादाप्यं तदाप्यमेवेत्यादिस्वजात्यपरित्यागः, रसस्तु क्षीरमधुरत्वं परित्यज्याम्लतां यातीत्यनुसरणींयं, जातिश्चेह मित्यादिजातिभेदो नोद्भवनीयः ।

** डल्हणः- स्वस्यां पार्थिवादिजातावस्थितत्वादित्यर्थः । अन्यभावं न गच्छति आप्यादिजातिं न गच्छति ।

२. पञ्चेन्द्रियग्रहणाच्च, पञ्चभिरिन्द्रियैर्गृह्यते द्रव्यं न रसादयः य़ (सु.सू. ४०/३)

* चक्रपाणिः- .....पञ्चभिरिन्द्रियैर्द्रव्यं गृह्यते इति चक्षुषा स्पर्शनेन तावद्व्यग्रहणमविवादसिद्धमेव; घ्राणरसनाश्रोत्राणामपि सुरभि चन्दनं, मधुरः कोषकारः, तथा सुस्वरा वीणेत्यादि समानाधिकरणज्ञानेन द्रव्यग्रहणं प्रति स्फुटतर-व्यापाराद् द्रव्यग्रहकत्वं ज्ञेयम् ।

** डल्हणः- द्रव्ये गृहीते तदाश्रया गुणा गृहीता भवन्ति, गुणाश्च शब्दस्पर्शरूपरसगन्धाः। द्रव्ये शब्दोऽप्यस्ति, यथा- पार्थिवेद्रव्ये कटकटाशब्दः, आप्ये खलखलाशब्दः,वैजसे तटटाशब्द इत्यादिकः। वायव्यमाकाशाद्रव्यं चानुमानग्राह्यममूर्तत्वात् । न रसादय इति रसगुणनीवीर्यविपाकास्तु न पञ्चेन्द्रियग्राह्या इत्यर्थः ।

३. सर्वेन्द्रियोपलब्धेः .....। (र.वै.१. सू. १०१)

*भाष्यं:-...सर्वैः श्रोतादिभिरिन्द्रियैर्द्रव्यं गृह्यते, रसादयो ह्येकेन्द्रियग्राह्याः।...एकमनेकेन्द्रियग्राह्यत्वात् प्रधानं द्रव्यमिति ।

(5) Asrayatwa: ***(Host for properties)***

Only dravya can act as the host for other constituents like rasa, guna, virya etc., vice versa is not possible. There fore dravya is considered as important[1,2].

(6) Arambhasamarthya: ***(Initiation of action)***

Initiation of a specific pharmacological action is possible only by using the dravya. It is not possible to pick up the constituents (rasa, guna etc.) and use in the treatment. Hence dravya is supreme.[3,4]

(7) Sastra Pramanya: ***(Classical references)***

All the ancient Ayurvedic classics have mentioned different medicines or drugs on the basis of dravya only. Different ganas are explained on the basis of dravya but not Rasa etc. Even though we find the reference about Rasa skandha. They are also represented by group of dravyas but not by rasa. Hence dravya is superior[5,6].

(8) Kramapekshitatwa: ***(Degree of maturity of drug and qualities)***

The properties depend upon the state of the dravya. When a drug is tender then the properties will remain incomplete, and when the drug matures all the properties will be present in it. That means

---

१. आश्रायत्वाच्च, द्रव्यमाश्रिता रसादय: । (सु.सू. ४०/३)

* चक्रपाणि:- आश्रयत्वाच्चेति रसादीनां द्रव्यमाश्रय:, तेनाश्रित रसादय: परतन्त्रत्वादप्रधाना:, आश्रयस्तु प्रधानमित्यर्थ: ।

** डल्हण:- आश्रय इति द्रव्यं रसादीनाम् ।

२. अधिष्ठानादाश्रयात् .... । (र.वै. १. सू. १६६)

* भाष्यं:- द्रव्यमाश्रय आश्रयिणो रसादय: इति । आश्रयभूत: प्रधान: स्वामी दृष्ट इति ।

३. आरम्भसामर्थ्याच्च, द्रव्यमाश्रित आरम्भ:, यथा- 'विदारिगन्धादिमाह्य संक्षुद्य विपचेत्' इन्येवमादिषु न रसादष्विारम्भ: (सु.सू. ४०/३)

* डल्हण:- आरम्भसामर्थ्यात् उपक्रमसामर्थ्यादित्यर्थ: ।

४. आरम्भसामर्थ्यात् .... । (र.वै. १. सू. १०४)

* भाष्य:- आरम्भश्चिकित्सायां क्रियारम्भ: मूलमाहरेतेत्यादि तस्मिन् द्रव्यस्यैव सामर्थ्यं न रसादीनामारम्भसामर्थ्यम् । अविकलेन्द्रिय: पुरुष: प्रधानो दृष्ट: पङ्गोरिति ।

५. शास्त्रप्रामाण्याच्च, शास्त्रे हि द्रव्य प्रधानमुपदेशे योगानां , यथा- 'मातुलुङ्ग- अग्निमन्थौ च' इत्यादौ न रसादय उपदिश्यंते । (सु.सू. ४०/३)

६. शास्त्रोपदेशसामर्थ्यात् .... । (र.वै.अ. । सू. १०७)

* भाष्यं:- आगमादित्यर्थ:। शास्त्र एवोपदिश्यते हि- 'य एव हि गुणा द्रव्ये शरीरेष्वपि ते स्मृता:। तान् द्रव्यैस्तद्गणैरेव प्रयोगेणाभिवर्धयेत् ।' इति सामान्यप्रयोगवचते विशिष्टेन प्रयोगो निर्दिश्यते इति ।

the degree of maturity of drug and its properties are directly proportional. Therefore dravya is caimed to be important[1,2].

(9) Ekadesa sadhyatwa: ***(Utility through part used)***

Dravya can be utilized in the treatment by using a part of it. Whereas rasa, virya etc., can not be used partly e.g., the latex of Snuhi can be used in many diseases but its taste can not be. Therefore dravya is more important.[3,4]

Badhanta Nagarjuna mentioned three more factors. They are:

(10) Taratama yoganupalabdhi ***(Non-availability of grading)***

Gunas and rasas can be used according to the grading like mild, moderate and severe (Taratama Yoga). However this type of grading is not possible for dravya. Though the constituents vary in their nature dravya remain stable. Hence it is important[5].

(11) Vikalpa samarthya: ***(Possibility of pharmaceutics)***

Dravya can be made into different forms of pharmaceutics viz., kalka, kashaya, swarasa, churna etc. But the constituents like rasa, guna etc, can not be utilized for the same purpose.

---

१. क्रमापेक्षितत्वाच्च रसादीनां, रसादयो हि द्रव्यक्रममपेक्षन्ते, यथा- तरुणे तरुणाः संपूर्णा इति। (सु.सू.४०/३)
   * डल्हनः तरुणे तरुणा इति अभिनवे अभिनवा इत्यर्थः ।

२. तदनुविधानाच्चेतरेषाम् ....।
   भाष्यंः इतरेषां रसादीनां द्रव्यस्यानुवधिनात्। द्रव्यमनुवर्तन्ते हि रसादयः, तारुण्ये तरुणाः, संपत्तौ संपन्नाः, विपत्तौ विपन्ना भवन्तीति ये यमनुवर्त्तन्ते ते तस्मादप्रधाना दृष्टाः । तद्यथा, गुरोः शिष्या इति।

३. एदेशसाध्यत्वाच्च, द्रव्याणामेकदेकशेनापि व्याधयः साध्यन्ते, तथा- महावृक्षक्षीरेणेति, तस्माद्द्रव्यं प्रधानं, न रसादयः, कस्मात्? निखयवत्वात् ।
   * चक्रपाणिः- कस्माद्रसादीनामेकदेशेन व्याधयो न साध्यन्त इत्याह- निरवयवत्कादिति।

४. अवयेव सिद्धेः............। (र.वै.अ.।सू.१०८)
   * भाष्यः- अवयवेन एकदेशेन प्रदेशेन सिद्धेः, प्रयोगेषु इति वाक्यशेषः यथा मूलत्वागादिना अवयवेन यः साधयति स प्रधानो दृष्टः ।

५. तरतमयोगानुपलब्धेः.............।
   * भाष्यंः- तरतमयोगो रसादिषु दृष्टः ।........मधुरतरो, शीततरः, शीततमः, छर्दनीयतरं, छर्दनीयतमं लघुतरः, लघुतमः, कर्मतरं, कर्मतमम् इति। द्रव्येषु नास्ति यष्टिमधुकतरो यष्टीमधुकतमं इति। तस्मात् तरतमयोगाभावाद् रसादिभ्यो द्रव्यं प्रधानमिति।

Therefore dravya is stated to be superior.[1]

(12) Pratighata samarthya: ***(Malleability)***

Among the seven constituents of dravyaguna only dravya possess some shape and structure which is visible (i.e., Murtitwa). Therefore dravya can occupy some space while rasa etc, can not exhibit these qualities.[2]

From the above factors it is apparent that Dravya (drug) is foremost in dravyaguna and other preporties are constituted in it.

---

१. विकल्पसामर्थ्यात् ....।

* भाष्यं:- विविध: कल्पो विकल्प: कल्ककषायादिभेदेन, तस्मिन् विकल्पे सामर्थ्यात् तत् सर्वं द्रव्यस्यैव नान्यस्येति ।

२. प्रतीघातसामर्थ्यात् ....।

* भाष्यं:- प्रतीघात आवरणं तस्मिन् सामर्थ्यं द्रव्यस्यैव भवति, मूर्तिमत्त्वात् ।......प्रतीघातसमर्थ्यात् स्वस्थानेऽन्यस्यानवकाशदानात् इति । रसादय: संपृक्तास्तिन्तीति । आवरणार्थोऽपि दृष्ट: चक्रवर्तीति ।

Chapter- III

Classification of Dravya

Materials (dravya) having medicinal values may be classified into different group according to their source, evolution, utility, age and properties. The present chapter will deal with the classification of dravyas in Ayurveda.

1. Classification on the basis of activity: (सृष्टिक्रमानुसारेण)

All the substances in the universe are grossly divided into two groups viz., Chetana (animate) and Achetana (inanimate)[1]. They are other wise described as Sendriya (living) and Nirindriya (non-living)[2]. The chetana group are sub-divided into two classes viz., Antah chetana (with internal activity) and Bahirantah chetana (with both internal & external activities).

'Antah chetana' group covers all the plant kingdom which will have most of the activites hidden inside its body. 'Bahirantah chetana' group will cover all the animal kingdom which will possess both invisible internal activities and visible external activities also.

Dravya

Chetana (Sendriya or Sasana) — Achetana (Nirindriya or Anasana)

Chetana: Antah chetana (e.g.: Plants) — Bahirantah Chetana (e.g.: Animals)

In the vedic literature Chetana and Achetana are denoted as Sasana (साशन) and Anasana (अनशन) respectively.

१. ......तच्चेतनावदचेतनं च । (च.सू. १/२६)

२. सेन्द्रियं चेतनं द्रव्यं निरिन्द्रियमचेतनम् । (च.सू. १/४८)

Manusmriti mention about Antah chetana dravyas like herbs, shrubs, climbers, trees etc., which are covered by Tamas. Thence, their activity is invisible and hidden. Renowned scientist Sir Jagadish Chandra Bose proved about the internal activity of plants through his research, at later period.

Chakrapani is of the openion that this classification is applicable to Karya dravyas (Effectual materials) but not to the Karana dravyas (caụsal materials). He further quoted several examples for Antah chetanas or Sendriya dravyas:

1. Sun flower (Surya Bhakta) following the movement of sun.
2. Big lemon (Beeja Pura) fruiting after exposure to the fat of fox's muscle (Srigala Vasa).
3. Mango (Āmrā) yielding more fruits after spraying/sprinkling fish fat (Matya Vasa) on it.
4. Lavali starts fruiting after listening to the roar of clouds.

2. Classification on the Basis of Cause & Effect: (कार्यकारणभेदेन)

Entire creation may be divided into two groups i.e., Kārana dravyas (causal materials) and Karya dravyas (effectual materials).

There are nine Kārana dravyas through which creation was possible viz., sabda tanmatra, sparsa tanmatra, rupa tanmatra, rasa tanmatra, gandha tanmatra, Atma, Manas, Kala & Disa[1].

The second group i.e., Kārya dravyas are made up of panchabhutas and are innumerable. e.g.,- Guduchi, Vacha, Shatavari, Godhuma, Yava etc.

3. Classification on the Basis of Evolution (उत्पत्तिभेदेन)

All the dravyas used in the treatment are made up of Pancha Bhutas (five elements)[2]. However, Sushrita clarified that the main characteristic of a dravya is decided on the basis of the major bhuta in it[3]. On this basis dravyas are of five types namely,(1) Ākasiya

१. खादीन्यात्मामनः कालो दिशश्च द्रव्यसंग्रहः । (च. सू. १)
२. सर्वं द्रव्यं पाञ्चभौतिकमस्मिन्नर्थे । (च. सू. २६)
३. व्यपदेशस्तु भूयसा । (सु.सू. ४१)

(2) Vāyavīya (3) Āgneya (4) Jaliya and (5) Parthiva[1].

(1) Ākasiya Drvya

Substances which have the properties like:Mridu (smooth), Laghu (lighter), Sukshma (minute), Vyavayi (stimulant first and depressant next), Slakshna (glisening), Visada(clear), Vivikta (seperate) and Avyakta rasa (unknown taste) etc., and substances which provides smoothness to body/skin etc., are known to be Akasiya dravyas. Sabda (sound) is its characteristic feature[2].

(2) Vāyaviya Dravya

Substances which have Laghu (lighter), Seeta (cold), Ruksha (non-unctuous), Khara (rough), Visada (clear), Sukshma (minute) etc., properties and having astringent taste are known as the Vayaviya dravyas. Sparsa (touch) is its characteristic feature[3].

(3) Āgneya Dravya

Substances which are having ushna (hot), Teekshna (stimulating), Sukshma (minute), Ruksha (non-unctuous), Khara (rough), Visada (clear) etc., properties and which acts as appetizer, which improves colour and complexion etc., is known as Āgneya dravya. Rupa (shape/colour/illumination) is its main characteristic feature. They will be mainly pungent with little bit salt cum sour taste. They exhibit a property of travelling in upward direction[4].

---

१. (i) मञ्चभूतात्मकं तत्तु क्ष्मामधिष्ठायजायते । अम्बुयोन्यग्नि पवन नभसां समवायतः॥ (अ. हृ. सू.९)
(ii) इह किं द्रव्यं पञ्चमहाभूतात्मकम् । तस्याधिष्ठानं- पृथिवी, योनिरुदकं,
समवायान्निर्वृत्तिविशेषाः। (अ.सं.सू. १७)

२. (i) मृदु लघु सूक्ष्म श्लक्ष्ण शब्दगुणबहुल्यकानि आकाशात्मकानि। (च.सू.२६)
(ii) श्लक्ष्ण सूक्ष्म मृदु व्यवायि विशद विविक्तं अव्यक्तरसं शब्दबहुलं आकाशीयं;
तन्मार्दव सौषिर्य लाघवकरमिति । (सु.सू. ४१)

३. (i) लघु शीत रूक्ष खर विशद सूक्ष्म स्पर्शबहुलानि वायव्यानि । (च.सू. २६)
(ii) सूक्ष्म सर शिशिर लघु विशदं स्पर्शगुणबहुलं ईषत्तिक्तं विशेषतः कषायमिति वायवीयं ।
(सु.सू. ४१)

४. (i) उष्ण तीक्ष्ण सूक्ष्म लघु रूक्ष विशद रूपगुणबहुलान्याग्नेयानि । (च.सू. २६)
(ii) उष्ण तीक्ष्ण सूक्ष्म रूक्ष खर लघु विशदं, रूपबहुलं ईषदम्ललवणं कटुरसप्रायं, विशेषतश्चोर्ध्व-
गतिस्वभावमिति तैजसं, तद्दहन-पाचन-दारण-तापन-प्रकाशन-प्रभावर्णकरमिति । (सु. सू. ४१)

(4) Āpya Dravya

Substances which have Drava (liquidity), Snigdha (unctuous), Seeta (cold), Manda (dull or slow acting), Mridu (smooth), Pichchila (sticky), Sāndra (turbid), Guru (heavy) etc., properties and which provides only appearance, nourishment, attachements inside the body, brings about fluidity etc., are known as Āpya or Jaliya dravyas. Rasa (taste) is its characteristic feature. They will be mainly sweet in taste with little bit of astringent, sour and salty tastes[1].

(5) Parthiva Dravya

Substances which have Guru (heavy), Khara (rough), Katina (hard), Manda (dull or slow acting), Sthira (stables), Visada (clear), Sandra (turbid), Sthula (bigger particle size) etc., properties and which provides strength, tonicity, attachements, growth etc., to body are known to be Parthiva dravyas. Gandha is its characteristic feature. They will be mainly sweet with little bit of stringent taste. They exhibit a property of spreading in downward direction[2].

4. Classification on the Basis of Source: (योनिभेदेन)

Dravyas are divided into three groups on the basis of their source of origin[3&4] viz.:

1. Jāngama (Animal source) e.g.: Kasturi (musk), Pearl (mukta) etc.
2. Oudbhida (Herbal source) e.g.: Yasthimadhu (liquoria), Visha (Aconite) etc.

---

१. (i) द्रवस्निग्ध शीत मन्द मृदु पिच्छिल रसगुणबहुलान्याप्यानि । (च. सू. २६)
(ii) शीत स्तिमित स्निग्ध मन्द गुरु सान्द्र मृदु पिच्छिलं रसबहुलमीषत्कषायाम्ललवणं मधुररसप्रायमाप्यम् तत् स्नेहन-ह्लादन-क्लेदन-बन्धन-विष्यन्दनकरमिति । (सु. सू. ४१)

२. (i) तत्र द्रव्याणि गुरू खर कठिन मन्द स्थिर विशद सान्द्र स्थूल गन्धगुण बहुलानि पार्थिवानि । (च. सू. २६)
(ii) तत्र स्थूल सान्द्र मन्द स्थिर गुरू कठिन गन्धबहुलं ईषत्कषायं प्रायशो मधुरमिति पार्थिवं । तत् स्थैर्य-बल-गौरव-संघात-उपचयकरं-विशेषतश्चाधोगतिस्वभावमिति । (सु. सू. ४१)

३. तत्पुनस्त्रिविधं प्रोक्तं जङ्गमौद्भिदपार्थिवम् । (च. सू. १/६८)

४. Sushrita considered only sthavara (plants) and Jangama (animals).
..... द्रव्याणि पुनरोषधयः । तासु द्विविधः -स्थावरा जङ्गमाश्च । (सु. सू. १/२८)

3. Parthiva or Bhouma (Mineral source) e.g.: Abhraka (mica), Parada (mercury) etc.

(1) Jāngamam

All the creatures which are able to walk or crawl (i.e., which are able to move) are considered as Jangama[1]. It is otherwise defined as those who have originated in the animal kingdom are known as Jangama[2]. These are sub-divided into four classes viz., (i) Jarayuja, (ii) Andaja, (iii) Swedaja & (iv) Udbhijja[3].

i. **Jarayuja:** animals which have placental birth e.g.: man, lion, tiger, cow, goat etc.

ii. **Andaja:** aves (birds) and reptiles etc., which have their birth through eggs e.g.: crow, snakes, lizards, fish etc.

iii. **Swedaja:** the creatures which have their birth in sweda (dirty water etc.) e.g.: flies, mosquitos, ants and worms found in the faces etc.

iv. **Udbhijja:** smaller creatures and animals which are born in the mud or clay e.g. frogs etc.

Dalhana enumerated certain exceptions in the above categories. Among birds Balaka (a crane variety) is Jarayuja as well as Andaja. Among snakes Ahipātaka (a snake) is Jarayuja only. Among Swedaja certain ants are Andaja as well as Udbhijja[4].

Charaka quoted the following items as animal products: honey, milk and milk products, bile, lard (vasa), bone narrow, blood, meat feces, urine, skin, semen, bone, ligaments, horns, nails, hoofs, hair, choliolyths, testes, urinary bladder etc[5].

---

१. गच्छतीति जङ्गमम् । (चक्रपाणि)

२. जङ्गमप्रभवं जाङ्गमम् । (योगेन्द्रनाथ)

३. जङ्गमा:खल्वपि चतुर्विधा: - जरायुजाण्डजस्वेदजोद्भिज्जा: । तत्र पशुमनुष्य-
व्यालादयो जरायुजा:; खगसर्पसरीसृपप्रभृतयोऽण्डजा:; कृमिकीटपिपीलिकाप्रभृतय:
स्वेदजा:; इन्द्रगोपमण्डूकप्रभृतय: उद्भिज्जा:।। (सु.सू. १/३०)

४. जरायुजादिषु पूर्वोक्तसंस्वेदजादिक्रमत्यागो योनिसंकरं बोधयति; तेन पक्षिषु
बलाका जरायुजा अण्डजा चेति, सर्पजातिषु अहिपताका जरायुजा, संस्वेदजेष्वपि
काश्चित् पिपीलिका अण्डजा उद्भिज्जाश्च । (डल्हण- सु.सू. १/३०)

५. (i) जङ्गमेभ्यश्चर्मनखरोमरुधिरादय: । (सु. सू. १/३१)
(ii) मधूनि गोरसा: पित्तं वसा मज्जाऽसृगामिषम् ।।

क्रमश: पृष्ठ २४ में........

Dalhana also made elaborate description of Jangama dravyas with several examples[1]. At later times other animal sources like Kasturi (musk), Puti (civet), Agnijara (amber) etc., are added to materia medica.

(2) Oudbhidam

Those which grows by sprouting through or piercing through the soil are known as oudbhida dravyas i.e., plants[2]. They are again divided into four classes viz., vanaspati (Apushpa), virudha, vānaspatya (vriksha or sapushpa) & oshdhi[3].

i. **Vanaspati:** These plants do not possess visible flowers. Hence called as 'Apushpa' (flower-less). They will themselves with fruits alone e.g. Udumbara (F. glomerata), vata (F. benghalensis) etc. These are mainly tall trees and therefore considered as the leaders/kings of forests[4].

पृष्ठ २३ से क्रमशः.............

विण्मूत्रचर्मरेतोऽस्थिस्नायुशृङ्गनखाः खुराः ।
जङ्गमेभ्यः प्रयुज्यन्ते केशा लोमानि रोचनाः ॥ (च.सू. १/६८-६९)

* चक्रपाणिः- संस्वेदजस्येह क्रिम्यादेर्जङ्गमेऽवरोधः, कुकुण्डकादेश्च औद्भिदे । जङ्गमशब्देन जङ्गमप्रभवं गोरसमध्वाद्यपि ग्राह्यम् । .... रोचना गोरोचना । डातच्च मध्वादि प्राय उपयोगित्वात् प्राधान्यादुक्तं,तेनाण्डबस्त्यादीनां च ग्रहणं बोद्धव्यम् ।

१. व्यालादय इति व्याला हिंस्रपशुव्याघ्रादयः, अन्ये तु पशुग्रहणादेव हिंस्रपशूनामपि ग्रहणमिति व्यालशब्देन सर्पविशेषमाहुः । ...... आदिग्रहणात् बलाकाजतुकादयः।...... खगसर्पेत्यादि खगाः पक्षिणः, सर्पा मन्दगामिनोऽजगरप्रभृतयः, सरीसृपाः शीघ्रगमिनः कृष्णसर्पादयः, मीनमकरादयो वा; प्रभृतिग्रहणं कूर्मनक्रादीनां ग्रहणं .....। कृमिकीटेत्यादि कृमयः कोष्ठपुरीषादिवाष्पसंभवाः, कीटा वृश्चिकषड्विन्दुप्रभृतयः, पिपिलिकाश्चटिकाः, प्रभृतिग्रहणादेवंविधा अन्येऽपि दृश्यन्ते । इन्द्रगोप इत्यादि इन्द्रगोपाः प्रावृट्कालजा अतिरक्तकृमयः 'इन्द्रवधू' इति लोके, प्रभृतिग्रहणादीदृशा अन्येऽपि । (डल्हण - सु. सू. १/३०)

२. उद्भिद्य पृथिवीं जायते इति औद्भिदम् । (चक्रपाणि- च. सू. १)

३. (i) ......औद्भिदं तु चतुर्विधम् । वनस्ततिस्तथावीरूद्वानस्पत्यस्तथौषधिः ॥ (च.सू.८/७१)
(ii) तासां स्थावराश्चतुर्विधा- वनस्पतयो, वृक्षा, वीरुध ओषधय इति । (सु. सू. १/२९)

४. (i) फलैर्वनस्पतिः ..... । (च. सू. १/७२)
(ii) फलैर्वनस्पतिरिति विनापुष्पैः फलैर्युक्ता वटोदुम्बरादयः । (चक्रपाणि)
(iii) तेषामपुष्पाः फलिनो वनस्पतय इति स्मृताः । (हारीत)
(iv) तासु, अपुष्पाः फलवन्तो वनस्पतयः । (सु. सू. १/२९)

क्रमशः पृष्ठ २४ में.......

ii. **Virudha:** Those plants which twin, crawl or climb are known as Virudhas[1]. These are sub-divided into two orders:

a. **Lata:** Climbers e.g. Vidari (Puraria tuberosa), Kapikachchu (Mucuna prurita) etc.

b. **Gulma:** Shrubs e.g. Atibala (Abutilon indicum), Saliparni (Desmodium gangeticum) etc.

iii. **Vānaspatya:** The plants which possess both the flowers and the fruits visibily are known as Vanaspatya or Vriksh or Sapushpa[2]. These are generally medium to big trees (not gaint trees like banyon etc.) yielding edible fruits e.g. Amra (mango),Jambu (Schyzizium jambosa) etc.

iv. **Oushadhi:** Those plants which die after yielding the fruits or after harvest are known as Oushadhis. These are usually annual herbs like paddy, pulses,wheat, maize etc[3].

पृष्ठ २४ से क्रमश:........

(v) अपुष्पा इति अविद्यमानपुष्पा: फलवन्त इति फलं येषामस्ति ते वनस्पतय इति .....प्लक्षोदुम्बरादय:। (डल्हण)

(vi) अपुष्पा इति पुष्पाणामतिसूक्ष्मतया पुष्पाधारकर्णिकया (peduncle) आच्छादितत्वाच्च अदृश्यपुष्पा इत्यर्थ:। (यादवजी त्रिकमजी- सु. सू. १/२९)

(Vii) वननां पाता पालयिता वा । (या. नि. ८/३)

१. (i) ..... प्रतानै: वीरुध: स्मृता: । (च. सू. १/७२)

(ii) वीरुध: ......वीरोहणात् । (या. नि. ६/३)

(iii) प्रतानशब्देन लता गुल्माश्च गृह्यन्ते । (चक्रपाणि)

(vi) लता गुल्माश्च वीरुध: । (हारीत)

(v) प्रतानवत्य: स्तम्बिन्यश्च वीरुध: । (सु. सू. १/२९)

(vi) प्रतानवत्यो विस्ताखत्य: वीरुध:, न केवलं प्रतानवत्यो वीरुध: स्तम्बिन्यश्च गुल्मिन्यश्च, गुल्म: पुन: वर्तुललतासन्ततिविटप:, ताश्च विदारीकोलवल्लीशालपर्णीपृश्निपर्णीप्रभृतय:। (डल्हण)

२. (i) .... पुष्पैर्वानस्पत्य: फलैरपि । (च. सू. १/७२)

(ii) पुष्पैर्वानस्पत्य: फलैरपि पुष्पानन्तरं फलभाज इत्यर्थ: । (चक्रपाणि)

(iii) वृक्षो व्रश्चनात् । वृत्वा क्षां तिष्ठति । (या. नि. १२/२९)

(vi) पुष्पफलवन्तो वृक्षा: । (सु. सू. १/२९)

(v) पुष्पफलवन्तो वृक्षा इति उभययुक्ता वृक्षा: ...... आम्रजम्बूप्रभृतय: । (डल्हण)

३. (i) औषध्य: फलपाकान्ता: .... । (च.सू. १/७२)

(ii) फलस्य पाकादन्तो विनाशो येषां तिलमुद्गादीनां ते फलपाकान्ता:, अत्र केचित् फलपाकान्ता:।

(vi) फलपाकनिष्ठा ओषधय इति । (सु. सू. १/२९)

क्रमश: पृष्ठ २६ में.......

Charaka quoted the following as the parthiva group: Mula (root), Twak (bark), Sara (sap or heart-wood), Niryasa (gum or resin), Nala (tubes), Swarasa (fresh juice), Pallava (tender leaves), Kshara (alkali), Kshira (latex), Phala (fruit), Pushpa (flower), Bhasma (ash), Taila (oil), Kantaka (spines, thorns), Patra (leaf), Sunga (galls terminal buds), Kanda (tubers), Praroha (ariel roots & climbing stems) etc[1].

(3) Parthivam or Bhoumam

Those substances which are available beneath the earth i.e., soil are known as 'Parthivam'[2]. Usually all the mineral ores, metals, salts, alkalies etc., are categorized as Parthiva dravyas[3]. Even

---

पृष्ठ २५से क्रमशः.......

(v) फलपाकनिष्ठा इति निष्ठा नाशः, फलपाकेन परणित्था नाशो यासां तास्तथोक्ताः; ते पुनर्गोधूमादयः। अन्ये तु निष्ठाशब्दं प्रत्येकं संबध्नन्ति, फलनिष्ठाः पाकनिष्ठा इति; तत्र फलनिष्ठा शालितिलकुलत्थादयः, पाकनिष्ठा कवकादयः । (डल्हण)

१. (i) मूलत्वक्सारनिर्यासनालस्वरसपल्लवाः । क्षाराः क्षीरं फलं पुष्पं भस्म तैलानि कण्टकाः ॥ पत्राणि शुङ्गाः कन्दाश्च प्ररोहाश्चौद्भिदो गणः । (च. सू. १/७३-७४)

(ii) तत्र स्थावरेभ्य स्त्वक पत्रपुष्पफलमूलकन्दनिर्यासस्वरसादयः प्रयोजनवन्तः। (सु. सू. १/३१)

२. पृथिवीविकारः पार्थिवम् । (चक्रपाणि- च. सू. १/६८)

३. (i) सुवर्णं समलाः पञ्च लोहाः ससिकता सुधा । मनःशिलायो मणयो लवणं गैरिकाञ्जने ॥ भौममौषधमुद्दिष्ठम् .... । (च. सू. १/)

* चक्रपाणिः- पञ्चलोहा इति ताम्ररजतत्रपुशीशकृष्णलोहानां ग्रहणम् । समला इति मलशब्देन शिलाजतूनि लोहमलरूपाणि गृह्यन्ते, तच्च सुश्रुतदर्शनात् सुवर्ण रजतादिभंव षङ्विधमेव गृह्यते, सुश्रुते हि षङ्विधमेव शिलाजतूक्तम् , इह तु रसायने चतुर्विधमुक्तं- ''चतुर्भ्यो धातुभ्यस्तस्य संभवः । हेम्नोऽय रजतात्ताम्राद्वरं कृष्णायसादपि'' (चि. अ. १) इति वचनात् । डातच्च वचनं रसायनाधिकारितां चतुर्विधस्य शिलाजतुनो दर्शयति, नतु षङ्विधशिलाजतुप्रतिषेधपरमिति न सुश्रुतेन समं विरोधः । किंवा सुवर्णं निर्मलं, समलास्तु रजतताम्रत्रपुशीसलोहाः (इति मिलित्वा पञ्चलोहाः।) शिलजतुपाषाणङ्कप्रभृतीनां तु ग्रहणमुद्दिष्टशब्देन सूचितम्; उद्देशो ह्यल्पकथनम् । सुधा गाङ्गेयिका। आलं हरितालम् । अञ्जनं सौवीराञ्जनम् ।

(ii) पार्थिवाः सुवर्णरजतमणिमुक्तामनःशिलामृत्कपालादयः ॥ (सु. सू. १/३२)

* डल्हणः- रसाधिकारिकमौवधिवर्गं स्थावरजङ्गमं प्रतिपाद्य, परिशिष्टं प्रतिपादयितुमाह- पार्थिवा इत्यादि। पृथिव्या विकाराः पार्थिवाः, रजतं रौप्यं, मणिः स्फटिकादिः, मुक्ता मौक्तिकं, मृत् मृत्तिका, कपालं कर्परम्। सुवर्णस्येह पार्थिवत्वमेवाङ्गीक्रियते गुरुत्वकाठिन्यस्थैर्यादिहेतुभिः सूत्रे आदिग्रहणाल्लोह-मल-सिकतासुधाहरि-ताललवणगैरिकरसाञ्जप्रभृतीनां ग्रहणम् । यद्यपि स्थितिशीलत्वात्तथा लोकद्वित्व-समाख्यानेऽपृथगुक्तत्वाच्च स्थावरशब्देनैव पार्थिवा उच्यन्ते, तथाऽप्यत्र प्रकरणाद्येष्वाहारोपयोगित्वं फलमूलद्यवयवेषु रसप्रधानतया तत्रैव चतुर्विधे वनस्पत्यादिगणे स्थावरशब्दो वर्तते न तु पार्थिवेष्वपि, तेषामाहारेषु प्रायेणानुपयोगात्; अन्यदपि समाधानान्तरमस्ति, तच्च विस्तरभयान्न लिखितम् ॥

Mukta, Pravala etc., were also considered as Bhauma dsavyas. But this view was not accepted by Yadavji.

Classification of sthavara dravyas or parthiva dravyas indicates the knowledge of Rasa oushadhis in the ancient times before the development of Rasa-Sastra.

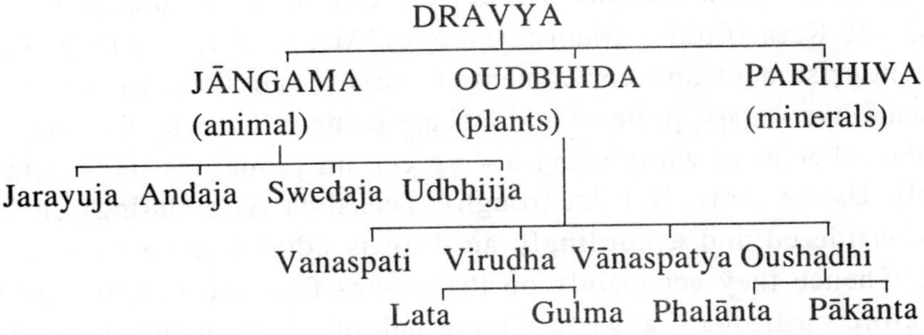

Though Suśruta accepted the classfication of Jangama, Oudbhida and Parthiva, he mainly divided the substances into two groups viz., Jangama and Ouddhida. Afterwards he seperately explained Bhouma dravyas i.e., metals and minerals.

5. Classification on the Basis of Utility: (प्रयोग भेदेन)

On the basis of the usage or utility, dravyas may be classified as oushadha dravyas (drugs) and Āhara dravyas (foods). Chakrapani proposed this concept while discussing about Yavagu (grue)[1]. According to him the drug important on the basis of potency (Virya) and food is important on the basis of taste (Rasa). Active principle and Primary metabolites of a herb are responsible for the above aspects respectively.

Usually drugs like Haritaki (T. chebula) Amalaki (E. officinalis), chitraka (P. zeylanica) are used for their respective therapeutic effects basing upon the potency. But food materials like Sali (rice), Mudga (green gram), Taila (gingely oil) are used as diet basing upon their primary metabolites viz., carbohydrates, proteins, fats. Over all, both Āhara and Oushadha are of equal impor-

१. यवागूसाधनद्रव्यं तावद् द्विविधं वीर्यप्रधानमौषधद्रव्यं रसप्रधानमाहारद्रव्यञ्च ।
(चक्रपाणि- च. सू. २१)

tance in the treatment. For example- Guduchi or Kirata tikta or Usiradi panaka are used as Jwara hara (anti-pyretic). At the same time Seetodaka (cold water), Yavagu (grue) etc., are indicated as diet. hence these two are inseperable aspects of treatment.

The major difference between Oushadha and Ahara dravyas will be that 'Ahara dravyas will act directly upon the dhatus (tissues) like Rasa (fluids), Mamsa (muscle), Medas (fat) and helps in their nourishment and enrichment. In this process the food constituents like sugars, proteins and fats are being utilized by the body. On the other hand while using a drug certain properties like Seeta (cold), Ushna (hot), Ruksha (rough), Teekshna (stimulating) etc., are considered and accordingly an drug is administered to a patient. Thence they act mainly on the doshas first and dhatus next. Therefore oushadha dravyas are more helpful in the mangement of the diseases.

A suitable example will be Pushkaramula (Inula racemosa). Inulin a carbohydrate/starch is used as food and its active principles (triterpenoids) are used as drugs. The former ingredient is primary metabolite and the later ingredient is secondary metabolite.

Chakrapani sub-divided the oushadha dravyas into three classes viz., Tikshna (severe), Madhyama (moderate) & Mridu (mild) viryas[1].

DRAVYA

- Oushadha (Drug)
  - Tikshna (Severe)
  - Madhyama (Moderate)
  - Mridu (Mild)
- Ahara (Food)

6. Classification on the Basis of Teste: (रसभेदेन या रसस्कन्ध)

On the basis of six tastes (Shad Rasa), Acharyas of Ayurveda classified the dravyas into six groups viz.,

(1) Madhura Skandha– drugs which are mainly sweet in taste e.g. grapes, honey, Yashti, Madhu etc.

१. त्रिविधं वीर्यभेदात् तीक्ष्णवीर्यं, मध्यवीर्यं, मृदुवीर्यं चेति । (चक्रपाणि- च. सू. २१)

(2) **Amla Skandha–** drugs which are mainly sour in taste e.g. lemon, pomegranate, tamarind etc.

(3) **Lavana Skandha–** drugs which are mainly salt in taste e.g. normal salt, rock salt etc.

(4) **Katuka Skandha–** drugs which are mainly pungent in taste e.g. pepper, ginger etc.

(5) **Tikta Skandha–** drugs which are mainly bitter in taste e.g. neem, bitter gourd etc.

(6) **Kashaya Skandha–** drugs which are mainly astringent in taste e.g. chebulic fruit, Ficus sps etc.

* **Note:** The important ingredients of individual groups have been tabulated, vide: (Table No.I) Page No. 30.

(7) Classification on the Basis of Potency: (वीर्यभेदेन)

Most of the drugs mentioned under Ayurvedic materia medica are denoted as either Sita or Ushna virya dravyas. We come across the classification of dravyas on the basis of potency (virya) in the CCIM syllabus and also in the text book of Acharya P.V. Sharmaji. Chandanadi varga dravyas and Agurvadi varga dravyas were described as the examples of 'Sita virya' and 'Ushna virya' dravyas respectively.

However the above two groups are mentioned for Taila preparation under Kashaya kalpana. Therefore scholars like Dr. K. Nisteswar do not agree with the above concept because:

1. Chandanadi varga dravyas contain certain Ushna virya dravyas like Atmagupta, sravani etc.
2. Āgruvadi varga dravyas contain certain Sita virya dravyas like Bala, Ati bala etc.

Above all, one can not find any classical reference for the virya based drug classification. But the 120 main drugs which are present in CCIM Syllabus may be classified into two groups:

(a) Seeta Virya Dravyas

(1)*Ativisha (2) Arjuna (3) Ashoka (4) Āmalaki (5) Āragwadha (6) Udumbara (7) Useera (8) Ela (9) Kanchanāra (10) Katuka (11)

Table No. I

Classification of Dravyas on the basis of taste (Rasa)

Madhura Skandha	Amla Skandha	Lavana Skandha	Katuka Skandha	Tikta Skandha	Kashaya Skandha
Kakoli, Kshira, Kakoli, Jivaka, Rishabhaka, Mudga parni, meda, Maha, Meda, Guduchi, Karkata Sringi, Kshira, Riddhi, Vriddhi, Sringataka, Jivanti, Yashti madhu, Ghrita, vasa, Majja, Sali, Sashtika dhanya, Yava, Godhuma, Masha, Kaseruka, Trapusha, Ērvaruka, Karkaru, Ālabu, Kālinda, Kataka, Priyala, Padma beeja, kashmarya, Madhuka, Draksha, Kharjura, Tala, Narikela, Vidari, Ikshu, Kapikachchu, Gokshura, shatavari, Saliparni, Prisniparni, Sata pushpa, Mundi, Aswagandha, Bala, Punarnava, Parushaka Sariva etc.	Dadima, Āmalaka, Bija pura, Āmra, Amrataka Badara, Karamarda, Kapitha, Raja badara, Prachinamalaka, Tintidika, Kōsamra, Bhavya, Pāravata, Lakucha, Amlavetasa, Jambira, Dadhi, Takra, Sura, Sukta, Souviraka, Tushodaka, Dhanyamla, Iravata, vrikshamla, Dhanvana, Asmantaka, Changeri etc.	Sanidhav lavana, Souvarcha lavana, Kāla lavana, Vida lavana, Samudra lavana, oudbhida lavana, Yava kshar, Sarja kshar etc.	Pippali, Gaja pippali, Pippali mula, Chavya, Chitraka, Sunthi, Maricha, Ajamoda, Ārdraka, Vidanga, Dhanyaka, Pilu, Tejohva, Ela, Kushta, Bhallataka, Hingu, Devadaru, Mulaka, Sarshapa, Lasuna, Karanja, Sigru, Madhu sigru, Tulasi, Kshara, Mutra, Pitta, Karpura, Bakuchi, Guggulu, Mustaka, Langali etc. Single herb's and Pippalyadi gana, Surasadi gana, Sāla saradi gana ingredients mostly.	Chandana, Vsira, Krita mala, Naktamala, Nimba, Tumburu, Kutaja, Haridra, Daru haridra, Musta, Murva, Kirata tikta, katu rohini, Kebuka Trayamana, Karavella, Kara Veera, Punarnava, vasa, Manduka Parni, Vārtaka, Kākamachi, Ativisha, Kakodumbara, Patola, Pāta, Guduchi, Vikankata, Bakula, Katphala, Sapta parna, Jāti, Arka Vacha, Tagara, Agaru, Varuna, Indra-Yava, Brihati, Kantakari, Trivrit, yava tikta, kritavedhana, Sankhapushpi etc., and Āragwadhadi gana, Guduchyadi gana ingredients mostly.	Priyangu, Syonaka Pata, Amrosthi, Lodhra, Mocha Rasa, Lajjalu, Dhataki pushpa, Sirisha, Sinsipa, Sweta, khadira, Tinduka, Priyala, Khadira, Kadara, Aswakarna, Tinisa, Arjuna, Asana, Arimeda, Elavaluka, kadamba, kaivarta mustha, Sallaki, Jingini, Kaseru, Kat phala, vamsa, Padmaka, Asoka, Sāla, Dhava, Sarja, Bhurja, Sana pushpi, Sami, Kataka, Madanaphala, pāshana bheda, kovidara etc., and Nyagrodhadi gana, Ambashtadi gana, Rodhradi gana, Triphala, Salasāradi gana ingredients mostly.

Karpura (12) Kiratatikta (13)* Kutaja (14) Kupilu (16) Kushmanda (17) Khadira (18) Gokshura (19) Chandana (20) Jambu (21) Jatamamsi (22) Nāga bala (23) Nimba (24)* Patha (कै. नि) (25)* Pippali (Ardra) (26) Bala (27) Brahmi (28) Mandukaparni (29) Madhu yashti (30) Misreya (31) Mustaka (32) Yavasa (33) Lavanga (34) Lodhra (35) Vāsa (36) Sankha pushpi (37) Shatavari (38) Sariva (39) Shala (40) Shalmali.

(b) Ushna Virya Dravyas

(1) Agaru (2) Agnimantha (3) Ajamoda (4)* Ativisha (6) Apamarga (7) Arka (8) Aswagandha (9) Ahiphena (10) Indravaruni (11) Eranda (12) Kantakari (13) Kapikachchu (14) Karanja (15) Karaveera (16) Karkata sringi (17) Kupilu (18) Kushta (19) Krishna jiraka (20) Gandha prasarini (21) Gambhari (22) Guggulu (23) Guduchi (24) Changeri (25) Chitraka (26) Jati phala (27) Jeeraka (28) Jyotishmati (29) Talisa patri (30) Tulasi (31) Tuvaraka (32) Tejohva (33)Trivrit (34) Twak (35) Danti (36) Dadima (37) Daru haridra (38) Deva daru (39) Drona pushpi (40) Dhattura (41) Dhātaki (42) Dhānyaka (43) Naga kesara (44) Nimbuka (45) Nirgundi (46) Patala (47) Palasa (48) Patola (49)* Patha (50) Pārasika yavani (51)* Pippali (Sushka) (52) Punarnava (53) Pushkarmul (54) Prisni parni (55) Bākuchi (56) Bilva (57) Brihati (58) Bhangā (59) Bhallataka (60) Bhārangi (61) Bhringa raja (62) Manjishta (63) Madanaphala (64) Maricha (65) Yavani (66) Rasna (67)Latakaranja (68) Vacha (69) Vatsanabhi (70) Varuna (71) Vidanga (72) Vibhitaki (73) Satapushpi (74) Sarapunkha (75) Saliparni (76) Shigru (77) Syonaka (78) Sapta parna (79) Sarpagandha (80) Haridra (81) Haritaki (82) Hingu (83) Kutaja (रा. नि) (84) Sirisha (अनुष्णवीर्य).

Note— *Marked herbs have Seeta or Ushna Virya according to different texts/part used.

8. Classification on the Basis of Effect on the Humors: (दोषकर्मानुसारेण)

Dravyas are classified into three major groups on the basis of their activity over the humors (Tridoshas) viz.,

(1) Dosha Sāmaka- drugs used to subside the aggravated doshas.

(2) Dosha Prakopaka- drugs used to stimulated the doshas.

(3) Swastha Hita- drugs used in the preventive medicare[1].

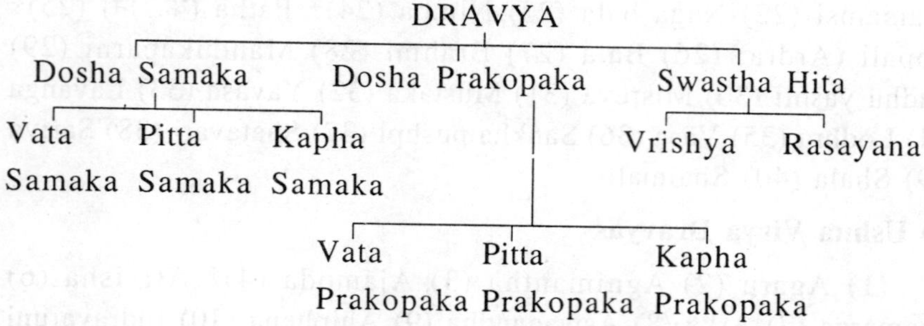

After going through diferent concepts of drug classifications, the author proposes the following comprehensive classfication of dravya.

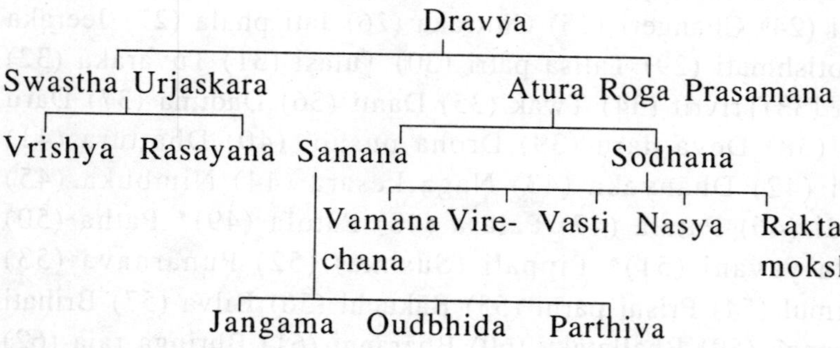

Samsodhana Dravyas

There is another group described seperately on the basis of their effect on the doshas again. These are known as "Dosha Samsodhana Dravyas" i.e., drugs used to expel or eliminate the vitiated doshas completely. They are described under three subgroups viz.,

(1) Urdhwa Bhagahara (elimination in upward direction)- i.e., vamana (emesis) e.g. Madana phala.

(2) Adho Bhagahara (elimination in downward direction)- i.e., Virechana (purgation) e.g. Snuhi ksheera.

१. (i) किञ्चिद्दोषप्रशमनं किञ्चिद्धातुप्रदूषणम् ।
स्वस्थवृत्तौ मतं किञ्चित्रिविधं द्रव्यमुच्यते ॥ (च. सू. १)

(ii) शमनं-कोपनं-स्वस्थहितं द्रव्यमिति त्रिधा ॥ (अ. सं. सू. १)

(iii) स्वस्थस्योर्जस्करं यत्तु तद्वृष्यं तद्रसायनम् ॥ (च. चि.। अ.।पा.)

(3) Ubhaya Bhagahara (elimination in both direction)- i.e., Vamana & Virechana e.g. Ikshwaku[1].

(1) Swastha Hita Dravyas

There are two groups of drugs which are generally prescribed even in the healthy state. They are: Rasayana and Vajikarana. A part from these, under Oushadha and Āhara of Swastha (vide: Swastha Vritta Niyama), many foods and drugs are deliniated. In this context it is essential to high-light the concept of Agrya Oushadhas and Pathya tama dravyas of Charaka Sutra 25th chapter[2,3].

They are: Rakta Sali, Mudga, Antarikshodaka, Saindhava, Jivanti Saka, Ena mamsa, Lāva mamsa, Godha mamsa, Rohita matsya, Goghrita, Tila taila, Varaha vasa, Paka hamsa vasa, Kukkutavasa, Aja medas, Sringavera, Mridvika, Sarkara, Dadima, Āmalaka etc.

(2) Dosha Samaka Dravyas

(i) **Vata Samaka-** Madhura-Amla-Lavana rasas; Ushna-Snigdha guna, Ushna virya; Guru (Madhura) vipaka[4,5,6,7,8] etc. Drugs like- Devadaru, Varuna, Sallaki, Bharangi etc.

---

१. तत्रं दोषहरणं ऊर्ध्वभाग वमनसंज्ञकं, अधोभागं विरेचन संज्ञकं ।
उभयं वा शरीरमलरेचनात् विरेचनमिति संज्ञां लभते । (च. क.)

२. लोहितशालयः शूकधान्यानां पथ्यतमत्वेन श्रेष्ठतमा भवन्ति, मुद्गाः शमीधान्यानाम्, आन्तरिक्षमुदकानां, सैन्धवं लवणानाम् , जीवन्तीशाकं शाकानाम् , डोणेयं मृगमांसानां, लावः पक्षिणां, गोधा बिलेशयानां, रोहितो मत्स्यानां, गन्यं सर्विः सर्पिषां, गोक्षीरं क्षीराणां, तिलतैलं स्थावरजातानां स्नेहानाम्, वराहवसा आनूपमृगवसानां, चलुकीवसा मत्स्यवसानां, पाकहंसवसा जलचरविहंगवसानां, कुक्कुटवसा विष्किर-शकुनिवसानां, अजमेदः शखादमेदसां, शृङ्गबेरं कन्दानां, मृद्वीका फलानां, शर्करा इक्षुविकाराणामिति प्रकृत्यैव हिततमानामाहारविकाराणां प्राधान्यतो द्रव्याणि व्याख्यातानि भवन्ति । (च. सू. २५)

३. यदाहारजातमग्निवेश, समांश्चैव शरीरधातून् प्रकृतौ स्थापयतीति विषमाँश्च समीकरोतीत्येतद्धितं विद्धि विपरीतमहितमिति । (च. सू. २५)

४. रूक्षः शीतो लघुः सूक्ष्मश्चलोऽय विशदः खरः । वीपरीतगुणैर्द्रव्यैर्मारुतः संप्रशाम्यति ।।(च. सू. । अ.)

५. तत्र भद्रदारूकुष्ठ हरिद्रा वरुण मेषशृङ्गी बलातिबलार्तगल कच्छुरा शल्लकी कुबेराक्षी वीरतरु सहचर अग्निमन्थ वत्सादनी डारण्ड अश्मभेदक अलर्क अर्क शतावरी पुनर्नवा वसुक वसिर काञ्चनक भार्ङ्गी कार्पासी वृश्चिकाली पत्तूर बदर यव कोल कुलुत्थ प्रभृतीनि विदारिगन्धादिश्च द्वे चाद्ये पञ्चमूल्यौ समासेन वातसंशमनो वर्गः । (सु.सू. ३९)

६. तत्र मधुराम्ललवणा वातघ्नाः । (सु. सू. ४१)

७. गुरुपाको वातपित्तघ्नः । (सु. सू. ४१)

८. तत्र उष्णस्निग्धौ वातघ्नौ । (सु. सू. ४१)

(ii) **Pitta Samaka–** Madhura-Tikta-Kashaya rasas; Seeta-Mridu-pichila gunas; Seeta virya; Guru (Madhura) vipaka. Drugs like-Chandana, Usira, Murva, Sariva, Manjishta[1,2,3,4] etc.

(iii) **Kapha Samaka–** Kata-Tikta-Kashaya rasas; Ushra-Ruksha gunas; Ushna virya; Laghu (Amla or Katu) vipaka. Drugs like- Aguru, Langali, Rasna, Haridra[5,6,7,8] etc.

(3) Dosha Prakopaka dravyas

(i) **Vata Prakopaka–** Sushka Saka, Sushka Mamsa, Syamaka, Mudga, Masura, Jambu, Tinduka, Kalaya etc[9].

(ii) **Pitta Prakopaka–** Tila taila, Keulatha, Sarshapa, Matsya mamsa, Aja mamsa, Musta, Sura, Kshara, Mutra, Kanjika, Pilu, Langali, Maricha etc.[10]

(iii) **Kapha Prakopaka–** Yavaka, Masha, Godhuma, Dadhi, Dugdha, Ikshu vikara, Anupa mamsa, Sringataka, Pruthuka, Bhavya, Kharjura, Narikela etc[11].

---

१. सस्नेहमुष्णं तीक्ष्णं च द्रवमम्लं सरं कटु । विपरीतगुणैः पित्तं द्रव्यैराशु प्रशाम्यति ॥ (च. सू.१)

२. चन्दन कुचन्दन ह्रीबेर उशीर मञ्जिष्ठा पयस्या विदारी शतावरी गुन्द्रा शैवाल कह्लार कुमुद उत्पल कन्दली दूर्वा मूर्वा प्रभृतीनि काकोल्यादिः सारिवादिः अञ्जनादिः उत्पलादिः न्यग्रोधादिः तृणपञ्चमूलमिति समासेन पित्तसंशमनो वर्गः । (सु. सू. ३९)

३. मधुरतिक्तकषायाः पित्तघ्नाः । (सु. सू. ४१)

४. शीतमृदुपिच्छिलालः पित्तघ्नाः । (सु. सू. ४१)

५. गुरुशीतमृदुस्निग्धमधुरस्थिरपिच्छिलाः । श्लेष्माणः प्रशमं यान्ति विपरीतगुणैर्गुणाः ॥ (च. सू. १)

६. कालेयक अगुरु तिलपर्णी कुष्ठ हरिद्रा शीत शिव शतपुष्पा सरल रास्ना प्रकीर्या उदकीर्या इङ्गुदी सुमनः काकादनी लाङ्गलकी हस्तिकर्ण मुञ्जातक लामज्जक प्रभृतीनि वल्लीकण्टकपञ्चमूल्यौ पिप्पल्यादिः बृहत्यादिः मुष्ककादिः वचादिः सुरसादिः आरग्वधादिरिति समासेन श्लेष्मसंशमनो वर्गः ।(सु. सू. ३९)

७. कटुतिक्तकषायाः श्लेष्मघ्नाः । (सु. सू. ४१)

८. लघुपाकः श्लेष्मघ्नः । (सु. सू. ४१)

९. तत्र .... कटुतिक्तकषायरूक्षलघुशीतवीर्यशुष्कशाक वल्लूर वराक उद्दालक कोरदूष श्यामाक नीवार मुद्ग आढकी हरेणु कन्नाय निष्पाव......वेगविघातादिभिर्विशेषैः वायुः प्रकोपमापद्यते ।(सु. सू. २१)

१०. तत्र......कट्वम्ललवणतीक्ष्णोष्णघुविदाहि तिलतैल पिण्याक कुलत्थ सर्षप अतसी हरितशाक गोधामत्स्याजाविकमांस दधि तक्रकूर्चिका मस्तु सौवीरक सुराविकार अम्लफलकट्वरप्रभृतिभिः पित्तं प्रकोपमापद्यते । (सु. सू. २१)

११. तत्र.....मधुराम्ललवणशीतस्निग्धगुरुपिच्छिलाभिष्यन्दि हायनक यवक नैषध इत्कट माष महामाष गोधूम तिलपिष्टविकृति दधि दुग्ध कृशरा पायस इक्षुविकार आनूपौदकमांसवसा बिस मृणाल कसेरूक शृङ्गाटक मधुरवल्लीफल.....प्रभृतिभिः श्लेष्मा प्रकोपमापद्यते । (सु. सू. २१)

9. Classification on the Basis of Vipaka

Like virya classification this is also not mentioned in any of the classical texts. Acharya Priyavrata Sharmaji grouped certain drugs into three groups viz.,

(1) **Madhura Vipaka-** Madhura & Lavana rasa dravyas mainly.

(2) **Amla Vipaka-** Amla skandha dravyas mainly.

(3) **Katu Vipaka-** Katu-Tikta-Kashaya dravyas mainly. The 120 drugs of CCIM syllabus may be arranged into the following three groups on the basis of vipaka:

(1) Madhura Vipaka

(1) Aswagandha (2) Āmalaki (3) Aragwadha (4) Ārdraka (5) Eranda (6) Ela (7) Kapikachchu (8) Kūshmanda (9) Guduchi (10) Gokshura (11)* Dadima (12) Dhanyaka (13) Naga bala (14) Pippali (15) Prisniparni (16) Bala (17) Brahmi (18) Bhallataka (19) Manduka parni (20) Madhu yashti (21) Misreya (22) Vibhitaka (23) Sankhapushpi (24) Shatavari (25) Sāriva (26) Shali parni (27) Shalmali (28) Haritaki.

(2) Amla Vipaka

(1) Chāngeri (2) Dadima (3) Nimbuka (4) Bhavya

(3) Katu Vipaka

(1) Aguru (2) Agnimantha (3) Ajamoda (4) Ativisha (5) Aparajita (6) Apamarga (7) Arka (8) Arjuna (9) Ashoka (10) Ahiphena (11) Indravaruni (12) Udumbara (13) Useera (14) Kantakari (15) Kānchanāra (16) Katuka (17) Karanja (18) Karavira (19) Karkata sringi (20) Karpura (21) Kirata tikta (22) Kutaja (23) Kupilu (24) Kumari (25) Kushta (26) Krishna jiraka (27) Khadira (28) Gandha prasārini (29) Gambhari (30) Guggulu (31) Chandana (32) Chitraka (33) Jambu (34) Jatamamsi (35) Jatiphala (36) Jeeraka (37) Jyotishmati (38) Talisa pathri (39) Tulasi (40) Tuvaraka (41) Tejohva (42) Trivrit (43)Twak (44) Danthi (45) Dāru haridra (46) Deva daru (47) Drona pushpi (48) Dhattura (49) Dhataki (50) Naga kesara (51) Nimba (52) Nirgundi (53) Patola (54) Palasa (55) Patala (56) Patha (57) Parasika yavani(58) Punarnava (59) Pushkaramula

(60) Bakuchi (61) Bilva (62) Brihati (63) Bhanga (64) Bharngi (65) Bhringa raja (66) Manjishta (67) Madana phala (68) Maricha (69) Mustha (70) Yavani (71)Yavasa (72) Rasona (73) Lavanga (74) Lata karanja (75) Lodhra (76) Vacha (77) Vatsanabha (78) Varuna (79) Vāsā (80) Vidanga (81) Sata Pushpa (82) Sarapunkha (83) Shala (84) Shigru (85) Sirisha (86) Syonaka (87) Sapta parni (88) Sarpa gandha (89) Haridra (90) Hingu.

10. Classification of Dravya on the Basis of Evolution, Class, Shape and Age

Actually, most of these aspects are already discussed under different heads in the present chapter. Some of the modern aspects of classification are discussed in the XI chapter also.

Classification on the basis of evolution (Utpatti bhedena) is discussed in this chapter under 3rd point.

Classification on the basis of shape include trees, shrubs, climbers and herbs.These are discussed in this chapter under 4th point.

Classification on the basis of class, order, family, species etc, will be discussed in the XI chapter.

Classification on the basis of age deals with (i) Annuals (ii) Biennials and (iii) Perennials. Oshadhis and Vanaspatis will be the examples of annuals and perennials respectively.

11. Comparative knownledge of the groups of the Dravyas Quoted by Charaka, Suśruta and Vagbhata

In the ancient Ayurvedic treatises drugs have been grouped into either 'Vargas' or 'Ganas'. This grouping or classification was based upon their pharmacological properties as well as dietary use. Etymologically,Varga and Gana will provide the same meaning.

(i) **Varga*-** is a group of limited number of herbs having similar pharmacological properties.

---

* वर्गः = वृज्यते इति वर्गः । 'वृजि' वर्ज्जने । स्वजातीयसमूहः । (श. क. द्रु.)
= सजातीय समूहः । यथा मनुष्यवर्गः, पशुवर्गः ।
समानधर्मिभिः प्राण्यप्राणिभिः कृते ॥ (वाचस्पत्यम्)

(ii) **Gana****– is a group of large number of herbs having similar pharmacological properties.

(iii) **Skandha*****– is a group of drugs

From the above references it is clear that varga, gana and skandha denote a group of drugs described with similar pharmacological properties. Some scholars did mention that varga contain few drugs while gana contains many. But we do not find any such tendency in the treatises. For example Panchamula, Triphala etc., mentioned under ganas have very few drugs.

On review of literature it is observed that Charaka mainly concentrated upon a group of 10 drugs having one common indication e.g. Balya Varga, Hridya Varga, Daha prasamana varga, Krimighna varga etc. While Sushrita concentrated upon the multiple indications of a group of drugs e.g. Varunadi gana is indicated in Sirha sula, Gulma, Abhyantara vidhradi etc.; Surasadi gana is indicated in Krimi, Pratisyaya, Aruchi, Swasa-kasa, Varna etc. Another major difference between Charaka and Suśruta is that the former named the groups on the basis of its pharmacological action and the later named the groups on the basis of first ingredient. Over all, Charaka mentioned about 50 vargas and Suśruta quoted about 37 vargas[1,2,3,4].

Vriddha Vagbhata (author of Ashtanga Sangraha) accepted both the views of Charaka and Suśruta. He described 45 out of 50

** गण = गण समूहे । संग्रहविशेषे । सर्वसमिष्टि: । अथवा गण संख्याने । (वाचस्पत्यम्)
= गण्यते गणयति वा । समूहः । (श. क. द्रु.)

*** स्कन्धः = समूहे । (वाचस्पत्यम्)

१. (i) समासेन सप्तत्रिंशद् द्रव्यगणा भवन्ति । (सु. सू. ३८)
(ii) त्रयस्त्रिंशदिति प्रोक्ता वेर्गास्तेषु त्वलाभतः । (अ. हृ. सू. १५)

२. एतावन्तो ह्यलमल्पबुद्धीनां व्यवहाराय, बुद्धिमतां च स्वलक्षण्यानुमानयुक्तिकुशलानामनुक्तार्थज्ञानाय। (च.सू.४)
समस्तं वर्गमर्धं वा यथालाभमथापि वा । प्रयुञ्जीत भिषक् प्राज्ञो यथोद्दिष्टेषु कर्मसु ॥ (सु. सू. ३७)

३. समीक्ष्य दोषभेदाँश्च गणान् भिन्नान् प्रयोजयेत् ।
पृथक्मिश्रन् समस्तान् वा गणं वा व्यस्तसंहतम् ॥ (सु. सू. ३८)

४. प्रोक्तमपि यद्द्रव्यं भवेद् व्याधावयोगिकम् । तदुद्धरेद्यौगिकं तु प्रक्षिपेदप्यकीर्तितम् ॥ (सु.चि. १)

vargas of Charaka in the sutra sthana 15th chapter. The remaining 5 vargas are found in the 14th chapter. Among these five there is a little change since vagbhata mention:

Vamaka gana in place of Vamanopaga of Charaka,
Virechaka gana in place of Virechanopaga of Charaka,
Niruhopaga gana in place of Asthapanopaga of Charaka,
Sirvirechanopaga gana is common with Charaka,

Anuvasanopaga gana of charaka replaced with Ubhayabhaga hara gana. At the same time he also accepted the classification of Suśruta. But only 25 vargas are described under sutra sthana 16th chapter. He described Triphala, Trikatu, Trijataka, Pancha-mula etc., smaller groups seperately.

Laghu Vagbhata accepted only Suśruta's classification. Hence 33 vargas (out of 37 of suśruta) are described in Ashtanga Hridaya. Out of these 33 ganas, first 26 are the ganas based up-on Suśruta Sutra sthana 38th chapter and remaining 7 are accepted from the 39th chapter.

Among the ganas of Suśruta, Brihatyadi gana is not mentioned by both Vagbhatas. Nyagrodhadi gana is not quoted by Vriddha Vagbhata only. While Suśruta did not mention Vatsakadi gana which is commonly described by both Vagbhatas. Utpaladi and Sālasāradi ganas of Suśruta are replaced by Padmakadi and Asanadi ganas in Vagbhata; Trikatu, Triphala etc., are mentioned seperately in another context by Vriddha Vagbhata. He specially added a new group called "Dhumopayoga varga". Jivaniya Panchamula, Madhyama Panchamula, Trijataka & Chaturjataka are the new groups added by Vriddha Vagbhata.

The ganas of Suśruta, Vriddha Vagbhata and Laghu Vagbhata are tabulated (vide: Table No. II)

The missing ganas in Suśruta when compared to vagbhata are: (1) Vatsakadi & (2) Niruhana. Modified ganas are: (1) Utpaladi as Padmakadi (2) Kakolyadi as Jivaniya and (3) Salasaradi as Asanada. However the ingredients are different among them.

Table No. II

Comparision between Suśruta & Vagbhata classifications

Suśruta	Ashtanga Sangraha		Ashtanga Hridaya	
	S.N.	Order No.	S.N.	Order No.
1. Vidarigandhadigana	1. Vidāryadi gana	1	1. Vidaryadi	9
2. Aragwadhadi gana	2. Aragwadhadi	7	2. Aragwadhadi	16
3. Salasaradi gana	3. Asanadi	24	3. Asanādi	17
4. Varunadi gana	4. Varunādi	8	4. Varunādi	18
5. Viratarwadi gana	5. Viratarwadi	10	5. Viratarwadi	20
6. Rodhradi gana	6. Rodhradi	11	6. Rodhradi	21
7. Arkadi gana	7. Arkādi	12	7. Arkādi	22
8. Surasadi gana	8. Surasadi	13	8. Surasādi	23
9. Mushkakādi gana	9. Mushkakadi	14	9. Mushkakadi	24
10. Pippalyadi gana	10. Pippalyadi	22	–	
11. Eladi gana	11. Elādi	20	10. Elādi	32
12. Vachadi gana	12. Vachadi		11. Vachadi	26
13. Haridradi gana	13. Haridradi		12. Haridradi	27
14. Shyamadi gana	14. Shyamadi		13. Shyamadi	33
15. Brihatyadi gana	–		–	
16. Patoladi gana	15. Patoladi5		14. Patoladi	14
17. Kākoalyadi gana	–		15. Jivaniya	8
18. Ushakadi gana	16. Ushakadi	9	16. Ushakadi	19
19. Sārivadi gana	17. Sarivadi	2	17. Sārivadi	10
20. Anjanadi gana	18. Anjanadi	4	18. Anjanadi	13
21. Parushakadi gana	19. Parushakadi	3	19. Parushakadi	12
22. Priyangwadi gana	20. Priyangwadi	17	20. Priyangwadi	28
23. Ambashtādi gana	21. Ambashtadi	18	21. Ambashtadi	29
24. Nyagradhadi gana	–		22. Nygrodhadi	31
25. Guduchyadi gana	22. Guduchyadi	6	23. Guduchyadi	15
26. Utpalādi gana	23. Padmakadi	23	24. Padmakadi	11
27. Mustadi gana	24. Mustadi	19	25. Mustadi	30

28. Triphala gana	–	–
29. Trikatu gana	–	–
30. Amalakyadi gana	–	–
31. Trapvyadi gana	–	–
32. ākshadi panch-amula	25. Vatsakadi 25	26. Vatsakadi 25
33. Laghu gana	–	
34. Brihat panch-amula	–	
35. Valli panch-amula	–	
36. Kantaka panchamula	–	
37. Trina panchamula		
38. Urdhwabhaga hara	26. Vamana 4	27. Vamana 1
39. Adho bhaga hara	27. Virechana 5	28. Virechana 2
40. Ubhaya bhaga hara	28. Ubhaya bhaga hara 8	-
41. Siro virechana	29. Siro virech-anopaga 7	29. Siro virechana 4
42. Vata samsamana	30. Vata samaka 1	30. Vayu nasaka 5
43. Pitta samsamana	31. Pitta sāmaka 2	31. Pitta nasaka 6
44. Kapha samsamana	32. Kapha sāmaka 3	32. Kapha nasaka 7
	33. Dhumopayoga 9	33. Niruhana 3
	34. Niruhopaga 6	

Note: * 1 to 37 items of Suśruta are from sutra. 38th chapter and 38to 44 are from 39th chapter.

** 1 to 25 items of As. Sangraha are from Sutra 16 chapter and 26 to 34 are from 14th chapter.

*** 1 to 33 items of As. Hridaya are described under one chapter only i.e., Sutra 15th chapter.

**** First order indicates serial number and second order indicates the original order numbers from the respective texts of vagbhata.

Table No. III

Comparision between Charaka & Vagbhata classifications

Sl. No.	Charaka Samhita	Sl. No.	Ashtanga Sangraha
1.	Jeevaniya	1.	Jeevaniya
2.	Brimhaniya	2.	Brimhaniya
3.	Lekhaniya	3.	Lekhaniya
4.	Bhedaniya	4.	Bhedaniya
5.	Sandhaniya	5.	Sandhaniya
6.	Deepaniya	6.	Deepaniya
7.	Balya	7.	Balya
8.	Varnya	8.	Varnya
9.	Kantya	9.	Kantya
10.	Hridya	10.	Hridya
11.	Triptighna	11.	Triptighna
12.	Arshoghna	12.	Arshoghna
13.	Kushtaghna	13.	Kushtaghna
14.	Kandughna	14.	Kandughna
15.	Krimighna	15.	Krimighna
16.	Vishaghna	16.	Vishaghna
17.	Kasa hara	17.	Kasaghna
18.	Swasa hara	18.	Swasa samana
19.	Swayathu hara	19.	Sotha hara
20.	Jawara hara	20.	Jwara samaka
21.	Srama hara	21.	Srama nashaka
22.	Dāha prasamana	22.	Daha hara
23.	Seeta prasamana	23.	Seeta samaka
24.	Udarda prasamana	24.	Udarda prasamana
25.	Angamarda prasamana	25.	Angamardaghna
26.	Sula prasamana	26.	Sula samaka
27.	Sonita sthapana	27.	Rudhira samsthapana
28.	Vedana sthapana	28.	Vedana sthapana
29.	Sanjna sthapana	29.	Sanjna sthapana
30.	Praja sthapana	30.	Garbha sthapana
31.	Vayah sthapana	31.	Vaya sthapana

32.	Chardi nigrahana	32.	Vamana nigrahana
33.	Trishna nigrahana	33.	Trishna nigrahana
34.	Hikka nigrahana	34.	Hikka nigrahana
35.	Mutra sangrahaniya	35.	Mutra grahana
36.	Purisha sangrahaniya	36.	Vit grahana
37.	Purisha virajaniya	37.	Vit virajana
38.	Mutra virajaniya	38.	Mutra virajana
39.	Mutra virechaniya	39.	Mutra virechaniya
40.	Stanya janana	40.	Stanya janana
41.	Stanya sodhana	41.	Stanya sodhana
42.	Sukra janana	42.	Sukra janana
43.	Sukra sodhdana	43.	Sukra Sodhana
44.	Snehopaga	44.	Snehopaga
45.	Swedopaga	45.	Swedopaga
46.	Vamanopaga	46.	Vamaka
47.	Virechanopaga	47.	Virechaka
48.	Asthapanopaga	48.	Niruhopaga
49.	Anuvasanopaga	49.	Ubhaya bhagahara
50.	Sirovirechanopaga	50.	Siro virechanopaga

Missing ganas in Vagbhatam when compared to Suśruta Samhita: (1) Brihatyadi (2) Kākolyadi (in As. Sangraha) (3) Nyagrodhadi (4) Triphala (5) Trikatu (6) Āmalakyadi (7) Trapvyadi (8) Lakshadi (9) Laghu panchamula (10) Brihat panchamula (11) Valli panchamula (12) Kantaka panchamula (13) Trina panchamula.

Similarly, there are certain differences between Charaka's kashaya vargas and those of Vriddha Vagbhata, 1 to 45 vargas are common in both the texts while 46-50 items of Charaka were mentioned in the 14th chapter of As. Sangraha sutra sthana. (1 to 45 are described in 15th chapter.) Another difference between both the Acharyas is Charaka quoted about Vamanopaga & Virechanopaga while Vagbhata mentioned them as Vamaka & Virechaka. Asthapanopaga & Anuvasanopaga are replaced by Niruhopaga & Ubhayabhagahara. Sirovirechanopaga is common in both the texts. The vargas of Charaka and Virddha Vagbhata are tabulated (vide: table No. III).

Coming to Āhara dravyas, Charaka classified Āhara dravyas in to 12 vargas in the 27th chapter of Sutra sthana. Suśruta mentioned Ahara dravyas mainly into two groups viz., Drava dravya and Anna dravya. The fomer group contains 10 vargas and the later contains 11 vargas. Under Anna dravyas- Dhatu varga, Ratna varga, Lavana varga, Kshara varga, Pushpa varga, & Kanda varga are newly described by Suśruta. He also mentioned Taila varga, Madhu Varga, Mutra varga under Drava dravyas (Su.Su. 45 & 46 chapter). In Astanga Sangraha both Drava & Dravya vargas are described under 12 vargas (As san Su 6&7 chapter). In Ashtanga Hridaya Sutra sthana 5th & 6th chapters 5 vargas for Drava dravyas and 7 vargas for Anna dravyas were described. The respective classifications are tabulated (vide: Table No. IV)[1,2,3,4].

Other details of classification of dravyas in Brihat-tryai are discussed under chapter XV.

Table No. IV

Classification of Ahara dravyas in Brihat-trayi

Charaka **च.सू. २७ अ.**	**Suśruta** **सु.सू. ४५ अ.**	**Vagbhata-I** **अ.सं.सू. ६ अ.**	**Vagbhata-II** **अ.हृ.सू. ५ अ.**
1. Jala varga	1. Pāniya varga	1. Jala varga	1. Toya varga
2. Gorasa varga	2. Ksheera varga	2. Ksheera varga	2. Ksheera varga
-	3. Dadhi varga	-	-
-	4. Takra varga	-	-
-	5. Ghrita varga	-	-
-	6. Taila varga	3. Taila varga	3. Taila varga
-	7. Madhu varga		- -
3. Ikshu varga	8. Ikshu varga	4. Ikshu varga	4. Ikshu varga
4. Madya varga	9. Madya varga	5. Madya varga	5. Madya varga
-	10. Mutra varga	6. Mutra varga	-
	सु.सू.४६.अ.	अ.स.सू.७.अ.	अ.हृ.सू.६.अ.
5. Sukadhanya varga	11. Sāli varga	7. Suka dhanya	6. Suka dhanya

१. अत्र वर्गशब्देन प्रकरणात् समानक्रियाण्णं समूहे उच्यते....समानकार्या वर्गाः । (चक्रपाणि-च.सू.४)

२. व्याधिप्रशमनादौ कार्ये येषां येषां भेषजानां क्षमत्वं तानि वर्गीकृत्याभिधातुं द्रव्यसंग्रहणीयेऽभिधीयते । (चक्रपाणि)

३. अत्रौषधानां मिश्रीकृत्य गणरूपतयाऽभिधानादस्य मिश्रकसंज्ञा । (चक्रपाणि-सु.सं.)

४. गणायन्त इति गणाः समूहाः । (डल्हण-सु.सू. ३८)

6. Sami dhanya varga	12. Kudhanya	7. Simbi dhanya varga	7. Simbi dhanya
7. Mamsa varga	13. Mamsa varga	9. Mamsa varga	8. Mamsa varga
8. Phala varga	14. Phala varga	10. Phala varga	9. Phala varga
9. Saka varga	15. Sāka varga	11. Sāka varga	10. Sāka varga
	-	16. Pushpa varga	- -
	-	17. Kanda varga	- -
		18. Lavana varga	- -
10. Kritanna varga	19. Kritanna varga	12. Kritanna varga	11. Kritanna varga
11. Āharopayogi varga	20.Bhakshya varga	-	-
	21. Anupana varga	-	-
12. Harita varga	-	-	12. Oushadha varga

12. Classification methods of other Nighantus

As the number of drugs gradually increased from the early times to medieval period where many lexicons were written, the drugs are arranged into different groups.

1. Dhanwantari Nigantu possess 7 vargas. Among these vargas Guduchyadi contain drugs which act as appetizers (Agni-dipana) and tonic (Balya) etc., properties. Satapushpadi varga possess drugs with several indications.
2. Sodhala Nighantu possess 27 vargas.
3. Sidha Mantra contain 8 vargas on the basis of the drugs and their effects on doshas.
4. Madhava dravya guna contain 29 vargas-mainly food materials are discussed.
5. Dravya Guna Sangraha of Chakrapani possess 15 vargas.
6. Raja Nighantu & Bhava prakasa contain 23 vargas.
7. Kaiyadeva Nighantu has 9 vargas. The last group (Nanartha varga) deals with different synonyms of herbs.

A detailed notes on the nighantus and their respective classification methods etc., is provided in the xvi chapter.

✸

Chapter-IV

Concept of Guna

1. Etymology of Guna

Guna is defined as the characteristic by which people are attracted towards a particular substance[1]. In other words guna is meant as quality, mode, property, predicament etc. The auther personally of the openion that Guna in this context shall be considered as 'physical property' since all the other constituents of the dravya i.e., Rasa, Virya, Vipaka & Prashava will denote mainly the 'chemical properties'. In general sense guna may be considered as property.

2. Characteristics of Guna

Charaka defined guna as the character or property which will remain in a dravya with inherent relationship. At the same time it will remain inactive and maintain a non-inherent relation (Asamavaya Karana) with the action/effect (Karma)[2&3].

The difference between dravya and guna is that the former is the seat of both guna and karma while the later is not[4]. As the guna is inactive in nature, it can not perform association (Samyoga) or dissociation (Vibhaga) reactions like karma. This is the significant difference between karma & guna. However both Guna & Karma will have inherent relationship with the dravya[5].

Badhanta Nagarjuna had considered the innumerable number

---

१. (i) गुण आमन्त्रणे । गुण्यते आमन्त्र्यते लोक अनेन इति गुणः । (वाचः)
(ii) गुण्यतेऽप्रधानत्वेनामन्त्र्यतेऽपेक्षते प्रधानेनेति गुणः । (गुणपरिज्ञान)
(iii) गुण्यते समवेतत्वेनामन्त्र्यते द्रव्येणेति गुणः यद्वा गुणयति आमन्त्र्यते समवायित्वेन द्रव्यं इति गुणः । (गुणपरिज्ञान)

२. समवायी तु निश्चेष्टः कारणं गुणः । (च. सू. १)

३. अथ द्रव्याश्रितः ज्ञेया निर्गुणा निष्क्रिया गुणाः । (कारिकावली-६८)

४. द्रव्यं गुणकर्माश्रयः, गुणस्तुगुणकर्मानाश्रयः इति द्रव्यतो भेदः । (योगेन्द्रनाथ)

५. द्रव्याश्रय्यगुणवान् संयोगविभागेष्वकारणमनपेक्ष इति गुणलक्षणम् । (वै. द. अ. ।. सू. १६)

of qualities or properties of different substances as gunas[1].

Boudha Darsana concluded that guna means a group of characters or qualities or properties[2].

Jaina Darsana used the term guna as synonymous to Dravya since dravya is known through certain properties only[3].

In the end it may be concluded that it is really difficult to draw a clear definition of guna on the base of exact characteristics. It is because, rasa can be assessed by rasanendriya (रसनेन्द्रियग्राह्यो रसः); virya is assessed by it action (कर्मलक्षणं वीर्य) and vipaka is denoted by change in original form (परिणामलक्षणो विपाकः). However guna can not be assessed like the above factors since it is linked with different senses. For example- cold & hot (Seeta & Ushna) are known through touch (स्पर्शनेन्द्रियग्राह्यः); unctuous & non-unctuousness (Singdha & Ruksha) are known through sight (चक्षुर्ग्राह्याः).

There fore it appears that Badanta Nagarjuna's definition of guna appears to cover a broader area. We understand various materials only because of their properties or qualities (gunas) as these impress us through our senses. The qualities of compounds reflect those of their molecules. The qualities of molecules are determined not only by those of the atoms that compose them but also the manner or mode in which they combine in substances. Their qualities are mutually determining. In other words, the qualities implicit in the elemental substances which are designated as the karma or cause, become actualised in the kārya or effect i.e., the substances which arise as the result of the combination and permutation of 'Paramanus'. This is based on the principle, "The properties that exist in the causative factor are seen to manifest in the resultant factor"[4,5].

१. विश्वलक्षणाः गुणाः । (र. वै. । सू. १६८)

* भाष्यं:- गुणानामेवमेकलक्षणावरोधो नास्ति.......तस्मादेवतेषामतुल्यं विकीर्णलक्षत्वमेव लक्षणम् इति ।..... लक्षणलक्षितेष्वलक्षणलक्षितत्वाल्लक्षणप्रसिद्धिरिति ।

२. लक्षण कूटोगुणः । (बौद्ध. दर्शन)

३. गुणपर्यायवद् द्रव्यम् । (जै. द.)

४. कारण गुण पूर्वकः कार्यगुणो दृश्यते ।

कारणगुणपूर्वकं कार्यं दृष्टमकारणगुणपूर्वकं च दृष्टम् । (अरुणदत्त- अ.हृ.सू.)

5. Dwarakanath C.; The fundamental principles of Ayurveda Part III Mysore: The Bangalore Press Bran-' 1954 pp. 46-47.

3. Classification of gunas & number of gunas

Charaka mentioned 41 gunas totally. They are: 5 Indriyarthas (qualities of five senses), 20 Gurvadi gunas (Guru, Laghu, Ushna, Tikshna etc.) and 10 Paradi gunas (Paratwa, Aparatwa etc.)[1].

Chakrapani classified gunas into mainly three groups viz;[2&3].

1. Vaisēhika gunas (specific qualities of senses)[4]
2. Sāmanya gunas (general qualities used in treatment)[5]
3. Ātma gunas (qualities of the soul)[6]

Out of these the Sāmānya gunas are again sub-divided into two classes i.e.;

i. Gurvadi gunas or Sareeraka gunas (qualities of human body)
ii. Paradi gunas or Chikitsopayoga gunas (qualities related to treatment)

Gurvadi gunas will denote the common properties of tissue (dhatus) of human body as well as the drugs (dravyas). Hence they are termed as Sariraka gunas by Kaviraja Gangadhara.

Paradi gunas are very essential during administration of the drugs. Therefore may be considered as Chikitsopayoga gunas.

Both these groups are representing the general qualities of Panchabhutas. Thus they are called as "Samanyagunas". However, sabda, sparsa, rupa, rasa & gandha are the specific qualities/properties of each bhuta individullay. Hence are known as "Vaisēṣhika gunas."

Both Sāmānya and Vaisēṣhika gunas are related to the physical or material world and are know as 'Ādhi-bhoutika gunas' where

१. सार्थागुर्वादयो बुद्धिः प्रयत्नान्ता परादयः । गुणाः प्रोक्ताः ....।। (च. सू.। अ.)
२. अनेन त्रिविधा अपि वैशेषिकाः सामान्याः आत्मगुणाश्चोद्दिष्टाः । (चक्रपाणि)
३. तस्य गुणाः शब्दादयो गुर्वादयश्च द्रवान्ताः । (च. सू. २६)
४. एते च वैशेषिकाः, यतः आकाशस्यैव शब्दः प्राधान्येन, वायोरेव स्पर्शः प्राधान्येन, एवमन्यादिषु रूपादयः । (चक्रपाणि)
५. एते च सामान्यगुणाः पृथिव्यादीनां सामान्यत्वात् । (चक्रपाणि)
६. इच्छाद्वेषः सुखं दुःखं प्रयत्नश्चेतना धृतिः । बुद्धिः स्मृतिरहंकारो लिङ्गानि परमात्मनः।। (च.शा.।अ.)
* चक्रपाणिः- बुद्धिः ज्ञानम्, अनेन च स्मृति- चेतना-धृत्यहंकारादीनां बुद्धिविशेषाणां ग्रहणम् । इह चेतनादीनां बुद्धिग्रहणेनैव ग्रहणम् ।........प्रयत्नोऽन्ते येषां ते प्रयत्नान्ताः, एतेन चेच्छा द्वेषसुखदुःखप्रयत्नानां ग्रहणम् ।

as the Ātma gunas are beyond the physical world and are related to the spiritual world. Hence they are known as 'Ādhyatmika gunas'.

GUNA

Ādhi-bhoutika Ādhyatmika

Sāmānya Visiṣhta Icha Dvesha Sukha Duhkha Prayatna Buddhi

Gurvādi Parādi Sabda Sparsa Rupa Rasa Gandha

(20 gunas) (10 gunas)

There are totally 41 gunas accepted by the Acharyas commonly. They are:

Adhyatma gunas	-	6
Gurvadi gunas	-	20
Paradi gunas	-	10
Visishta gunas	-	5
Total	=	41 gunas

To these qualities Yogendranath had added 'Manas' and therefore 42 gunas according to his view[1].

Sankhya philosophy proposed Tri-gunas or Tri-vidha Ahamkaras as the cause of creation[2&3]. But these are the Gunas of Karana dravyas. As already discussed earlier dravya-guna deals with karya dravyas and therefore physical properties of various drugs are considered under guna. Various qualities and properties of drugs are considerd as gunas in this context[4].

4. Detailed knowledge on Gurvadi Gunas

Gurvadi gunas are mainly 20 in number and are otherwise known as Sariraka gunas[5]. These 20 are arranged in 10 pairs[6].

१. मनो मनोऽर्थो बुद्धिरात्माचेत्यध्यात्म । द्रव्यसंग्रह: (च. शा. । अ.)

२. सत्त्वरजस्तमसां साम्यावस्था प्रकृति: । (सां. दं)

३. प्रकृते: क्रियमाणानि गुणै: कर्माणि सर्वश: ।
अहंकारविमूढात्मा कर्ताहमिति मन्यते ॥ (भगवद्गीता ३/२७)

४. विश्वं विकीर्णं भिन्नं लक्षणं येषां ते विश्वलक्षणा: गुणा: । (भाष्य)

५. गुणा य उक्ता द्रव्येषु शरीरेष्वपि ते तथा । (सु. सू.)

६. स (आहार:) विशंतिगुण: गुरुलघुशीतउष्ण स्निग्धरूक्षमन्द तीक्ष्ण मृदुकठिन विशद
पिच्छिल स्थिर सर शलक्ष्ण खर सूक्ष्म स्थूल सान्द्र द्रवानुगमात् । (च. सू. २५/३६)

Each pair consists of two gunas which have opposite qualities to each other. eg. Guru-Laghu; Seeta-Ushna etc.

Badanta Nagarjuna quoted that there are 10 potential gunas (Visishta Samarthya Sampanna gunas)[1]. Out of these ten gunas, again Visada and Pichchila are left out to denote eight potencies (Ashta vidha viryas).

On review of literature we come across a common view between Charaka[2,3,4], Vriddha Vagbhata[5] and Laghu Vagbhata. But Suśruta and Bhavamisra have expressed some different view. Suśruta divided 20 qualities into two categories[6]. The first group consists of 10 potential gunas of Badhanta Nagarjuna and the second group consists of remaining 10 gunas.

The views of diferent Acharyas in this regard are presented in the table No. V

Another important feature of Suśruta's view is that certain properties mentioned in the earlier texts are replaced with new properties. They are:

i. Drava - Sandra.
ii. Slakshna - Khara.
iii. Sugandha - Durgandha.
iv. Sara - Manda
v. Āsukari - Sukshma

A part from these, Mridu and Tikshna are mentioned in place of Manda-Tikshna.

१. रूक्षादयां भावप्रधानाः तेन रूक्षत्वादयो गुणाः मन्तव्याः । (चक्रपाणि- च. सू. १२/४)

२. तत्र इमे शरीरधातुगुणाः संख्यासामर्थ्यकराः, तद्यथा-गुरुलघु शीत उण स्निग्ध रूक्ष मन्द तीक्ष्ण स्थिर सर मृदु कठिन विशदपिच्छिल श्लक्ष्ण खर स्थूल सूक्ष्म सान्द्र द्रवाः ॥ (च. शा. ६/२०)

३. गुर्वादयस्तु, गुरूलघुशीतोष्णस्निग्धरूक्षमन्दतीक्ष्ण स्थिरसरमृदुकठिनविशदपिच्छिल-श्लक्ष्णखरस्थूलसूक्ष्मसान्द्रद्रवाः विंशतिः । (चक्रपाणि)

४. गुरुमन्दहिमस्निग्धश्लक्ष्णसान्द्रमृदुस्थिराः ।
गुणाः ससूक्ष्मविशदा विंशतिः सविपर्ययाः ॥ (अ.सं.सू. १)

५. दशाद्याः कर्मतः प्रोक्तास्तेषां कर्मविशेषणैः ।
दशैवान्यान् प्रवक्ष्यामि द्रवादींस्तान्निबोध मे ॥ (सु. सू. ४६)

* हारणचन्द्रः- तदिदानीं पूर्वाचार्यप्रसिद्धेन क्रमेण द्वेधा विभज्यं कर्मतः शीतादीन् गुणानुपदिदिक्षति । तेषां व्याचिख्यासितानां गुणानां मध्ये आद्याः पूर्वाचार्यैरदावुपदिष्टाः ..... ।

Suśruta also mentioned another two new properties Vyavayi and Vikasi. However total number of Gurvadi gunas are restricted to same old number of twenty. The difference between Charaka's view and that of Suśruta is that Katina-Sthula is mentioned instead of Sukshma-Sthula.

Table No. V

Number of Gunas according to different texts

Charaka	Suśruta	Vagbhata -I	Vagbhata -II	Rasa Vaiseshika	Bhavamishra
1. Guru	Guru	Guru	Guru	Guru	Guru
2. Laghu	Laghu	Laghu	Laghu	Laghu	Laghu
3. Seeta	Seeta	Seeta	Seeta	Seeta	Seeta
4. Ushna	Ushna	Ushna	Ushna	Ushna	Ushna
5. Snigdha	Snigdha	Snigdha	Snigdha	Snigdha	Snigdha
6. Ruksha	Ruksha	Ruksha	Ruksha	Ruksha	Ruksha
7. Manda	Manda	Manda	Manda	-	Manda
8. Tikshna	Tikshna	Tikshna	Tikshna	Tikshna	Tikshna
9. Pichchila	Pichchila	Pichchila	Pichchila	Pichchila	Pichchila
10. Visada	Visada	Visada	Visada	Visada	Visada
11. Sthula	Sthula	Sthula	Sthula	-	Sthula
12. Sukshma	Sukshma	Sukshma	Sukshma	-	Sukshma
13. Mridu	Mridu	Mridu	Mridu	Mridu	Mridu
14. Katina	-	Katina	Katina	-	Slakshna
15. Slakshna	Slakshna	Slakshna	Slakshna	-	
16. Khara	Karkasa	Khara	Khara	-	Karkasa
17. Sthira	-	Sthira	Sthira	-	Sthira
18. Sara	Sara	Sara	Sara	-	Sara
19. Sāndra	Sāndra	Sandra	Sandra	-	Sushka
20. Drava	Drava	Drava	Drava	-	Drava
-	Sugandha	-	-	-	-
-	Durgandha	-	-	-	-

-	Vyavāyi	-	-	-	-
-	Vikasi	-	-	-	-
-	Āsukari	-	-		Āsu

Qualities like Sugandha, Durgandha, Vyavayi, Vikasi & Āsukari are also new to Charaka. Suśruta accepted the following new pairs:

i. Mridu - Tikshna for Manda - Tikshna
ii. Manda - Sara for Sthira - Sara
iii. Slakshna - Karkasa for Slakshna - Khara

Bhava mishra[1] changed the order of Suśruta and arranged them in the following order: Guru-Laghu; Snigdha-Ruksha[2]; Tikshna-Slakshna, Sthira-sara; Pichchila-Visada; Seeta-Ushna; Mridu-Karkasa; Sthula-Sukshma; Drava-Sushka; and Asu-Manda. Though he claimed that he is following Suśruta's classification of Gunas, there is some change in the order compared to the earlier.

The difference we fined between are Suśruta and Bhava mishra are: Mridu-Tikshna are replaced by Tikshna-Slakshna. Vyavayi-Vikasi and Sugandha-Durgandha are not mentioned by Bhava mishra. But he added 'Suskha' as opposite to Drava.

Similarly Bhava mishra diviated from Charaka's view in the following way:

(i) Mridu- Karkasa for Mridu- Katina
(ii) Sushka- Drava for Sandra- Drava
(iii) Manda- Asu for Manda- Tikshna

The variation in the pairs of Gunas are tabulated (vide: Table No. VI).

Dalhana and Hemadri expressed their view that these Gurvadi gunas can be only twenty.[3,4] Even though there are different view expressed by different authors, finally these qualities will fall

१. सुश्रुते तु गुणाः प्रोक्ता विंशतिस्तान् ब्रुवे श्रुणु । (भा. प्र.)
२. शीतोष्णस्निग्धरूक्षविशदपिच्छिलगुरुलघुमृदुतीक्ष्ण गुणाः कर्मण्याः । (र. वै. अ. ३ सू. १११)
३. केचिदत्र संख्याभङ्गभयाद् व्यवायिविकास्याशुकारिणमपाठमेव मन्यन्ते । (डल्हण)
४. य एतेऽतिरिक्ता गुणा दर्शिताः ते विंशतावेवान्तर्भूताः । (हेमाद्रि)

Table No. VI

List of pairs of Gurvadi gunas according to diferent Acharyas

S.N.	Charaka	Suśruta	Vagbhata	Badhanta Nagarjuna	Bhava mishra
1.	Guru-Laghu	Guru-Laghu	Guru-Laghu	Guru-Laghu	
2.	Seeta-Ushna	Seeta-Ushna	Seeta-Ushna	Seeta-Ushna	
3.	Snigdha-Ruksha	Snigdha-Ruksha	Snigdha-Ruksha	Snigdha-Ruksha	
4.	Manda-Tikshna	Mridu-Tikshna	Manda-Tikshna	Mridu-Tikshna	
5.	Sthira-Sara	Manda-Sara	Sthira-Chala (?)	Manda-Sara	
6.	Mridu-Katina	Sugandha-Durgandha	Mridu-Katina	-	
7.	Visada-Pichchila	Visada-Pichchila	Visada-Pichchila	Visada-Pichchila	
8.	Slakshna-Khara	Slakshna-Karkasa	Slakshna-Khara	-	Slakshna-Karkasa
9.	Sthula-Sukshma	Sthula-Sukshma	Sthula-Sukshma	-	
10.	Sandra-Drava	Sandra-Drava	Sandra-Drava	-	
		* Vyavayi, Vikasi & Asukari			

under the above 20 properties only[1].

The newer properties may be accommodated under the 20 properties. For example-

Vyavayi	=	Sara (Drava by Hemachandra)
Vikasi	=	Tikshna (Khara by Hemachandra)
Sugandha	=	Manda
Durgandha	=	Tikshna
Āsukari	=	Chala
Prasanna	=	Sthula
Suchi or Vimala	=	Visada
Visra	=	Tikshna

Some consider that Gurvadi Gunas are innumerable. However Ayurvedic classics considered them as 20 only. In the context of Madya, Chakrapani explained that-though Vikasi-Asukari-Vyavayi are gunas, they can not be included into Gurvadi gunas since they do not fall under twenty gunas.

From the above we conclude that there is Niyata Guna Sankhya vada and Aniyata Guna Sankhya vada (definite and infinite number of properties).

(1) Guru Guna: ***(Heaviness or Physical mass)***

The quality which is responsible for the force of gravity[2].

---

१. (i) गुर्वादय इति एते आविष्कृततया एव यज्जः पुरुषीये उक्ताः, तेन गुणाश्नामसंख्येयत्वादन्येऽपि ज्ञेयाः । अत एव प्रमेहे श्लेष्मगणेषु अच्छत्वादयो गुणाः पठ्यन्ते । (शिवदासः)

(ii) एते विकासित्वादयो गुणा यद्यपि विंशतिगुणगणनायां न पठिताः, तथाप्यसंख्येयतया गुणानामेषामपि गुणत्वं सिद्धम्; ये तु तत्र पठितास्ते तावदाविष्कृततमाः ज्ञेयाः । (चक्रपाणि)

(iii) अधिकायामपि गुणविंशतावुक्तायां गुणा विंशतिरुक्ताः, न चात्र नियमो विंशतिरेवेति; व्यवायि-विकास्याशुकारिणां तु स्वतन्त्रे च परतन्त्रे च दर्शनात् पादो न्याय्य एव । (डल्हण)

२. (i) गुरुत्वं जलभूम्योः पतनकारणम् । (प्र. पा. भा.)

(ii) यस्य द्रव्यस्य बृंहणे कर्मणि शक्तिः स गुरुः । (हेमाद्रि)

(iii) गौरवं पार्थिवमाप्यञ्च । (र. वै. अ. ३सू. ११६)

(iv) सादोपलेप बलकृत् गुरुस्तर्पण बृंहणः ।

* डल्हण- सादोऽङ्गग्लानिः, उपलेपो मलवृद्धिः, बलं श्लेष्मा, तर्पणः तृप्तिजनकः, बृंहणो देहे वृद्धिकरः ।

(v) गुरुर्वातहरः पुष्टिश्लेष्मकृत् चिरपाकी च । (भा. प्र.)

Mass and gravitational force are directly proportional. Substances possessing high molecular weight like proteins may have guru guna e.g. Masha, Godhuma etc.

Guru guna acts as vata hara and kapha vardhaka (reduces vata and aggravates kapha); it nourishes all the dhatus (Brimhana); it increases malas (increases quanity of excreta) and coats the srotas (Srotopalepa); under goes Guru pāka (Madhura vipaka).

Virechana, Balya, Brimhana, Vrishya etc., are pharmacological actions exerted by Guru guna.

However, it may cause digestion disturbances owing to its quality of heaviness. Substances with higher mol. wt. and lower mol. wt. may under go delayed and easy digestive changes respectively in the stomach e.g.

Masha - Swabhava guru, Mātra guru.

Mugda - Swabhava laghu, Mātra laghu.

On the Psyche (Manas) it may impose inhibitory effects on receptive capacity. e.g. Glani, Avasāda etc.

Guru guna is the main feature of Prithvi and Jala bhutas[1]. It is responsible for Madhura rasa, Madhura vipaka and Seeta virya.

(2) Laghu guna: ***(Lightness)***

The quality which results in very light weight or which reduces weight is known as laghu[2]. Substances possessing lower molecular weight may have Laghu guna e.g. Mudga, Laja etc.

It acts as kapha hara and vata vardhaka (reduces kapha and aggravates vata); it reduces the tissue weights (Langhana); it reduces malas (decrease quanity of excreta) and clears the channels

---

१. पृथ्वीजलवृत्तिः (आ. द. अ.३ आ. २ सू. ५)

२. (i) लघुस्तद्विपरीतस्याल्लेखनो रोपणस्तथा । (सु. सू. ४६/४२०)

* डल्हणः- लघुस्तद्विपरीत इति असादानुपलेपादिकृत् कफहरश्चेत्यर्थः । लेखनः पत्तलीकरणः।

(ii) लङ्घने लघुः । (हेमाद्रि)

(iii) लघुपथ्यं परं प्रोक्तं कफघ्नं शीघ्रपाकि च । (भा. प्र.)

(iv) उल्वावयवत्वं लघुत्वं । (आ. द. अ. ३ आ. २ सू. ६)

(v) अग्निवायू हि लघू लघुत्वाच्च तान्यूर्ध्वमुत्तिष्ठन्ति । (सु. सू. ४१।९)

of the body (Sroto Sodhana), it under goes Laghu pāka (Katu or Amla Vipaka).

Vamana, Lekhana, Pachana etc., are the pharmacological actions exerted by Laghu guna.

It improves the digestion being easily digestible.

On the psyche (manas) it has positive effects by improving activeness and providing inspiration.

Laghu guna is the main feature in Ākasa, Vayu and Agni bhutas. It is responsible for Katu-Kashaya Rasas, Katu Vipaka and Ushna Virya.

(3) Seeta guna: *(Cold)*

The quality which reduces the body temperature is known as Seeta guna[1]. It helps to check the flow of water and fluids. e.g.- Chandana, Usira etc.

It subsides, pitta and aggravates vata-kapha; improves tissues; acts as diuretic and controls sweating and purgation. This quality is helpful in the mangement of Murcha,Trishna, Daha etc. Pitta states.

It produces pleasant fealing to mind. Jala bhuta and vayu bhuta are seeta in nature.

Among the Rasas Madhura- tikta-kashaya are Seeta in nature. Madhura vipaka is also cold in nature.

(4) Ushna guna: *(Hotness)*

The quality by which body temperature is increased or the

---

१. (i) स्तम्भनो हिमः । (हेमाद्रि)
(ii) ह्लादनः स्तम्भनः शीतो मूर्च्छातृट्स्वेददाहजित् । (सु. सू. ४६/४१५)
* डल्हणः- ह्लादनः सुखकारीत्यर्थः, तृट्स्वेदमूर्छादाहजिदित्यर्थः ।
(iii) शीतस्तु ह्लादनः स्तम्भी मूर्च्छातृट्स्वेददाह नुत् (भा. प्र.)
(iv) दाहनाशकत्वं शीतत्वम् । (आ. द. अ. २ सू. १०)
(v) सलिलानिलधरालमोवृत्तिः । (आ. द.अ. ३ आ. २ सू. ११)
(vi) शीत-मधुररसप्रायमाप्यम् । (सु. सू. ४१/४-६)
(vii) द्रव-शीत-रसगुणबहुलमौदकम् । (अ. सं. सू. १७)

property which results in sweating is known as Ushna guna[1].

Ushna guna acts as Vata-Kapha hara and pitta vardhaka (reduces vata kapha and increases pitta); it results in heamorrhage and has adverse effects on dhatus; it reduces the quantity of urine and increases that of Sweat & Stools.

It produces pharmacological action like Pachana, Deepana, Swedana, Langhana etc. It is useful in conditions like: Agnimandya, Pratisyaya, Kapha vikaras etc.

Ushna guna is the main feature of Agni bhuta. It is responsible for katu rasa, katu vipaka and Ushna virya e.g. Chitraka, Chavya etc.

(5) Snigdha guna: ***(Unctuousness)***

The quality which provides oily appearance or unctuousness is known as Snigdha. It will provide smoothness, moisture and oily nature to the body[2].

It subsides vata and aggravates kapha; provides tonicity to tissues; regularize the movement of malas; acts as Vajikarana.

Balya, Vrishya, Snehana, Varnya etc., are the pharmacological actions of Snigdha guna.

Snigdha guna is the specific feature of Jala bhuta e.g. Ghrita, Sigru etc.

It is found in Madhura-Amla-Lavana rasas; and Madhura vipaka. It is useful in vata vyadhis, pada dari, vata predominant skin problems like Kitibha, Mandala etc.

---

१. (i) उष्ण: तद्विपरीत: स्यात् पाचनश्च विशेषत: । (सु. सू. ४६/४१५)
* डल्हण:- पाचनो व्रणादीनां ।
(ii) स्वेदने उष्ण: । (हेमाद्रि)
(iii) तैजसमौष्ण्यं तैक्ष्ण्यं च । (र. वै. ३ सू. ११३)
(iv) उष्णो भवति शीतस्य विपरीतश्च पाचन: । (भा. प्र.)
(v) दाहजनकत्वमुष्णत्वम् । (आ.द.अ. ३ आ. २ सू. १४)
(vi) तत्र मृदुशीतोष्णा: स्पर्शग्राह्या: । (सु.सू. ४१/१८)

२. (i) यस्य क्लेदने शक्ति: स स्निग्ध: । (हेमाद्रि)
(ii) स्नेहमार्दवकृत् स्निग्धो बलवर्णकरस्तथा । (सु. सू. ४६/४१६)
*डल्हण:- स्नेहेत्यादि स्निग्धो गुण: स्नेहादिकारण इत्यर्थ: ।
(iii) स्निग्ध वातहरं श्लेष्मकारि वृष्यं बलावहम् । (भा. प्र.)
(iv) स्नेहोऽपां विशेषगुण: । (प्र.पा.भा.)

(6) Ruksha guna: ***(Dryness or non-unctuousness)***

The property which is responsible for dryness or which results in absorption of moisture is known as Ruksha[1].

It subsides kapha and aggravates vata; it will have negative effect on most of the dhatus; reduces the quantity of excreta.

Ruksha guna results in Sthambhana, Soshana, Rukshana, Avrishya actions.

Ruksha guna is mainly related with vayu bhuta. But there are references about Agni and Prithvi also possessing rukshatwa.

It is found in Katu-Tikta-Kashaya rasas and Katu Vipaka. It is useful in Sotha, Prameha, Swasa Medo roga, Āma dosha, Urusthambha etc.

(7) Manda guna: ***(Dullness or Mildness)***

The property which is responsible for the slow activity or delayed response of a substance is known as Manda guna[2]. It is otherwise defined as the quality which will subside the vitiated doshas or which is helpful in the palliative treatment of diseases. This activity makes the drug to travel through the body for a long time.

It aggravates kapha and subsides vata; it strengthens the tissues; does not help in the expulsion of excreta.

Vata-pitta samaka, Mala bandhaka, Chira paka etc; are its

---

१. (i) शोषणे रूक्ष: । (हेमाद्रि)
(ii) रूक्षस्तद्विपरीत: स्याद्विशेषात् स्तम्भन: खर: ॥ (सु. सू. ४६/४१६)
* डल्हण:- रूक्षो गुणस्तद्विपरीतो रौक्ष्यकाठिन्यकर इत्यर्थ: । स्तम्भन: अतीसारादीनाम् । खर: कर्कश:।
(iii) रूक्षं समीरणकरं परं कफहरं मतम् । (भा. प्र.)
(iv) तद् (स्नेह) विपरीतत्वं रूक्षत्वम् । (आ.द.अ.३ आ.२.सू.२१)
(v) रूक्ष-वायव्यं । (अ.सं.सू. १७)

२. (i) मन्दो यात्राकर: स्मृत: । (सु.सू. ४६/४२२)
* डल्हण:- यात्राकर: इति शरीरस्थायित्वाद्देहस्य यात्रां वर्तनं करोति ।
(ii) यस्य शमने शक्ति: स मन्द: । (हेमाद्रि)
(iii) चिरकारित्वम् मन्दत्वम् । (आ.द.अ.३.आ.२.सू. २३)
(iv) मन्द: सकलकार्येषु शिथिलोऽल्पीऽपि जायते । (भा. प्र.)
(v) धरणीसलिलवृत्ति । (आ.द.अ.३आ.२ सू. २४)

actions. It is mainly related to prithvi and Jala bhutas. e.g. Guduchi, Amalaki, Ati visha etc.

Madhura-Tikta-Kashya Rasas; Seeta virya and Madhura vipaka are results of Manda guna.

(8) Tikshna guna: ***(Sharpness or Fast-acting)***

It is the quality which is responsible for the quick activity of a drug or sharpness of a drug. It is otherwise known as the property which will expel the doshas completely i.e., it is helpful in curative treatment of discases[1].

This property usually stimulates through irritation etc. Where as Manda guna depresses the activities.

Tikshna guna acts as pitta vardhaka and Kapha-vata hara; it reduces tissue weights; enhances the excretion of malas.

It is useful in Vamana (emesis) and Virechana (purgation). It also produces Dāha, Pāka and Srāva.

Tikshna guna is mainly related to Agni bhuta. This property is used in Apasmara, Mada, Sanyasa, Swasa etc., conditions e.g. Bhallataka, Maricha, Danti etc.

(9) Sthira guna: ***(Immobility)***

The quality which brings about immobility or firmness is known as sthira guna. It mainly restricts the falling of Kesa (hair), Smasru (mustach), Roma (bodily hair), Asthi (bone), Nakha (nails), Danta (teeth), Sira (veins),Snāyu (ligaments) Dhamani (arteries) & Sukra (Semen). That means it provides strength to many of the tissues and skin sppendages etc[2].

१. (i) शोधने तीक्ष्ण: । (हेमाद्रि)
(ii) दाहपाककरस्तीक्ष्ण: स्रावणो । (सु.सू. ४६/४१८)
(iii) तीक्ष्णं पित्तकरं प्रायोलेखनं कफवातहृत् । (भा. प्र.)
(iv) शीघ्रकारित्वम् तीक्ष्णत्वम् । (आ.द.अ.३आ.२सू.२५)
(v) तेजोवृत्ति । (आ.द.अ.३आ.२सू.२६)

२. (i) धारणे स्थिर: । (हेमाद्रि)
(ii) केशश्मश्रुलोमास्थिनखदन्तसिरास्नायुधमनीरेत: प्रभृतीनि स्थिराणि । (सु. शा. ३)
(iii) स्थिरो वातमलस्तम्भी । (भा.प्र.)
(iv) क्षिति वृत्ति: । (आ.द.अ.३.आ.२.सू.२८)
(v) चलरहितत्वम् स्थिरत्वम् । (आ.द.अ.३.आ.२.सू. २७)

It acts as kapha vardhaka and subsides vata; strengthens all the dhatus; controls faeces and flatus etc.

It is the quality mostly related with Prithvi bhuta. It is useful in conditions like: Khālitya, Asthi Sosha, Danta chalana, Sira saithilya, Dhamani saithilya, Sukra meha etc. e.g.: Balā, Sukti, Atibalā etc.

It is responsible for Madhura-Tikta rasas; Seeta Veerya and Madhura vipaka.

(10) Sara guna: ***(Mobility)***

The quality by which a substance spreads all over the body very easily or very quickly is known as Sara guna[1]. It is otherwise defined as the property which stimulates different movements e.g. Haritaki, Trivrit.

It usually aggravates vata and through that other malas or doshas are stimulated. It reduces the tissue weights and enhances the movement of excreta (malas).

Though Sushrita considered it as a quality of Jala bhuta, it appears to be predominantly vata property.

Some people consider 'Chala' guna in place of Sara guna.

This quality is useful in the vitiation of Kapha, Medo roga, etc.

(11) Mridu guna: ***(Softness or Fragility)***

The property which brings about softness or fragility to the body is known as Mridu[2].

---

१. (i) प्रेरणे चलः । (हेमाद्रि- अ.हृ.सू. १/१८)
(ii) यस्य प्रेरणे शक्तिः स सरः । (द्र. गु. वि.)
(iii) सरोऽनुलोमनः प्रोक्तः । (सु. सू. ४६/४२२)
* डल्हणः- अनुलोमनो वातमलप्रवर्तनः ।
(iv) सरस्तेषां (वातमलानां) प्रवर्तकः । (भा. प्र.)
(v) सर्वतः प्रवृत्तिशीलत्वम् सरत्वम् । (आ.द.अ. ३ आ. २ सू. २९)
(vi) सलिलवृत्तिः । (आ. द.अ.३ आ. २ सू. ३०)

२. (i) श्लथने मृदुः । (हेमाद्रि)
(ii) मांसशोणितमेदो मज्जाहृन्नाभियकृत्प्लीहान्त्रगुदप्रभृतीनि मृदूनि। (सु. शा. ३)
(iii) मृदुरन्यथा । (सु. सू. ४६/४१८)
* डल्हणः- दाहेत्यादि अन्यथा इति- अदाहपाककरोऽस्रावण इत्यर्थः ।
(iv) मार्दवमान्तरिक्षमाप्यं च । (र. वै. ३ सू. ११५)
(v) शिथिलावयवत्वं मृदुत्वम् । .... अप्रतीघातकत्वं वा । (आ.द.अ.३ आ. २ सू. ३१-३२)

Mamsa (muscle), Rakta (blood), Medas (fatty tissue), Majja (bone marrow), Hridaya (heart), Nabhi (umbilicus), Yakrit (liver) etc., organs are considered as soft in nature by Sushrita.

It aggravates kapha and subsides vata-pitta; it brings about fragility to the tissues; liquifies the excreta.

It is useful in reducing Dāha (burning), Pāka (inflamnation) and Srava (secretions)

Mridu guna is mainly related to Ākasa bhuta. e.g. Godhuma, Eranda taila, Yashti madhu etc.

(12) Katina guna: ***(Hardness)***

The quality which gives rise to the feeling of hardness and rigidity is known as Katina[1].

It aggravates vata but provides hardness or strength to dhatus also. It however dries up the excreta.

Prithvi bhuta mainly bears this quality. Examples of Katina guna dravyas are: Aswagandha, Shatavari, Pravala etc.

Kaṭina guna is used in Sandhimukta, Kanda bhagna etc.

(13) Visada guna: ***(Clearness)***

It provides transparant nature or clearness to the subjects. That means this quality provides clean and clear state of the tissues[2].

The property which washes away the dirt is also called as Visada. It makes the dhatus free from impurities etc. e.g.: Nimba, Mamsa rohini etc.

---

१. (i) दृढीकरणे कठिन: । (हेमाद्रि)
(ii) कठिनत्वम् पार्थिवम् । (र. वै. २ सू. ५८)
(iii) संघातोऽवयवानाम् काठिन्यम् । (आ.द.अ.३ आ. २ सू. ३४)

२. (i) क्षालने विशद: । (हेमाद्रि)
(ii) विशदो विपरीतोऽस्मात् क्लेदाचूषणरोपण: । (सु. सू. ४६/४१७)
*डल्हण:- विपरीतोऽस्मात् इति असन्धानीऽजीवनोऽश्लेषी च ।
क्लेदाचूषण:-आर्द्रीभावविनाशकर इत्यर्थ: ।
(iii) क्लेदच्छेदकर: ख्यातो विशदो व्रणरोपण: । (भा. प्र.)
(iv) क्लेदनाशकत्वं विशदत्वम् । (आ.द.अ. ३. आ. २ सू. ४६)
(v) धरानिलानलवृत्ति: । (आ.द.अ. ३. आ. २ सू. ३७)

It aggravates vata and subsides kapha; it does mala soshana; acts as lekhana and vrana ropana.

Visada guna is seen with Prithvi, vayu, Agni and Ākasa.

(14) Pichchila guna: ***(Stickyness or Sliminess)***

The quality which is responsible for stickyness of a substance is known as Pichchila. It will have a coating effect (lepana) over the tissues[1].

It aggravates kapha and subsides vata; it improves the dhatus and causes stickyness to the excreta. e.g.: Asthi Samharaka, Bhallataka etc.

It also results in actions like: Jeevaniya, Balya, Sandhanakara etc. Mainly useful in Asthi bhagna and Sandhi mukta.

Pichchila guna is mainly related to the Jala bhuta.

(15) Slakshna guna: ***(Smoothness)***

The quality which provides smoothness is known as slakshna. It helps in soothing (ropana) process[2]. e.g. Haridra, Abhraka etc.

It acts as Kapha-Pitta vardhaka and vata hara; provides dhatu vriddhi; causes expulsion of malas.

Charaka quoted it as Ākasa guna while Nagarjuna considered as Agni guna. Sushrita described it as equivalent to Pichchila guna.

---

१. (i) लेपने पिच्छिल: । (हेमाद्रि)
(ii) पिच्छिलो जीवनो बल्य: सन्धान: श्लेष्मलो गुरु: । (सु. सू. ४६/४१७)
* डल्हण:- पिच्छिलो गुण:- जीवन: प्राणधारण: । सन्धानो भग्नस्य ।
(iii) पिच्छिलस्तन्तुलो बल्य: सन्धान: श्लेष्मलो गुरु: । (भा. प्र.)
(iv) पिच्छिलत्वमाप्यम् । (र. वै ३. सू. ११२)
(v) सान्द्रचिक्कणत्वं पिच्छिलत्वम् । चकचकायमानं वा । (आ.द.अ. ३. आ. २ सू. ३८-३९)

२. (i) रोपणे श्लक्ष्ण: । (हेमाद्रि)
(ii) श्लक्ष्ण: पिच्छिलवत् ज्ञेय: । (सू. सू. ४६)
*डल्हण:- श्लक्ष्णो गुण: पिच्छिलवत् ज्ञेय: । जीवन: श्लेष्मसन्धानकृदित्यर्थ: ।
(iii) श्लक्ष्ण: स्नेहं विनाऽपि स्यात् कठिनोऽपिहि चिक्कण: । (भा. प्र.)
(vi) तैजसं श्लक्ष्णत्वं नाम । (र. वै. अ. २ सू. ५८)
(v) अपरुषत्वं श्लक्ष्णत्वम् । (आ.द.अ. ३ आ. २ सू. ४१)

(16) Khara guna: ***(Roughness)***

The quality responsible for roughness of a substance is known as Khara[1]. e.g.: Vacha, Silajatu, Karkoti etc.

It will have lakhana property; acts as vata-vardhaka; reduces the dhatu levels; also reduces the quantity of malas.

This is otherwise mentioned as 'Karkasa' by Sushrita. Its functions are claimed to be same as Visada.

Khara or Karkasa is the quality mainly seen with Vayu and Agni.

(17) Sukshma guna: ***(Fineness or Microscopic nature)***

The quality through which a drug can penetrate through the minutest channels of the body is known as Sukshma. Therefore it is defined as the fineness of a Substance[2].

It aggravates vata and subsides kapha; it reduces tissue weights; also reduce the quantity of excreta and under goes Laghu paka.

Vasodilatation may be the result of this property. Agni, Vayu, Akasa are all posessing Sukshma guna. e.g. alcohal (Madya), Lavana (salt) etc.

(18) Sthula guna: ***(Bulkiness)***

It is the quality which brings about bulkiness and delay in desintigration of a drug[3]. e.g.: Dadhi, Pinyaka, etc.

---

१. (i) लेखने खरः । (हेमाद्रि)
(ii) कर्कशो विशदो यथा । (सु. सू. ४६/४२१)
* डल्हणः- विशदो यथा इति- अजीवनोऽश्लेषी च, तथाऽसन्धानकार्श्यकृच्च ।
(iii) कर्कशत्वं वायव्यः । (र. वै. अ. २ सू. ६०)
(iv) परूषत्वं खरत्वम् । (आ. द. अ. ३ आ. २ सू. ४३)

२. (i) विवरणे सूक्ष्मः । (हेमाद्रिः)
(ii) सौक्ष्मयात् सूक्ष्मस्तु सूक्ष्मेषु स्रोतःस्वनुसरः स्मृतः । (सु. सू. ४६/४२४)
(iii) अवयवानां संकोचः सूक्ष्मत्वम् । (आ.द.अ. ३ आ. २ सू. ४५)
(iv) देहस्य सूक्ष्मछिद्रेषु विशेद्यत्सूक्ष्ममुच्यते । (भा. प्र.)
(v) अनलानिलाम्बर तमोवृत्तिः । (आ.द.अ. ३ आ. २ सू. ४६)

३. (i) संवरणे स्थूलः । (हेमाद्रिः)
(ii) स्थूलः स्थौल्यकरो देहे स्रोतसामवरोधकृत् । (भा. प्र.)
(iii) प्रसृतावयवत्वं स्थूलत्वम् । (आ.द.अ. ३ आ. २ सू. ४७)
(iv) क्षितिवृत्ति । (आ.द.अ. ३ आ. २ सू. ४८)

It results in Guru paka and causes Sorotorodha (obstruction to channels of the body). It acts as Kapha vardhaka and vata-pitta Samaka.

It increases the tissue weights and also increases the quantity of Malas there by helping in their expulsion.

It is main feature of Prithvi bhuta. It is used in Vata Vyadhis.

(19) Sāndra guna: ***(Solidity or Turbidity)***

The quality which provides solidity or turbidity to any substance is known as Sāndra guna[1]. In other words it is described as the property by which different parts of the body are strengthened or nourished (Prasadana).

It aggravates kapha and subsides vata; increases the tissue functions & structure; solidifies the excreta.

Sāndra is the characteristic feature of Prithvi bhuta. e.g. butter, milk-cream etc. This property is responsible for Brimhana, Bandhana, Prasadana etc. effects.

Bhava Mishra mentioned **Sushka** in place of Sandra (as opposite to Drava). It is because of Prithvi, vayu, Agni bhutas.

(20) Drava guna: ***(Fluidity)***

The property which is responsible for fluidity is known as Drava[2]. It is the main feature of Jala bhuta. We find the utility of Drava guna is Snehana, Swedana & Sthambhana.

It aggravates Kapha-pitta and subsides vata; improves liquid

---

१. (i) यस्य प्रसादने शक्तिः स सान्द्रः । (हेमाद्रिः)

(ii) सान्द्रः स्थूलः स्याद्बन्धकारकः । (सु. सू. ४६/४२०)

* डल्हणः- सान्द्रो गुणः । बन्धकारक उपचयकारक इत्यर्थः । द्रव प्रक्लेदनो व्यापी शुष्कः स्याद्बन्ध-कारकः इति केचित् पठन्ति । शुष्को गुणः बन्धकारकः शुष्कस्य शोषणत्वेना-वयवापृथक्त्वमित्यर्थः ।

(iii) निविडावयवत्वं सान्द्रत्वम् । (आ.द.अ. ३. आ. २ सू. ४९)

२. (i) द्रवः प्रक्लेदनः परः .... । (सु. सू. ४६/४२०)

* डल्हणः- द्रवो गुणः । प्रक्लेदन आर्द्रभावकरः । .....द्रवः प्रक्लेदनो व्यापी ....।

(ii) यस्य विलोडने शक्तिः स द्रवः । (हेमाद्रिः)

(iii) सांसिद्धिकं द्रवत्वं स्यात्, नैमित्तिकमथापरम् ।
सांसिद्धिकं तु सलिले द्वितीयं क्षितितेजसोः ॥
नैमित्तिकं वह्नियोगात्तपनीयघृतादिषु । (कारिकावली)

dhatus like Rasa, Rakta etc.; also increases the quantity of excreta. e.g. Jala (water), Ksheera (milk) etc.

It is two types: (i) Sansiddhika (natural) e.g. water (ii) Naimittika (artificial) e.g. ghee, oil etc.

Drava guna is useful in conditions like Atisara, Jwara, Trishna etc.

Comparision between Guru and Laghu gunas

S.N.		Guru	Laghu
1.	Panchabhuta Composition	Prithvi + Ap	Angi + Vayu
2.	Rasa	Madhura Amla, Kashaya	Tikta, Lavana, Katu
3.	Physical character	Heaviness	Lightness
4.	Vipaka	Madhura (Guru)	Amla,Katu (Laghu)
5.	Effect on doshas	Kapha Vardhaka Vata Samaka	Vata Vardhaka Kapha Samaka
6.	Effect on dhatus	Dhatu Vriddhi	Dhatu Kshaya
7.	Effect on Malas	Mala Vriddhi	Mala Kshaya
8.	Effect on Agni	Delays Digestion	Easy Digestion
9.	Utility in treatment	Snehana & Brimhana	Rukshana & Langhana

Comparision between Seeta and Ushna Gunas

S.N.		Seeta	Ushna
1.	Pancha bhuta composition	Vayu + Ap	Agni
2.	Rasa	Tikta-Madhura-Kashaya	Lavana-Amla-Katu
3.	Physical character	cold	hot
4.	Vipaka	Madhura	Katu
5.	Effect on doshas	Kapha-Vata Vardhaka	Pitta Samaka
6.	Effect on dhatus	Dhatu vriddhi	Dhatu kshaya
7.	Effect on Malas	Mala vriddhi	Mala kshaya
8.	Effect on Angi	Angnimandya	Agni Vardhaka
9.	Utility in treatment	Snehana & Sthambhana	Rukshana & Swedana

Comparision between Snigdha and Ruksha gunas

S.N.		Snigdha	Ruksha
1.	Panchabhuta composition	Prithvi + Ap	Agni + Vayu
2.	Rasa	Madhura-Amla-Lavana	Katu-Tikta-Kashaya
3.	Physical character	Unctuous	non-unctuous
4.	Vipaka	Madhura	Katu
5.	Effect on doshas	kapha-pitta vardhaka, vata hara	kapha-pitta hara, vata vardhaka
6.	Effect on dhatus	Dhatu vardhaka	Dhatu kshaya
7.	Effect on Malas	Mals Vriddhi	Mala Kshaya
8.	Effect on Agni	Agni Vardhaka	Agni mandyakara
9.	Utility in treatment	snehana, Brimhana	Rukshana, Langhana

Comparision between Mridu and Tikshna gunas

S.N.		Mridu	Tikshna
1.	Panchabhuta composition	Ap & Akasa	Agni & Vayu
2.	Rasa	Madhura-Tikta-Kashaya	Amla-Lavana-Katu
3.	Physical character	mild	stimulant
4.	Vipaka	Madhura	Katu
5.	Effect on doshas	Kapha Vardhaka, vata hara	Pitta Vardhaka, vata hara
6.	Effect on dhatus	Dhatu Vriddhi	Dhatu Kshaya
7.	Effect on Malas	Mala Vardhaka	Mala Kshaya
8.	Effect on Agni	Agni Vardhaka	Agni Vardhaka
9.	Utility in treatment	Snehana,Brimhana & Sthambhana	Rukshana, Langhana & Swedana.

The other gunas which are not covered under twenty types of Gurvadi gunas are further discussed here:

Sugandha–

The quality which is responsible for good smell & taste; mrudu & sukshma; generates pleasant feeling is known as Sugandha[1].

Durgandha–

It is exactly opposite to Sugandha. It is the quality which results in foetid or unpleasant smell etc[2].

Every one will experience the effect of pleasant and foefid smell. Pungent smell etc, are quoted as the causative factors of Chardhi (Dwishta gandhaja chardi). Ugra gandha of Vacha is known for its utility as Nasya in Apasmara. However, Gandha guna shall be considered under Vaiseshika gunas but not under Gurvadi gunas.

Other gunas viz., Vyavayi, Vikasi and Asukāri will be discussed in connection with Karma in the coming chapters.

5. Detailed knowledge on Parādi Gunas-

For the successful implimentation of the treatment procedures ten important qualities/properties have been deleniated by charaka. These are known as Parādi gunas which are very essential factors for the treatment. They are: (1) Paratwa (priority) (2) Aparatwa (posteriority) (3) Yukti (logic) (4) Sankhya (numbering) (5) Samyoga (integration) (6) Vibhaga (disentigration) (7) Prithaktwa (severality) (8) Parimana (dimension) (9) Samskara (changing original property) (10) Abhyasa (regular use)[3].

Though Chakrapani quoted that these properties are not of primary importance in the treatment[4], Charaka clearly mentioned

---

१. सुखानुबन्धी सूक्ष्मश्च सुगन्धो रोचनो मृदुः ॥ (सु. सू. ४६/४२१)
* डल्हणः- सुखानुबन्धी सुखोत्पादक इत्यर्थः । सूक्ष्मोऽवगाहकः । सुगन्धो गुणः ।

२. दुर्गन्धो विपरीतोऽस्माद्‌हल्लासारुचिकारकः ।
* डल्हणः- हल्लासारुचिकारक इति पुनररुचिग्रहणं द्विविधारुचिप्रापणार्थं, तेनाहारं न काङ्क्षति क्रियामाणाच्च विरसीभवति; हल्लासः थूत्करणं छर्दिरित्यन्ये ।

३. परत्वापरत्वे युक्तिश्च संख्या संयोग एव च ।
विभागश्च पृथक्त्वं च परिमाणमथापि च ॥
संस्कारोऽभ्यास इत्येते गुणा ज्ञेयाः परादयः ।
सिद्ध्युपायाश्चिकित्साया लक्षणैस्तान् प्रचक्ष्महे ॥ (च. सू. २६)

४. एते सामान्यगुणा अपि नात्युपयुक्तत्वात्तथा बुद्धिप्राधान्याच्चान्ते प्रोक्ताः । (चक्रपाणि)

their significance by mentioning that treatment is not possible without the knowledge of Parādi gunas[1].

(1) Partwam: ***(Priority or Superiority)***

Paratwa means priority or superiority of a substance over the other innumerable substances[2]. When there are many dravyas and gunas indicated in a specific disease, picking up a drug on priority basis is known as Paratwa, e.g. Amla rasa as Hridya, Eranda mula as Vata hara, Khadira as Kushtaghna etc.

Though there are many drugs available for the above purposes, specific drugs are mentioned on the basis of specificity. Even under the modern pharmacology we come across the concept of "drug of choice". For typhoid ciproflaxacin, chloramphenicol, cotrimoxizole are conisedred as the drugs of choice in chronology purely on the basis of priority or superiority over other anti-biotics. Similarly we have very good drugs like Bakuchi, Bhallataki, chakramarda etc., which are all useful in skin conditions. However Khadira is considered as the best on the basis of Paratwa. Hence the concept of 'Agryaoushadhas' in the Ayurvedic treatises.

Yogendranath Sen accepted Paratwa as the quality which decides about the close relation of a material or substance in the treatment[3]. Things like Desa, Kala, Mana, Virya etc., are considered under this.

(2) Aparatwam: ***(Posteriority or inferior quality)***

This quality is exactly opposite to Paratwa. Aparatwa denotes the inferior quality of a drug or its constituents etc[4].

The same is depicted in the form of Ahita padarthas (harm-

---

१. इति स्वलक्षणैरुक्ता गुणाः सर्वे परादयः ।
चिकित्सा यैरविदितैर्न यथावत् प्रवर्तते ॥ (च. सू. २६)

२. (i) तच्च परत्वं प्रधानत्वम् । (चक्रपाणि- च. सू. २६/३५)
(ii) परत्वं सन्निकृष्टत्वम् उपयोगितायामासन्नत्वम् । (योगेन्द्रनाथ)

३. (i) अपरत्वं अप्रधानत्वम् । (चक्रपाणि- च. सू. २६/३५)
(ii) तद्विपर्ययः अपरत्वम् । (योगेन्द्रनाथ)

४. एकदिक्काभ्यामेककालाभ्यां सन्निकृष्टविप्रकृष्टाभ्यां परमपरं च । (वै. द.)

ful substances) by Charaka e.g. Chilichima in Matsya, Sarshapa Saka in saka etc. In modern pharmacology we find a list of drugs which are mentioned on the similar lines e.g. Brufen in asthama patients, NSAIDS in pepticulcer patients, cholesterol for obese and hypercholesteraemic patients etc.

It is a well known fact that posteriority has more value in medical research than a positive result. Aparatwa gives us a change to know about harmful aspects to health.

Examples of Paratwa & Aparatwa

Vaiseshika darsana quoted that any thing which is close to utility in the treatment is known as Paratwa and away from utility is known as Aparatwa[1].

Charaka opine that both Paratwa & Aparatwa are more related to- Desa (place), Kāla (time), Āyu (aga), Māna (measurement), Pāka (metabolism), Virya (potency), Rasa (taste) etc., which are of practical importance in the management of diseases[2]. Ayurveda darsana also expressed similar view[3].

Chakrapani mentioned about the following examples for Paratwa & Aparatwa:

Paratwa– Vayu bhumi, Visarga kāla; Taruna vayah; usual measurements for body; respective ras, virya, vipaka etc.

Aparatwa– Ānupa desa; Ādāna kala etc., opposite aspects for the above examples.

Ayurveda darsana concluded by stating that if the cause is superior, the effect is also superior and vice versa.

---

१. देशकाल वयो मान पाक वीर्यरसादिषु परत्वापरत्वे .... । (च. सू. २६,.अ)
*चक्रपाणि:- तत्र देशो मरु: पर:, कालो विसर्ग: पर: वयस्तरूणं परम्, मानं च शरीरस्य यथावक्ष्यमाणं शरीरे परम्, पाकवीर्यरसास्तु ये यस्य योगिनस्ते तं प्रति परा: । ......आदिग्रहणात् प्रकृतिबलादीनां ग्रहणम् ।.....तत्रानूपोऽपर:, आदानमपर:, अपरमितरत्, ततोऽन्यदपरम् अयोगिका-स्त्वपरा: । ....वय: प्रभृतिषु परत्वापरत्वं यथासंभवं कालदेशकृतमेवेहोपयोगादुपचरितमप्यभिहतं, वतो न गुणे मनादौ गुणान्तरसंभव: ।

२. देशकालवयोमानपाकवीर्यरसादिषु उत्कर्षापकर्षाभ्यां परत्वापरत्वम् । (आ.द.अ. ५ आ. । सू. १)

३. (i) कारणपरत्वापरत्वाभ्यां कार्यपरापरत्वे । (आ.द.अ. ५ आ. । सू. २)
(ii) धरणीसलिलानलानिलगगनतमोवृत्ति: । (आ.द.अ. ५ आ. । सू.४)

(3) Yukti: ***(Logic)***

A drug must be selected with logic in a given condition by assessing the doshas and dushyas[1] Chakrapani stated that administration of a drug without scientific reasoning or logic is worst than not administering it e.g.: to a person who is not having a son.

While administering a medicine-Samyoga (combination), Parimana (dose), Samskara (modification) etc., are to be planned very carefully. By preparing a specific combination or medicament even poison can be used as medicine or it can be vice versa. It is also said that there is no material without medicinal value in this world. Only we need a person with proper descritory power to utilize them in therapeutics.

Even in Dravyaguna sastra emphasis is laid on Yuktijna than on the Nama rupajna. This Yukti is considered as one of the faculties of Buddhi.

(4) Samkhya: ***(Number)***

It is the quality by which we are able to count, Doshas, Rogas, dravyas etc. They are all mentioned with their number even samprapti is explained on the basis of number. It is very essential

---

१. (i) युक्तिश्च योजना या तु युज्यते । (च. सू. २६)
* चक्रपाणि:- योजना दोषाद्यपेक्षया भेषजस्य समीचीनकल्पना ।
या कल्पना यौगिकी भवति सा तु युक्तिरुच्यते, अयौगिकी तु कल्पनाऽपि सति युक्तिर्नोच्यते, पुत्रोऽप्यपुत्रत्वात् ।
युक्तिश्चेयं संयोगपरिमाणसंस्काराद्यन्तर्गताऽप्यत्युपयुक्तत्वात् पृथगुच्यते ।

(ii) अमन्त्रमक्षरं नास्ति, नास्ति मूलमनौषधम् ।
अयोग्य: पुरुषो नास्ति योजकस्तत्र दुर्लभ: ।। (चरक)

(iii) न नामज्ञानमात्रेण रूपज्ञानेन वा पुन: ।
ओषधीनां परां प्राप्तिं कश्चिद्वेदितुमर्हति ।।
योगविन्नामरूपज्ञस्तासां तत्त्वविदुच्यते । (च. सू. १ अ.)

(iv) बुद्धि: पश्यति या भावान् बहुकारणयोगजान् ।
युक्तिस्त्रिकाला सा ज्ञेया त्रिवर्ग: साध्यते यया ।। (च. सू.)

(v) रोगसापेक्षा भेषजस्य समीचीनकल्पना युक्ति: । (आ.द.अ.५ आ. १ सू.५)

(vi) मात्राकालाश्रया युक्ति: सिद्धिर्युक्तौ प्रतिष्ठिता ।
तिष्ठत्युपरि युक्तिज्ञो द्रव्य ज्ञानवतां सदा ।। (च. सू. २/१६)

in treatment since one should know how many pills are to be given, how many times to be given etc[1].

(5) Samyoga: ***(Integration or Combination)***

Combination of two or more than two substances is known as Samyoga[2]. It is the quality through which two or more drugs are combined together temporarily. This union can be separated at later times. Therefore it is Anitya (temporary).

This Samyoga can be two types viz., Nitya and Anitya. The combination of dravya and gunas is permanant (Nitya) but the combination of two different dravyas is always temporary (Anitya).

On the basis of cause (kāraṇa) Samyoga is of three types:

(i) Dwandwa Karmaja
(ii) Sarva Karmaja
(iii) Eka Karmaja

(i) In this combination union of both the dravyas will take part in the effect e.g.: Dwandwaja rogas like vata kapha jwara etc.

---

१. (i) संख्या स्याद् गणितम् । (चक्रपाणि- च. सू. २६)
(ii) गणितं गणनाव्यवहारहेतुरेकद्वित्र्यादिसंख्या । (योगेन्द्रनाथ)
(iii) सम्यक् ख्यायतेऽनया इति संख्या । (द्र. गु. वि.)
(iv) सर्वद्रव्यवृत्ति । (आ.द.अ. ५. आ. । सू. १२)

२. (i) संयोगः पुनर्द्वयो र्बहूनां वा द्रव्याणां संहतीभावः । (च. वि. ए. १/२७)
(ii) योगः सहसंयोगः उच्यते, द्रव्याणाम् ....। (च. सू. २६)
(iii) अप्राप्तयोस्तु या प्राप्तिः सैव संयोग ईरितः । (द्रव्य परिज्ञान)
(iv) समवायोऽपृथग्भावो भूम्यादीनां गुणैर्मतः । स नित्यः......। (च. सू. १)
(v) द्रव्याणां द्वन्द्वसर्वेककर्मजोऽनित्य एव च । (च. सू. २६)
* योगेन्द्रनाथः- स च संयोगो द्रव्याणां द्वन्द्वसर्वैककर्मजः । द्वद्वस्य द्वयोः, सर्वेषां बहूनाम्, एकस्य च कर्मणः, जायते तेन त्रिविधः ।
(vi) वैशेषिकास्त्वाहुः- अन्यतरकर्मजः उभयकर्मजः संयोगजश्च संयोगः (वै. द. ७२/९२)
(vii) संयोगज संयोगो यथा- अङ्गुलीतरूसंयोगात् शरीरतरूसंयोगः । (योगेन्द्रः)
(viii) अम्लेन सह संयुक्तः स तीक्ष्ण लवणो रसः ।
माधुर्यं भजतेऽत्यर्थं तीक्ष्णभावं विमुञ्चति ॥ (सु. सू. ११)
(ix) प्रकृत्या हेतुभूतया समः कारणानुरूपः समवायः कार्यकारणभावसंबन्धः प्रकृतिसमसमवायः करणानुरूपं कार्यमित्यर्थः, यथा शुक्लतन्तुसमवायारब्धस्य पटस्य शुक्लत्वम् । विकृत्या हेतुभूतया विषमः कारणानुरूपः समवायः विकृतिविषमसमवायः यथा हरिद्राचूर्ण-संयोगे लौहित्यमिति । (मधुकोशः)

(ii) In this combination union of all the dravyas will take part in the effect e.g.: Tridoshaja rogas like Sanipata jwara etc.

(iii) In this combination domination of one dravya will subside the others e.g.: Ekadoshaja rogas like Vata jwara etc.

Vaiseshika philosophy mentioned about Samyoga under three different varieties viz., Anyatara Karmaja, Ubhayakarmaja and Samyogaja.

Modern scientific community accepts only two types of combinations: They are:

(i) Physical combination - mixture

(ii) Chemical combination - compound

We find the same in the ancient texts where churnas and gutikas are the examples of mixtures. While, Asavas and lehyas etc., are the examples for compounds. Sushrita deleniated on example by quoting that a combination of Amla and Lavana will lead to Madhura.

Acharya P.V. Sharma consider that 'Prakritisamasamavaya' and 'Vikriti Vishama samavaya' are the equivalents of physical and chemical combinations respectively. When a particular combination produces an action corresponding to its cause it is known as Prakriti sama Samavaya, e.g.: union of white threads forming a white cloth. If the cause and effect have no similarity then it is known as Vikriti Vishama Samavaya e.g.: when calcium hydroxide and Turmeric are mixed, red colur is produced.

[The author is of the openion that there are certain exceptions to the above view].

(6) Vibhaga: ***(Disentigration)***

Division of a particular substance or division of a combination is known as vibhaga[1]. It is also temporary (Anitya). This is also three types like Samyoga:

---

१. (i) विभागस्तु विभक्तिः स्याद्वियोगो भागशो ग्रहः । (च. सू. २६)

* चक्रपाणि:- विभागशो विभक्त्वेन ग्रहणं यतो भवतीति भावः, तेन विभाक्तिरित्येषा भावरूपा प्रतीतिः, न संयोगाभावमात्रं भवति किं तर्हि भावरूपविभाग गुणयुक्तो इत्यर्थः ।

(ii) प्राप्तिपूर्विका अप्राप्तिः विभागः । (योगेन्द्रनाथ)

(iii) नतु संयोगाभाव एव विभागः, तथात्वे गुणकर्मणोरपि विभागव्यवहारप्रसंगः स्यात्।(योगेन्द्रनाथ)

(i) Dwandwa Karmaja
(ii) Sarwa Karmaja
(iii) Eka Karmaja

But Vaiseshikas consider vibhagaja vibhaga in place of sarwa karmaja vibhaga e.g.: falling leaves are seperated from the tree.

Some scholars consider it as the Abhava (non-existant) can feel the existance of Vibhaga.

This Vibhaga is explained in three steps

(a) Vibhakti- cutting Guduchi into pieces to prepare decoction.
(b) Viyoga- using Brihati alone instead of Brihati dwaya.
(c) Bhagoso graha- obtaining Sattwa from Guduchi.

Examples of Samyoga & Vibhaga

These two are almost similar to association and dissociation reaction dealt under karma. The main difference between guna and karma in this context are karma mainly deals with chemical aspects while guna mainly deals with physical aspects.

Samyoga and Vibhaga are inseperable aspects of treatment because preparation of a medicine is based upon either of these two processes. For example, Guduchi is used in the form of Amritarishta or Amritadi kashaya on the basis of Samyoga. Similarly Guduchi is used in the form of Guduchi Swarasa or Guduchi Sattwa on the basis of Vibhaga.

(7) Prithaktwa: ***(Severality or Seperateness)***

It is the quality by which one substance is differentiated or seperated from the other[1]. e.g. Haritaki is different from Amalaki.

---

१. (i) पृथक्त्ववसंयोगो वैलक्षण्यमनेकता (च. सू. २६)
(ii) इदं द्रव्यं पटलक्षणं घटात् पृथक् इत्यादिका बुद्धिर्यतो भवति तत् पृथक्त्वम् । (चक्रपाणि)
(iii) इदमस्मात् पृथक् अर्थान्तरमिति पृथक्प्रत्ययनिमित्तं पृथक्त्वम् । (योगेन्द्रनाथ)
(iv) अपोद्धाव्यवहारे कारणं पृथक्त्वम् । (आ.द.अ.५आ.।सू.२१)
(v) तत् त्रिविधमसंयोगो वैलक्षण्यमनेकता । (आ.द.अ.५आ.।सू. १२)
(vi) यत्सर्वथा असंयुज्यमानयोरिव मेरूहिमालययो: पृथक्त्वं, एतद् असंयोग इत्यनेनोक्तम् । तथा संयुज्यमानमपि पृथक्त्वं विजातीयानां महिषवराहादीनां, तदाह वैलक्षण्यमित्यादि विशिष्टलक्षण

क्रमश: पृष्ठ ७३ में...........

The quality or qualities differentiating these two is (are) known as Prithaktwa.

Prithaktwa is of three types viz.,

(i) **Asamyoga lakshana–** difference in the qualities of substance in two different places or in two different seasons e.g.:Chandana of Meru parvata is different from that of Himalayas.

(ii) **Vailakshanya rupa–** difference between two classes e.g.: difference between buffalo and pig.

(iii) **Anekata rupa–** difference between the substances belonging to same category e.g.: seven types of Haritaki, each having individual qualities differenting one from the other.

There is a debate over the issue that 'Anyonyabhava' and 'Prithaktwa' are same. But they are different. For example, through Anyonyabhava we can establish that Ghata (pot) is not Pata (cloth) wherein 'Abhava' is expressed. However through Prithaktwa we differentiate between Pata and Ghata which is expression of Bhava. The former is non-existant feature while the later is existing feature.

In treatment Prithaktwa may be used to differentiate between the quality of two drugs e.g. difference between Guduchi Swarasa and Sattwa; or difference between Amritadi kwath and Amritarishta.

(8) Parimana: *(Measurement)*

The quality by which measurement of various things is possible is known as Parimana[1]. Parimana is basically two types:

पृष्ठ ७२ से क्रमशः...........

-युक्तत्वलक्षितं विजातीयानां पृथक्त्वमित्यर्थः । एकजातीयेषु हि संयुक्तेषु न वैलक्षण्यं नाप्यसंयोगः अथचानेकता पृथक्त्वरूपा भवति । (चक्रपाणि)

(vii) अन्योऽन्याभावतो नास्यचरितार्थ च मिष्यते ।अस्मात्पृथग्घगिदं नेति प्रतीतिह विलक्षणा ।। (कारिकावली)

१. (i) परिमाणं पुनर्मानं । (च. सू. २६)

* चक्रपाणिः- मानं प्रस्थाढकादि तुलार्मयम् ।

** योगेन्द्रनाथः- परिमितिव्यवहारकारणं परिमाणं मानं प्रस्थाढकादि ।

(ii) परिमाणं भवेन्मानव्यवहारस्यकारणम् । (कारिकावली)

(i) Dairghya māna - measurement of dimension
(ii) Gurutwa māna - measurement of weight

(a) Dairghya māna ***(Measurement of lenght or dimension)***

This is Nitya (eternal) for Nitya dravyas like Paramana and Anitya (temporary) for Anitya dravyas like Dwyanukas etc. The later is of three types again:

(i) Sankhya janya - dwaynuka etc.
(ii) Parimana janya - ghata (pot) etc.
(iii) Parchaya janya - cotton etc.

This measurement is based on Anguli, Hasta, Aratni etc. Dairghya mana may be of another four varieties viz., Anu (invisible), Dirgha (very long), Mahat (huge) and Hraswa (small)[1].

(b) Gurutwa māna: ***(measurement of volume and weight)***

This is also two types i.e.; Nitya and Anitya. It is measured by means of Parstha, Ādhaka etc. with the help of vessels and balance.

In Amara kosa we come across three types of measurements-

(i) Poutava - measurement by weight
(ii) Drivaya - measurement by volume
(iii) Payya - measurement of lenght etc[2].

(9) Samskara: ***(changing the original quality)***

The quality through which some change is brought to the original properties of a dravya is known as Samskara[3]. e.g. Rice is made

---

१. (i) अनित्ये तदनित्यं स्यान्नित्ये नित्यमुदाहृतम् ॥
संख्यात: परिमाणच्चप्रचयादपि जायते ।
अनित्यं, द्वयणुकादौ तु संख्याजन्यमुदाहृत्रम् ॥
परिमाणं घटादौ तु परिमाणजमुच्यते ।
प्रथम: शिथिलाख्यो य: संयोगस्तेन जायते ॥
परिमामं तूलकादौ .... । (कारिकावली)

(ii) अणु दीर्घं महद् ह्रस्वमिति तद्भेद ईरित: । (कारिकावली)

२. पौतवं द्रवयं पाय्यमिति मानार्थकं त्रयम् ।
मानं तुलांगुलिप्रस्थै: । (अ.को.२/९/८५)

३. (i) संस्कार: करणं मतम् । (च. सू. २६)
संस्कारो हि गुणान्तराधनमुच्यते । ते च गुणास्तोयाग्निसन्निकर्षशौचमन्थनदेशकालवशेन भावनादिभि: कालप्रकर्षभांजनादिभिश्चाधीयन्ते । च.वि.१.अ.)

क्रमश: पृष्ठ ७५ में.......

into different forms with different properties through Saṃskara (ōdana, Lāja etc.) Similarly Parada (mercury) is provided with the best qualities through different Samskaras.

Vaiseshika philosophy quoted three types of Samskara.

(i) Vega - impulse
(ii) Sthiti sthapakata - elasticity
(iii) Bhāvana - impression

(10) Aḅhyāsa: *(Continuous usage)*

Regular usage of any thing over a period of time is known as Abhyasa. It is other wise known as seelana and Satata Kriya[1].

It is very important quality in the treatment because continuous usage of a drug can only yield good results. Similarly exercises etc., may also provide beneficial results on regular practice.

To avoid some unwanted or unhealthy food and behavioural aspects we need some practice continuously. Therefore the healthy state is restored. This practice is also Abhyasa only[2]. It is also mentioned that the qualities which will increase or decrease the doshas and dhatus may be equal or opposite to them respectively. Their continuous usage through food or exercise over a period of time will maintain the healthy state[3]. Therefore Abhyasa is useful in the treatment.

पृष्ठ ७४ से क्रमशः......

(ii) करणं हि स्वाभाविकानां द्रव्याणां अभिसंस्कारः ।
सन्निकर्षशौचमन्थनदेशकालवशेन भावनादिभिः कालप्रकर्षभांजनादिभिश्चाधीयन्ते ।(च.वि.१अ.)
(iii) करणं गुणान्तराधकत्वं संस्करणमित्यर्थः । (चक्रपाणि)
(iv) संस्कारभेदो वेगोऽथ स्थितिस्थापकभावने । (कारिकावली)
(v) गुणाधान् दोषरहितो वा संस्कारः । (आ.द.अ. ५ आ. १ सू. ३७)

१. भावाभ्यसनमभ्यासः शीलनं सततक्रिया। (च.सू. २६)
* चक्रपाणिः- भावस्य यष्टिकादेर्व्यायामादेश्चाम्यसनमभ्यासः ।
** योगेन्द्रनाथः- भावानामभ्यसनं पुनः पुनरनुष्ठानं सातत्येन करणमभ्यासः ।

२. त्यागाद् विषमहेतूना समानां चोपसेवनात्। विषमा नानुबन्ध्नन्ति जायन्ते धातवः समाः॥(च.सू.१६)

३. (i) समानगुणाभ्यासो हि धातूनां वृद्धिकारणमिति । (च.सू. १२)
(ii) नर्त्ते सन्तर्पणाभ्यासाच्चिरक्षीणस्तु पुष्यति । (च.सू. २३)
(iii) रसदोषसन्निपाते तु ये रसा यैर्दोषैः समानगुणभूयिष्ठा वा भवन्ति ते तानभिवर्धयन्ति,
विपरीतगुणा विपरीतगुणभूयिष्ठा वा शमयन्त्यभ्यास्यमानाः । (च.वि. १)
(iv) धातवः पुनः शारीराः समानगुणैः समानगुणभूयिष्ठैर्वाऽप्याहारविहारैरभ्यस्यमानैर्वृद्धिं प्राप्नुवन्ति,
ह्रासं तु विपरीतगुणैर्विपरीतगुणभूयिष्ठैर्वैऽप्यस्यमानैः । (च.शा. ६)

As the natural products, exert an cumulative effect on the body, continuous administration or usage of drug is essential many times. Similarly, continous exercise in hemiplegia and other connective tissue problems will help a lot.

From the previous pages it is apparent that Paradi gunas are not simply qualities for academic interest. Actually they are the methods needed for scientific research. While providing treatment one has to think about- drug of choice (Paratwa), contrain-dicated drugs (Aparatwa), carefull assessment of patients condition and drug (Yukti); how many times the drug is to be administered (Sankhya); what are the possible combinations with one drug (Samyoga) or what are all to be avoided in a group of drugs (Vibhaga); selection of specific drug after differential diagnosis (Prithaktwa); the dose (quantity) to be administered (Parimana); modifying the original property of drug if requried e.g. boiling the fruit of Haritaki to treat diarrhoea (Samskara) and finally administering the drug for sufficient period of time like 30 days, 60 days etc; (Abhyasa).

Through these methods a given drug is studied experimentally as well as clinically in the present days. Therefore Paradi gunas may also be called as Chikitsopayoga gunas (i.e. qualities used in the treatment of a disease).

6. Knowledge on Vaiseshika Gunas

Guna is catagorized into Adhibhoutika and Adhyatmika. The former has two sub-groups viz., Sāmanya and Visesha. We have discussed in detail about Samanya gunas which are the general properties of dravyas which are made up of Panchabhutas. However the Pancha bhutas at the minutest level will have five individual properties[1]. They are

(1) Akasa (vacuum) - Sabda (sound)

(2) Vāyu (gas) - sparsa (touch)

---

१. (i) महाभूतानि खं वायुरग्निरापः क्षितिस्तथा ।
शब्दः स्पर्शश्च रूपं च रसो गन्धश्च तद्गुणाः ॥ (च.शा. १/२७)

(ii) खर द्रव चल उष्णत्वं भूजलानिलतेजसाम् ।
आकाशस्याप्रतीघातो दृष्टं लिङ्गं यथाक्रमम् ॥ (च. शा. १/२९)

(3) Agni (plasma) - rupa (luminiscense or colour or shape)
(4) Jala (liquid) - rasa (taste)
(5) Prithvi (solid) - gandha (small)

These properties will have physical effects on the body and are therefore helpful in the treatment.

(1) Sabda: ***(Sound)***

It is the quality of Ākasa and is recieved through the subdendriya (ear). Its practical utility is seen in Rasakshaya state where in the patient can not tolerate Sabda i.e.; the quality of Ākasa which is aggravated mut be reduced. Therefore Jaliya and Parthiva dravyas are given in the management of Rasa kshaya e.g. Ksheera, Mamsa rasa etc[1].

It is well documented that sound has its effect on disease states. Hence music-therapy is used for the management of psychiatric problems accroding to Ayurveda.

(2) Sparsa: ***(Touch)***

It is the quality of vayu and is percieved by skin (Sparsanendriya). It is of three varieties viz., Seeta, Ushna and Anushna Seeta (cold, hot and leukwarm)[2].

This is usued practically where Manidharana is advised or Oushadha dharana is advised in graha roga etc. Vedana sthapana dravyas are also meant for their effect on sparsanendriya.

(3) Rupa: ***(Colour or shape or luminiscence)***

It is the main quality of Agni and it is percieved through Chakshurindriya (eye). It provides the knowledge about the shape, size, colour etc. Its utility is observed in disease diagnosis and management[3]. Prameha and its 20 types are based upon colour only.

---

१. (i) शब्दबहुलमाकाशः।
(ii) रसक्षये......घट्टते सहते शब्दं, शब्दं नैवातिबुध्यते ।

२. (i) स्पर्शबहुलोवायुः ।
(ii) स्पर्शेस्त्वगिन्द्रियग्राह्यः । (आ. द.)
(iii) शीतोष्णोऽनुष्णशीतश्च । (आ. द.)

३. (i) रूपबहुलो अग्निः ।
(ii) तत्र रूपं चक्षुर्ग्राह्यम् । (आ. द.)
(iii) मूत्रवर्णादि भेदेन भेदोमेहेषु कल्प्यते । (मा. नि.)

Treatment of Rakta vikaras with Manjishta (which is red in colour) and treatment of Ojo kshaya with Kshira (which is white in colour) etc; are few examples.

(4) Rasa: ***(Taste)***

It is the specific quality of Jala and is percived by the tongue (Rasanendriya)[1].

*It is discussed elaborately under Rasa chapter.

(5) Gandha: ***(Smell)***

It is the main qualities of Prithvi and is percieved through Ghranendriya (nose). It is three types viz.,

(i) Sugandha (aroma) (ii) Durgandha (foetid smell) & (iii) Avyakta gandha (unknown smell). Therefore it is clear that Sugandha & Durgandha are the varients of visesha gunas but not Gurvadi gunas.

It is important to realize that gandha guna at Paramanu level is Nitya and that of Kārya dravya is Anitya.

This is mainly used in Nasya Karma, Dhupa and Dhuma pana etc.

Asātmyendriyartha Samyoga (Hina-mithya-Ati yougas) of these qualities will lead to diseases and they are to be rectified by administering drugs which will have opposite qualities e.g., Jala & Prithvi dravyas are used in Akasa-Vayu-Agni vriddhi states[2].

7. Knowledge on Ātma Gunas

Ayurveda deals with the physical and metaphysical creation with same importance. Along with the body health it advises the healthy state of mind (Manah) and soul (Ātma) also. Manas and Ātma are intricated factors being Kārayita and Chetayita respectively.

---

१. (i) रसबहुलमाप्यम् ।
(ii) रसनेन्द्रियग्राह्यो रसः ।
२. (i) गन्धबहुला पृथिवी ।
(ii) गन्धो घ्राणग्राह्यः । (आ. द.)

Aḍhyatma gunas belong to the second basic category among gunas. these qualities attributed to Ātma are metaphysical and spiritual. They are Ichcha, Dwesha, Sukha, Duhkha, Prayatna and Buddhi[1].

1. Ichcha: This quality provides a reasonable and positive desire towards a particular substance.

2. Dwesha: It provides aversion towards the factors responsible for sorrowness in life.

3. Sukha: The quality through which positive effects are obtained for the combination of Ātma-Manas-Indriyarthas, is known as Sukha.

4. Duhkha: The quality which results in pain-ful effects over the combination of Ātma-Manas-Indriyarthas is known as Duhkha.

5. Prayatna: The quality through which stimulus for useful activities is obtained is known as Prayatna.

6. **Buddhi:** The quality which provides exact and exquisite knowledge regarding various substance is known as Buddhi. It is five types again viz., (i) Buddhi (ii) Smriti (iii) Dhriti, (iv) Chetana and (v) Ahamkara.

8. Pharmacological activities of Guna

Under Dravya guna sastra we come across several drug actions based upon guna (physical property). They are usually considered to be the properties of Rasa[2]. Sushrita considered that the effect of guna can be assessed with the help of inference (Anumana Pramana)[3]. For example, if it is claimed that a particular herb is guru in nature, then

---

१. अर्थाः शब्दादयो ज्ञेया गोचर विषया गुणाः । (च. शा.१)

२. (i) सुखादिच्छा । (आ.द.अ. ४ आ. २ सू. १)

(ii) आत्मनेन्द्रियार्थमनः सन्निकर्षादिष्टानिष्टफल सुखदुःखे । (आ. द.)

(iii) दुःखनिमित्तेद्वेषः । (आ.द.अ. ४. आ. २ सू. १७)

(iv) प्रयत्नः संरम्भउत्साह इत्यनर्थान्तरम् । (आ.द.अ. ४ आ. २ सू. ३७)

(v) प्रयत्नादिकर्मचेष्टितमुच्यते । (च. सू. १/४९)

(vi) स्मृतिधृतिरहंकारः प्रत्यभिज्ञाचेतना चेति पञ्चविधा । (आ. द.)

३. गुणा गुणाश्रया नोक्तास्तस्माद्रसगुणान् भिषक् ।
विद्याद्द्रव्यगुणान् .... ॥ (च. सू. २६)

one can expect gurutwa (increase in weight) in the body on its administration.

But guna can not perform any action of its own in the microworld. Pancha bhutas with different properties are combining with each other to form many materials (plant as well as animal). Therefore the human body and drug constituents are all having the similar combosition of Panchabhutas. The drugs with respective qualities are used for either vriddhi (inrease) or kshaya (decrease) of the vitiated dosha-dhatu-malas[1]. Even maintanance of health is depending upon these gunas through which preventive medicine is provided.

It is well known factor that Sāmanya (similarity) is responsible for Vriddhi (increase) and Visesha (dissimilarity) is responsible for Kshaya. The Sāmanya is of three types:

(i) Dravya Sāmanya
(ii) Guna Sāmanya
(iii) Karma Sāmanya

All these three are ultimately based upon the gunas while they are used in the treatment.

Charaka rightly said that dravyas will exert their action through Dravya prabhava or Guna prabhava or Dravya-guna prabhava. Among these three last two aspects are linked with Guna and Dravya prabhava is linked with Prabhava[2].

Basing upon their pharmacological action gunas may result either in Santarpana & Apatarpana[3].

(1) Santarpana guna

(1) Guru (2) Manda (3) Seeta (4) Snigdha (5) Slakshna (6) Sandra (7) Katina (8) Sthira (9) Sthula (10) Pichchila

(2) Apatarpana gunas

(1) Laghu (2) Tikshna (3) Ushna (4) Ruksha (5) Khara (6) Drava (7) Mridu (8) Sara (9) Sukshma (10) Visada.

---

१. कर्मभित्वनुमीयन्ते नानाद्रव्याश्रया गुणाः ॥ (सु. सू. ४६/५१४)

२. गुणाः उक्ताः द्रव्येषु शरीरेष्वपि ते तथा ॥
स्थानवृद्धिक्षयास्तस्माद् देहिनां द्रव्यहेतुकाः ॥ (सु. सू. ४१/१४)

३. द्रव्याणि हि द्रव्यप्रभावात् गुणप्रभावात् द्रव्यगुणप्रभावाच्च कार्मुकाणि भवन्ति । (च. सू. २६/१२)

On the same basis 'Shadupakramas' (six basic procedures in treatment) are performed by considering the following qualities:

1. Brimhana : Guru-Seeta-Mridu-Snigdha-Sandra-Sthula-Pichchila-Manda-Sthira
2. Snehana : Guru-Seeta-Mridu-Snigdha-Drava-Sukshma-Pichchila-Manda-Sara
3. Sthambana : Laghu-Seeta-Mridu-Ruksha-Drava-Sukshma-Visada-Manda-Sthira
4. Langhana : Laghu-Ushna-Tikshna-Ruksha-Drava-Sukshma-Visada-Manda-Sara
5. Rukshana : Laghu-Ushna-Tikshna-Ruksha-Drava-Sukshma-Visada-Manda-Sthira
6. Swedana: Guru-Ushna-Tikshna-Snigdha-Drava-Sukshma-Visada-Manda-Sthira & Sara

[* **Note:** Seeta-Mridu-Manda are common in Santarpana.]

Ushna-Tikshna-Ruksha are common in Apatarpana.

These are the few examples for the utility of guna (physical properties) in therapeutics. Even in modern pharmacology and pharmacotherapeutics also we come across certain examples for the physical properties which are responsible for different drug actions. Some of them are discussed here.

Role of Physical Properties in Drug action

(1) Colour: ***(रूप: या वर्ण:)***

Adding a pleasant colour to a medicament may exert some psychological effect on the patient e.g. coating the tablets etc., with colourful sugar coating or encapsulating medicine with colourful capsules.

It is observed on trials with placebos that even the colour of the tablet/capsule is responsible for variation in response.

(2) Taste: ***(रस:)***

Taste will definitely have some local and systemic activity e.g.

tincture of Cardamomum is added to medicaments to provide pleasant taste and colour.

Compounds with a bitter taste may reflexly increase the flow of HCl in the stomach and improve the appetite e.g. quassia, chirata and gentian.

(3) Smell: *(गन्धः)*

Unpleasant smell of a drug may be masked with the substance with aroma. Hence smell is an important aspect with drug manufacturing. Usually volatile oils like pippermint oil etc., are used to cover the unpleasant smell of mixtures.

Even odour of the smelling salt is useful in unconcious states.

[* Note:- The above three properties mentioned under modern pharmacology are nothing but the supporting factors of the concept of Vaiseshika gunas.]

(4) Physical mass: *(गुरुः)*

Substances having guru guna are claimed to possess Adhogamitwa or Rechana activity (i.e., purgative property). Compounds like Agar and Psyllium seeds absorb water when administered orally and swell in size (e.g. Bulk purgatives). This initiates peristalisis and exerts a laxative action.

(5) Osmosis: *(द्रवः)*

Osmosis will result in diuresis etc. e.g., osmotic diuretics like mannitol; osmotic purgatives like Magnesium sulphate.

(6) Adsorbtion: *(रूक्षः)*

Kaolin and activated charcoal are employed in the treatment of diarrhoea on the basis of their adsorbant property.

(7) Soothing & Demulcent: *(श्लक्ष्णः, पिच्छिलः)*

These properties are in the preparation of pharyngeal demulcent syrups used in the treatment of cough. Another example is usage of calamine lotion in eczema.

Drugs may also produce their effects through the following processes

(a) Stimulation

Increase in the activity of specialized cells is called as 'stimulation'. However excessive stimulation may ultimately lead to depression. e.g. morphine stimulates the vagus and the occulomotor nuclei, and the CTZ but also depresses the vomiting and the cough centres.

Ayurvedic texts mentioned this property as 'Vyavayi guna'. These are the drugs which causes stimulation and ends with depression of CNS. e.g. Bhanga (cannabis), Ahiphena (opium) etc.

There are four qualities which may result in stimulation:

(i) Sara guna - प्रेरणे सरः ।

(ii) Sukshma guna - विवरणे सूक्ष्मः ।

(iii) Ushna guna - स्वेदने उष्णः ।

(iv) Tikshna guna - शोधने तीक्ष्णः ।

(b) Depression:

Decrease in the activity of specializes cells is called 'depression' e.g. Quinidine depresses the myocardium while barbiturates depress the CNS.

Madakari group of drugs which causes alteration in sensovarium may be suitable example for depression.

The following qualities may be considered as examples under depression:

(i) Sthira guna - धारणो स्थिरः ।

(ii) Sthula guna - संवरणो स्थूलः ।

(iii) Seeta guna - स्तम्भनो हिमः ।

(iv) Manda guna - शमने मन्दः ।

(c) Irritation

These drugs produce effects on the growth, nutrition and morphology of living tissues. This phenomenon is not restricted to specialized cells but can occur in all the body tissues. Irritation may produce changes in the cellular structure.

The qualities mentioned under stimulation (Sara, Sukshma, Ushna & Tikshna gunas) are capable of producing irritation also.

Vikasi dravya may be considered as suitable example for this. Drugs which cause stimulation and irritation may have cholinergic and Muscarinic activities.

(i) Arecholine, the alkoloid of Areca catechu (Kramuka) has cholinergic action and is used as an anthelmintic in veterivary practice.

(ii) Kodrava may possess muscarinic activity.

Other properties which can be attributed to physical properties are:

(1) Broncho-dilators - विवरणे सूक्ष्मः ।
(2) Vasoconstrictors - संवरणे स्थूलः ।
(3) Diuretics - विलोडमे द्रवः ।
(4) Anti-diuretic - शोषणे रूक्षः ।
(5) Anti-diarrhoeal - स्तम्भनो हिमः । etc.

If we can assess the pharmacological properties of some of the Ayuvedic drugs on the basis of physical properties, exact concept of guna can be understood. The following are some of the examples of drug action based upon guna:

S.N.	Drug name	Guna	Karma
1.	Agnimantha	Ruksha & Laghu	Vata Sothahara; Dipana-Pachana
2.	Ajamoda	Ruksha, Laghu & Tikshna	Dipana, Vidahi, Chardinigrahana
3.	Ativisha	Laghu & Ruksha	Dipana-Pachana, Grahi
4.	Aparajita	Laghu & Ruksha	Atisarahara, Sotha hara.

The utilization of guna is more emphatically advised in the management of Rakta pitta, Kāsa etc. In Urdwagata Rakta pitta Ruksha-Ushna are the causative factors and in Adhogata Rakta pitta Snigdha-Ushna are the causative factors. Therefore Virechana in the former and Vamana in the later are advised. Similarly in Vata-Kapha Kasa Snigdha is advised while in Kaphaja Kasa Ruksha in used.

Another suitable example for guna is Jwara. In Jwara, Swedāvarodha (loss of sweating) is observed which may be considered as because of obstruction than kshaya (deficiency or deplition). The Malagni i.e., Swedagni is in aggravated state and therefore Sweda is reduced. This agni can be suppressed with Seeta guna and that is the reason for Seet upakramas in jwara.

We find that Koshtagni is displaced to peripheries in the process of causation of fever. The Ushna guna of Agni is tacked with Seeta guna of dravya.

Many examples can be discussed on the same lines and management of every disease should be critically analzed on the basis of gunas.

9. Importance of Guna

Badhanta Nagarjuna mentioned ten factors supporting the importance of guna.

(1) Rasāḥhibhava: ***(Over coming the taste)***

Guna will suppress the rasa and exhibit its effect. e.g. water is Madhura in nature and usually aggarvates Kapha. But hot water reduces Kapha by means of physical property. Similarly, Pātala and Brihat Panchamula are bitter in taste but subsides vata. In this case also Ushna guna is the reason but not the Rasa. Hence guna is important[1].

(2) Rasanugraha: ***(Guna based rasa selection)***

Rasas are selected for a particular purpose on the basis of their physical properties only. e.g. Ghrita is considered as the best among dravyas having Madhura rasa since it undergoes Laghu vipaka and it will posses Seeta, Snigdha, Pichchila qualities. Among Amla dravyas Āmalaki is the best as it possess Mridu, Seeta gunas and Laghu vipaka. Same is the case with others. Hence guna is given

१. गुणाः प्रधाना इति केचित् । गुणाद रसानामभिभवात् । (र. वै. आ.। सू. १२१)
* भाष्यंः- रसानभिभूय गुणाः स्वकार्यं निर्वर्तयन्ति । यथा उष्णोदकं श्लेष्मणां हरति माधुर्यमभिभूये तथा पटोलश्च महत्पञ्चमूलं च तिक्तमौष्याद् वातं जयति। यद् येनाभिभूयते तस्मादप्रधानं दृष्टम् । यथा भानोर्नक्षत्रम् इति ।

more importance than rasa[1].

(3) Vipaka Karanatwa: *(Vipaka depends upon Guna)*

Vipaka is depended upon the physical properties of a dravya e.g.

Seeta, Snigdha, Guru, Picchila guna dravyas – Guru vipaka. Ushna, Ruksha, Laghu, Visada, Tikshna guna dravyas – Laghu vipaka.

It is said that final action of rasa will be decided by the Vipaka and Vipaka is depending upon Gunas. In this context a simile has been made between vata and guna basing upon their action of dosha-dhatumalas and vipaka etc; respectively. Hence guna is important among the drug constituent[2].

(4) Sankhya bahulya: *(Gunas are more in number)*

Gunas are multipe or innumerable in number than rasas e.g., there are 41 gunas and 6 rasas in the literature of Ayurveda. Considering the number of items guna is claimed to be superior than rasas[3].

(5) Prayoga bahulya: *(Multiple utilities)*

Gunas are used more frequently and through different channels than Raras. Infact Rasa can be used through only one channel, that is Rasanendriya (tongue). Where as, properties like Seeta, Ushna, Snigdha, Ruksha etc., are generally used for Abhyanga

---

१. गुणानुगृहीतानां रसानां प्राधान्यात् । (र. वै. अ. । सू, १२८)

*भाष्यं:- गुणै: शीतादिभिरनुगृहीता ये रसास्तेषां प्राधान्यदर्शनात् रसेभ्यो गुणा: प्रधाना: इति विद्म: । कथं शैत्यात् स्नेहान्मार्दवाच्च पैच्छिल्यादविभागत: । मधुराणां घृतं श्रेष्ठं विपाके लाघवेन च ॥ अविदा-हान्मृदुत्वाच्च कषायमधुरान्वयात् । अम्लेष्वामलकं श्रेष्ठं विपाके लाघवेन च ॥ नात्युष्णत्वान्मृदुत्वाच्च स्नेर्हनानुगमादपि। लवणानां स्मृतं श्रेष्ठमविदाहाच्च सैन्धवम् ॥ मृदुत्वाच्चगुरुत्वाच्च वातपित्तप्रकोपणात् । कटुकानां स्मृता: श्रेष्ठा: पिघल्यो गुणसंपदा ॥ वृष्यत्वाच्च गुरुत्वाच्च मारुतस्याप्रकोपणात्। तिक्तानां तु स्मृतं श्रेष्ठं पैच्छिलयेन च कूलकम् ॥ वृष्यत्वाद् बृंहणत्वाच्च हिक्कानां वातनिग्रहात् । कषायाणां स्मृतं श्रेष्ठं विविधैश्च गुणैर्मधु ।

२. विपाककारणत्वात् । (र. वै. अ. । सू. १२३)

* भाष्यं:- गुणा: विपाकयो: कारणं, शीतस्निग्धगुरुपिच्छिला गुरुविपाकस्य, लघुरूक्षविशदतीक्ष्णा-लघुविपाकस्येति ।.......रसानां कार्यनिर्वृत्ति: पाकायत्ता, स च पाकी गुणायत्ता इति। यदपेक्षयाऽन्यस्थ वृत्तिस्तस्मात् तस्य प्राधान्यं दृष्टम् । यथा वायोर्दोषधातुमलानाम् ।

३. बाहुल्यान् । (र.वै.अ.।सू. १२४)

* भाष्यं:- रसेभ्यो बहवो गुणा दृष्टा: रसा: षट्, गुणा: दशेति, अल्पेभ्यो बहवो विशिष्टा इति लोक-प्रसिद्धमेककर्मणि।

(oliation), Parisheka (bathing), Avagaha (tub-bath) etc. Therefore gunas are more Prominant than Rasas[1].

(6) Karma bāhulya: ***(Multiple effects)***

Guna results in many effects (Karma) since it is common for Rasa, Virya, Vipāka etc. All the effects of other drug constitnents are rejected by gunas. Hence guna is superior[2].

(7) Viṣhaya bāhulya: ***(Guna is more related to mind faculties)***

Many qualities of gunas are more concerned with the faculties of mind compared to those of sensory organs. Hence guna is important[3].

(8) Upadesa: ***(Emphasis by the elders)***

All the treatises and Acharyas of Ayurveda have emphasized about the superiority of gunas. Hence is important among the drug constitnents[4].

(9) Apadesa: ***(Introduction by means gunas)***

Any living or non-living creation is introduced by means of their properties e.g. a man can be introduced as he is furious (तीक्ष्णोऽयं पुरुषः) or a calm going (मृदुरयं पुरुषः). Therefore guna is superior[5].

(10) Anumana

Through cause i.e., guna the effect can be inferred. Through Seeta, Ushna etc. gunas, the effects like Pittaghna, Vataghna etc; are assumed respectively. Hence guna is important[6].

✵

---

१. बहुधोपयोगात् । (र.वै.अ । सू.१२५)
* भाष्यं:- किं च बहुधाऽभ्यङ्गपरिषेकावगाहरूपेण शीतादय उपयुज्यन्ते, रसास्तु मुखत एवेति गुणाः प्रधानाः, ये बहुधोपयोगं गच्छन्ति ते प्रधाना दृष्टा यथा कल्पवृक्षाः ।

२. अनेककर्मत्वात् । (र.वै.अ । सू. १२६)
* भाष्यं:- रसादिसहितास्तेषां तेषां तत्तत्कर्मणि साहचर्यकरणादनेककर्माण इति ।

३. महाविषयत्वात् । (र.वै.अ । सू. १२७)

४. उपदेशात् ....। (र.वै. अ. । सू. १२९)
* भाष्यं:- तेषां गुरूष्णस्निग्धा वातघ्नाः इत्यादिरूपदेशः ।

५. अपदेशात् ....। (र.वै.अ.। सू. १२९)
* भाष्यं:- अपदेशः- तीक्ष्णोऽयं पुरुषः, मृदुश्यं गीत इति ।

६. अनुमानात् । (र.वै.अ.। सू. १२९)

Further References about Guna

(1) Gotecha M.; Guna Parigyanam. 1958.

[M.D. dissertation, Dept. of Dravya Guna, IPGTR, Gujrat Ayu. University, Jamnagar]

(2) Srinivasa Rao T.; Panchabhoutic Guna (A study with special reference to Guru and Laghu). 1970.

[M.D. dissertation, Dept. of Dravya Guna, IPGTR, Gujrat Ayurveda University, Jamnagar].

(3) Suman S.N.; Snigdha Evam Ruksha Gunon ka Adhyayan. 1971.

[M.D. dissertaion, Dept. of Dravya Guna, IMS, Banaras Hindu University, Varanasi]

❋

Chapter-V
Concept of Rasa

1. Etymology of Rasa

Rasa or taste is something experienced by an individual while consuming a dravya[1].

2. Definition of Rasa

Rasa is the special sense known through the Rasana or Rasanendriya (tongue or taste buds)[2].

Modern physiology defines taste as the direct action of a drug on the nerve endings in the mucous membrance of the mouth.

In this context it is very essential to clarify about different meanings of Rasa. They are:

i. Rasa Dhatu- the body fluids including blood circulating throughout the body. This meaning is used in physiology[3].

ii. Rasa (Parada)- the element (mercury) which digests other metals like gold, silver etc. This meaning is used in Rasa sastra (alchemy)[4].

iii. Rasa (Swarasa)- the fresh juice extracted from a herb. This meaning is more suitable to Bhaishajya kalpana (pharmacy)[5].

Out of all those meanings, 'Rasa' in the context of Dravya guna satra is taste only.

---

१. रस आस्वादने । (वाचस्पत्यम्)

२. (i) रस्यते आस्वाद्यते रसनेन इति रस: । (द्र.गु.वि.)

(ii) रसो रसनाग्राह्य: । (प्रशस्तपाद:)

(iii) रसनेन्द्रियग्रह्यत्वात् रस: । (अरुणदत्त:- अ.हृ.सू. १/१४-१५)

(iv) तत्र रसनाग्राह्यो रस: । (हेमाद्रि- अ.हृ.सू. १/१४-१५)

३. तत्र रसगतौधातु:, अहरहर्गच्छतीत्यतो रस: । (सु. सू. १४)

४. (i) रसति भक्ष्यति सर्वान् लोहान् इति रस: । (द्र.गु.वि.)

(ii) रसनात् (भक्षणात्) सर्वधातूनां रसेन्द्र इति कीर्तित: । (र.र.स.)

५. आहतात्तत्क्षणाकृष्टाद्द्रव्यात्क्षुण्णात्समुद्धरेत् ।
वस्त्रनिष्पीडितो य: स रस: स्वरस उच्यते ॥ (शा.सं.म.खं. १/२)

3. Characteristics of Rasa

Taste perception is the characteristic feature of Rasa. It is basically provided by two bhutas viz., Jala and Prithvi[1]. The Indriyartha of Rasanendriya is also characterized as Rasa.

4. Analytical Determination of Number of Rasas

Generally it is accepted that Rasas are six in number (Shadrasa)[2]. From Charaka Samhita it is evident that Acharya Punarvasu Ātreya convened a symposium on Rasa sankhya (no of tastes) and finalized the tastes as six ultimately. The views of various Rishis is discussed below:

No. of Rasas	Their details	concept propose by
One	Apya (water)	Bhadrakapya
Two	Chedaniya or Langhana (wt. reducing) Upasamaniya or Brimhana (wt. increasing)	Sakunteya Brahmana
Three	above two + Sadharana (ordinary)	Purnaksha Moudgalya
Four	Swaduhita (liked and good) Swadahita (liked but not good) Aswaduhita (disliked but good) Aswadahita (disliked and bad)	Hiranyaksha Koushika
Five	Bhouma, Udaka, Agneya, Vayavya, Akasiya	Kumarasira Bharadhwaja,

---

१. (i) रसनार्थोरसस्तस्य द्रव्यमाप: क्षितिस्तथा । (च.सू. १/६४)

(ii) रसस्तु रसनाग्रह्यो मधुरादिश्नेकधा । (कारिकावलि)

(iii) रसनेन्द्रियग्राह्यो योऽर्थ: स रस: । (शिवदास:)

(iv) रसनेन्द्रियग्राह्यवृत्ति गुणत्वावान्तर जातिमत्वं रसत्वं । (शिवदास:)

२. (i) रसास्तावत् षट् - मधुराम्ललवणकटुतिक्तकषाया: । (च. सू. १)

(ii) षडेवरसा: इत्यूवाच आत्रेय: । (च.सू. २६)

(iii) षडेवरसा: नोनाधिका: । (इन्दुकर:)

(iv) षट् सूत्रकार प्रामाण्यादास्वाद्याच्च । (र.वै. ३५)

Six	Guru (heavy), Laghu (lighter) Seeta (cold), Ushna (hot), Snigdha (unchtuous), Ruksha (non-unchtuous)	Varyovida Raja
Seven	Madhura (sweet), Amla (sour), Lavana (salt), Katu (pungent), Tikta (bitter), Kashaya (astringent), Kshara (alkaline)	Nimi (king of videha)
Eight	above 7 + Avyakta (tastelessness)	Badisa Dhamargava
Inumerable	Indefinite no. of rasas are there	(Kankayana (physician from Bahlika desa).

All the Maharshis proposed these concepts are aged and highly knowledgeable. However Purarvasu Ātreya condemned and disagreed with their concepts. He proposed that the Rasas are six only viz., Madhura, Amla, Lavana, Katu, Tikta & Kashaya[1].

Ātreya provided the following reasons for not accepting the earlier theories:

---

१. षड्रेव रसा इत्युवाच भगवानात्रेयः पुनर्वसुः मधुराम्ललवणकटुतिक्तकषायाः । तेषां षण्णां रसानां योनिएदकं, छेदनोपशमने द्वे कर्मणी, तयोर्मिश्रीभावात् साधारणत्वं, स्वाद्वस्वादुता भक्तिः, हिताहितौ प्रभावौ, पञ्चमहाभूतविकारास्त्वाश्रयाः, प्रकृतिविकृतिविचारदेशकालवशाः, तेष्वाश्रयेषु द्रव्यसंज्ञकेषु गुणा गुरुलघुशीतोष्णास्निग्धरूक्षाद्याः, क्षरणात् क्षारः नासौ रसः, द्रव्यं तदनेकरस-समुत्पन्नमनेकरसं कटुलवणभूयिष्ठमनेकेन्द्रियार्थसमन्वितं करणाभिनिर्वृत्तम्; अव्यक्तीभावस्तु खलु रसानां प्रकृतौ भवत्यनुरसेऽनुरससमन्विते वा द्रव्ये; अपरिसंख्येयत्वं पुनस्तेषामाश्रयादीनां भावानां विशेषापरिसंख्येयत्वान्न युक्तम्, एकैकोऽपि ह्येषामाश्रयादीनां भावानां विशेषानाश्रयते विशेषापरिसंख्येयत्वात्, न च तस्मादन्यत्वमुपपद्यते; परस्पर संसृष्टभूयिष्ठत्वान्न चैषामभिनि-वृत्तेर्गुणप्रकृतीनामपरिसंख्येयत्वं भवति; तस्मान्न संसृष्टानां रसानां कर्मोपदिशन्ति बुद्धिमन्तः, तच्चैव कारणयपेक्षमाणाः षण्णां रसानां परस्परेणासंसृष्टानां लक्षणपृथक्त्वमुपदेक्ष्यामः ॥ (च.सू. २६/९)

एक एव रस इत्युवाच भद्रकाप्यः, यं पञ्चानामिन्द्रियार्थनामन्यतमं जिह्वावैषयिकं भावमाचक्षतें कुशलाः, स पुनरुदकादनन्य इति । द्वौ रसाविति शाकुन्तयो ब्राह्मणः छेदनीय उपशमनीयश्चेति। त्रयो रसा इति पूर्णाक्षो मौद्गल्यः, छेदनीयोपशमनीयसाधारणा इति । चत्वारी रसा इति हिरण्याक्षः कौशिकः, स्वादुर्हितश्च स्वादुरहितश्चास्वादुर्हितश्चास्वादुरहिश्चेति । पञ्च रसा इति कुमारशिरा भरद्वाजः, भौमोदकाग्नेयवायव्यान्तरिक्षाः षड्सा इति वार्योविदो राजर्षिः, गुरुलघुशीतोष्ण-स्निग्धरूक्ताः । सप्त रसा इति निमिर्वैदेहः, मधुराम्ललवणकटुतिक्तकषायक्षाराः । अष्टौ रसा इति बडिशो धामार्गवः मधुराम्ललवणकटुनित्तकषायक्षाराव्यक्ताः । अपरिसंख्येया रसा इति काङ्क्षायनो बाह्लीकभिषक्, आश्रयगुणकर्मसंस्वटविशेषाणामपरिसंख्येयत्वात् । (च. सू. २६/८)

(1) Bhadrakapyaś view is that Rasa and Jala are one and the same, there is no difference between them. But Jala is Adhara (basis) and Rasa is Adeya (ingredient). Thence it can not be considered as Rasa. It is well known that Ādhara and Ādheya are different from each other.

(2) Sakunteyaś view is that Chedaniya or Langhana (decreasing quality) and Upasamaniya or Brimhana (increasing quality) are the Rasas. It is not acceptable since both are considered as pharmacological properties but not as Rasas.

(3) Moudgalya included Sadharana guna (neither increasing nor decreasing quality i.e., ordinary character) to the above two properties and considered three Rasas. But they can not be treated as Rasas, since they are all pharmacological properties.

(4) Hiranyaksha proposed Swaduhita, Swadahita, Aswaduhita and Aswadahita as the four Rasas. But these can not be accepted as tastes since like & dislike, good & bad are only qualities and not Rasas.

(5) Kumarasira Bharadwaja proposed that Rasas are five on the basis of Pancha bhutas. This view does not withstand scientific discussion since Panchabhutas will form different substances which inturn, will have Rasa, Virya, Vipaka etc. Rasa alone can not possess any other quality like dravya. Therefore Rasa can not be five as described by Bharadwaja.

(6) Varyovidaś view is that six main gunas among Gurvadi gunas viz., Guru, Laghu, Seeta, Ushna, Snigdha & Ruksha are the six Rasas. His view is not correct since these six are qualities but not the tastes.

(7) Nimi proposed seven Rasas viz., Madhura, Amla, Lavana, Katu, Tikta, Kashya & Kshara. Among these seven, first six are tastes while Kshara is a part and porcel of Lavana. Therefore this theory is disagreed.

(8) Badisa Dhamargava expressed his view that Avyakta Rasa along with the previous seven tastes will make the number of tastes as eight. However, this concept is also not accepted since tastelessness can not be considered as taste. The Divya Jala or Antarikshodaka (pure water from clouds) is tasteless (Avyakta Rasa). Where as dif-

ferent tastes can be denoted as primary, secondary etc. On this basis Atreya disagreed with this concept as well.

(9) Kankayana from Persian Gulf proposed that tastes are of infenite numbers since their base, properties, action etc., are innumerable. His view is also found to be incorrect, since every taste should reside in its own Asraya or Guna or Karma.

(10) After contradicting various concepts/views proposed by other Acharyas, Punarvasu Ātreya concluded the symposium by confirming that the Rasas are six only.

Vagbhataś View

Vagbhata also concluded that Rasas are six only. He elaborately explain his view with certain examples. He quotes that the constituents of Madhura skandha viz., Ghrita, Taila, Guda etc., do not possess exactly similar sweetness[1]. The degree of sweetness varies from one another and there fore Rasas are innumerbable in number. This variation is because of the concerned bhuta dominance. Moreover combined effect of the rasas of a group of drugs can not be compared individually or seperately with each ingredient. Even the Gurvadi gunas do not have any difference on the basis of deegre of quality since their species or category remains the same (i.e.), Guru guna remains guru guna though there is Tara (better), Tama (the best) differentiation. Similarly Rasa also remain six only and there are no further categories among them.

Badhanta Nagarjunaś View

Nagarjunas substantiated the concept of six Rasa with the help of Pratyaksha Pramana and Aptopadesa. He mentioned that in day to day life one can experience only six tastes. Even the earlier Acharyas

---

१. गुर्वादीनां विशेषेऽपि स्वजातेरनतिक्रमात् ॥
संख्याभेदो यथा नास्ति रसानामपि स क्रमः । दृष्टं मुखोपलेपादि यत् सर्वेषु घृतादिषु ॥
न च तद्दाडिमाद्येषु षडेवातो रसाः स्मृताः । आनन्त्यैकत्वयोश्च स्यान्न विचित्रार्थतन्त्रणम् ॥ (अ.सं.सू. १४)
मधुरस्कन्धनिर्दिष्टघृततैलगुडादिषु । गुणास्वादादिभेदेन रसषट्कं न युज्यते ॥
अस्तुभेदादसंख्यत्वमैक्यं वाऽऽस्वादलक्षणात् । भूतोत्कर्षापकर्षेणा भेदो योऽल्पेन कल्प्यते ॥
संकीर्णत्वात् फलेचासौ तुल्यत्वान्न विवक्ष्यते ॥

have accepted the same. Therefore the Rasas are six only[1].

On review of literature (Brihat Trayee) we come across six tastes in the Ayurvedic texts viz., Madhura, Amla, Lavana, Katu, Tikta, Kashaya[2].

Modern View on Teste

Taste or gustatory function is closely interlinked with smell according to modern physiology. A common chemical sensibility is observed between smell and taste, in the nose and mouth respectively. The common chemical stimulus is carried by trigeminal nerve endings. In the absence of olfaction, taste sensation will be altered e.g. during rhinitis variation in gustation is experienced by every one.

Fig. No. 1

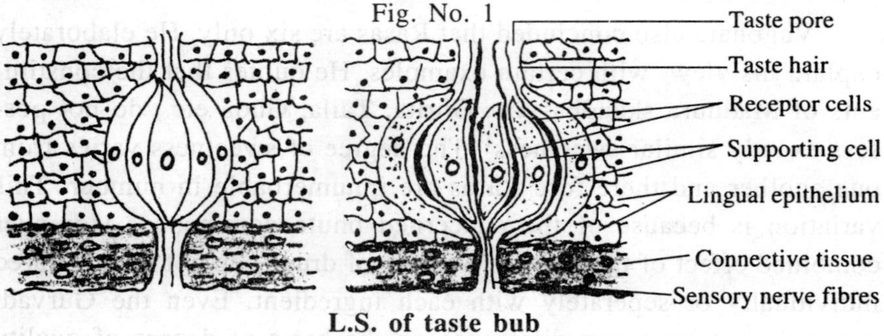

L.S. of taste bub

Fig. No. 2

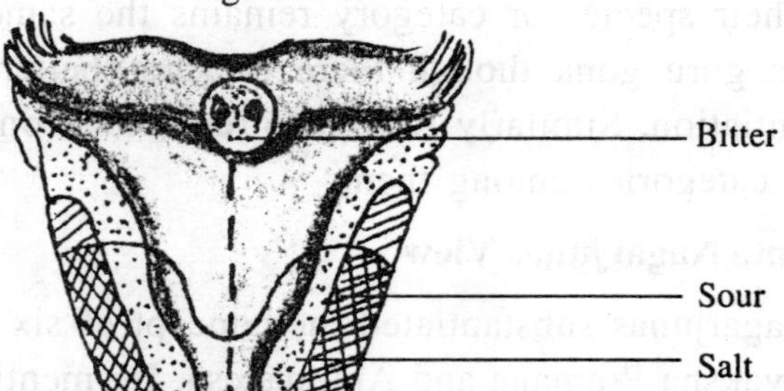

Areas of different tastes on tongue

---

१. षट्सूत्रकारप्रामाण्यादास्वादाच्च ॥ (र.वै. ३ सू. ५)

२. (i) स्वादुरम्लोऽथ लवण: कटुकस्तिक्त एव च ।
कषायश्चेति षट्कोऽयं रसानां संग्रह:स्मृत: ॥ (च.सू. १/६५)

(ii) स खल्वाप्यो रस: शेषभूतसंसर्गाद्विदग्ध: षोढाविभज्यते, तद्यथा मधुरोऽम्लो
लवण: कटुकस्तिक्त कषाय इति । (सु.सू. ४२/३)

(iii) रसा: स्वाद्वम्ललवण तिक्तोषणकषायका: ॥ षड्द्रव्यमाश्रितास्ते च यथा पूर्वं बलावहा: ।
(अ.सं.सू.।अ) (अ.हृ.सू. १/१४-१५)

Tongue is mainly concerned with taste. It bears the taste buds which are the end organs of taste. These are present in the mucosa of the epiglottis and pharynx and in the lateral walls of the fungiform and vallate papillae of the tongue. It is estimated that there are about 9000-10,000 taste buds in man. However their number decreases with age.

According to modern physiology there are four primary tastes viz., sweet, bitter, sour (acid) and salt. Others accept another two i.e. metallic and alkaline. Hence they are also six in modern medicine. But there are only four areas recognized for the perception of the tastes (vide: Figure No. 2).

The taste bud is about 70 μ in length and 50 μ in breadth. They are categorized into two group (1) gustatory or taste cells and (2) supporting or sustenticular cells. But they may be transitional in character. Taste cells are developed from the epithelial cells around the taste buds but they live for about 3-5 days. Each taste cell will have microvilli projecting into the taste pore. Each taste bud possess a number of receptor cells with their apical tips projecting through a pore on epithelial surface. The nerve fiber ending do not contain myelin sheath and they either invarigate the receptor cells or lie between them at the base of the taste bud.

Four types of nerve fibers are identified in cat with different action potentials when sweet, acid, salt and bitter substances are placed over the tongue.

It is important that the substance to be tasted must be in solution. Usually saliva acts as the solvent. Perhaps this is the reason why Acharyas of Ayurveda recognized Bodhaka sleshma for taste perception[1]. Taste according to Ayurveda has five aspects.

i. Rasanendriya dravya
ii. Rasanendriya Artha
iii. Rasanendriya Buddhi
iv. Rasanendriya Vishaya
v. Rasanendriya

१. रसबोधनात् बोधको इति संज्ञा ।

Taste receptors are considered as chemoreceptors that respond to substances dissolved in the oral fluids bathing them. There are specified areas are present for each taste on the tongue. They are:

1. Sweetness - is chiefly felt at the tip of the tongue.
2. Salt - on the dorsum anteriorly.
3. Sourness - at the sides.
4. Bitterness - at the back of the tongue.

* Mid-dorsum has no taste sensation.

From anterior two-thirds of tongue, taste sensations are carried by the facial nerve (VII crainal nerve) and from the posterior one-third by the glosso-pharyngeal nerve (IX cranial nerve).

5. Panchabhoutikata of Rasa and its evolution

Rasas have their evolution in a systematic fashion. It is believed that the water in the clouds (Antarikshodaka or Divyodaka) is devoid of any taste. As it gradually reaches the earth it will associate with other Panchabhutas in specific proportions and give rise to six tastes.

Different Acharyas proposed different configurations of bhutas in the formation of Rasas[1]. Their views are depicted in the following

१. (i) सौम्याः खल्वापोऽन्तरिक्षप्रभवाः प्रकृतिशीता लघ्व्यश्चाव्यक्तरसाश्च, तास्त्वन्तरिक्षाद् भ्रश्यमाना भ्रष्टाश्च पञ्चमहाभूतगुणसमन्विता जङ्गमस्थावराणां भूतानां मूर्तीरभिप्रीणयन्ति, तासु मूर्तिषू षडभिमूर्च्छन्ति रसाः। तेषु षण्णां रसानां सोमगुणातिरेकान्मधुरो रसः, पृथिव्यग्निभूयिष्ठत्वादम्लः, सलिलाग्निभूयिष्ठत्वाल्लवणः, वाय्वग्निभूयिष्ठत्वात् कटुकः, वाय्वाकाशातिरिक्तत्वात्तिक्तः, पवन पृथिवीव्यतिरेकात् कषाय इति। एवमेषां रसानां षट्त्वमुपपन्नं न्यूनातिरेकविशेषान्महाभूतानां, भूतानामिव स्थावरजङ्गमानां नानावर्णाकृतिविशेषाः; षड्तुकत्वाच्च कालस्योपपन्नो महाभूतानां न्यूनातिरेकविशेषः ॥ (च.सू.२६ अ.)

(ii) आकाश पवन दहन तोय भूमिषु यथासंख्यमेकोत्तरपरिवृद्धिः शब्द स्पर्शरूप रस गन्धाः, तस्मादाप्यो रसः। परस्परसंसगति, परस्परानुग्रहात् परस्परानुप्रवेशाच्च सर्वेषु सर्वेषां सान्निध्यमस्ति,उत्कर्षापकर्षात्तु ग्रहणम् । स खल्वाप्यो रसः शेषभूतसंसर्गादिदग्धः षोढा विभज्यते, तद्यथा-मधुरः, अम्लः, लवणः, कटुकः, तिक्तः कषाय इति । ते च भूयः परस्परंसंगात्रिषष्टिधा भिद्यते । तत्र, भूम्यबुगुणबाहुल्यान्मधुरः, तोयाग्निगुणबाहुल्यादम्लः, भूम्यग्निगुणबाहुल्याल्लवुणः, वाय्वग्निगुणबाहुल्यात् कटुकः, वाय्वाकाशगुणबाहुल्यात्तिक्तः, पृथिव्यनिलगुणबाहुल्यात् कषाय इति। (सु. सू.४२)

(iii) रसः खल्वाप्यः प्रागव्यक्तश्च । स षड्तुकत्वात् कालस्य महाभूतगुणैर्नातिरिक्तैः संसृष्टो विषमं विदग्धः षोढा पृथग्विपरिणमते मधुरादिभेदेन । तत्र भूजलयोर्बाहुल्यान्मधुरो रसः, भू-तेजसोरम्लः, जल-तेजसोर्लवणः, वाय्वाकाशयोस्तिक्तः, वायु-तेजसोः कटुकः, वायूर्व्योः कषायः । (अ.सं.सू.१८)

(iv) क्ष्माम्भोग्निक्ष्माम्बुतेजः खवाय्वग्न्यनिलगोनिलैः । द्वयोल्वर्णैः क्रमाद्भुतैर्मधुरादिरसोद्भवः ॥ (अ.हृ.सू. १०/१)

(v) तत्र पृथिव्यापां वाहुल्यान्मधुरं विद्यात् अम्लमपामग्नेश्च; लवणमग्नेरपां च, कटुकमग्नेर्वायोश्च, तिक्तं खस्य वायोश्च, कषायमग्नेर्वायोश्च । (र.वै.अ.३.सू. ३८-४३)

table:

S.N.	Rasa	Charaka	Suśruta	Vagbhata	Nagarjuna
1.	Madhura	Ap+Prithvi	Prithvi+Ap	Prithvi+Ap	Prithvi+Ap
2.	Amla	Prthvi+Agni	Ap+Agni	Prithvi+Agni	Ap+Agni
3.	Lavana	Ap+Agni	Prithvi+ Agni	Ap+Agni	Agni+Ap
4.	Katu	Vayu+Agni	Vayu+ Agni	Vayu+Agni	Agni+ Vayu
5.	Tikta	Vayu+Akasa	Vayu+ Akasa	Vayu+ Akasa	Akasa+ Vayu
6.	Kashaya	Vayu+ Prithvi	Prithvi+ Vayu	Vayu+ Prithvi	Agni+ Vayu

Commentators concluded that specific bhuta configurations can only form the six Rasas[1]. They consider nature (Swabhava) as the reason for this limited number and specific combinations.

Acharyas have differed in the combination of Amla, Lavana and Kashaya Rasas. Sushrita opine that Jala-Agni and Prthvi-Agni will result in Amla and Lavana Rasas. However others consider that it is vice versa. Badhanta Nagarjuna mentioned Agni+Vayu for Kashaya Rasa while others described it as Prithvi+Vayu.

The configuration of these Rasas (Bhoutika Nishpatti) may be assessed by inference[2]. For example, Kapha Vriddhi and Pitta Kshaya by Madhura rasa will indicate that Madhura rasa is composed of Prithvi and Jala bhutas. Scientific background of chemical configuration of different tastes is explained below:

As mentioned earlier the Panchabhutas will represent the elements and compounds. Acording to modern chemistry, the tastes are resultant from certain chemicals. For example, Madhura rasa in carbohydrates, Lavana Rasa in salts, Amla rasa in acids etc. If carefully evaluated the ancient concept will be matching with the present scientific views.

---

१. रसनार्थो रसस्तस्य द्रव्यमापः क्षितिस्तथा । निवृत्तौ च विशेषेण प्रत्ययाः खादयस्त्रयः ॥ (च.सू. १/६४)

२. ते निर्धार्यन्तेऽनुमानात् । (र.वै.)

1. Madhura Rasa– Sugar- $C_6H_{12}O_6$. $24H_2O$ (Prithvi + Jala) (in this combination Carbon is Prithvi and H_2O is Jala)
2. Amla Rasa– CH_3COOH (Agni + Jala)
3. Lavana Rasa– Salt- NaCl (Agni + Prithvi)

(luminiscent element sodium is Agni and chlorine with pungent smell is Prithvi. They together form salt. The above formula indicates anhydrous salt. If it is hydrated salt then NaCl + H_2O (Agni +Jala). Hence both the views of Charak and Suśruta regarding Lavana Rasa are correct).

4. Katu Rasa– NH + CH (Agni + Vayu)
5. Tikta Rasa– S (Akasa + Vayu)

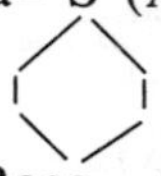

6. Kashaya Rasa - OH + COOH = astringent (Vayu + Prithvi)

Carbohydrates such as sucrose, glycogen and starch are sweet in taste. Sugars are soluble in water, crystalline compounds and are also sweet in taste. Tannins are soluble in water and have astringent taste. Volatile oils may have pungent taste e.g. Black mustard, bark of Cinnamomum etc. Alkaloids are generally bitter in taste. Glycosides possessing bitter taste are called bitter glycosides.

Structure function interrelation of molecules and the taste

(i) Salty tastes– are given by (a) inorganic and (b) ionizable substances. NaCl is the classical example. Of the ions , the cation (e.g. Na^+) is the chief determinant of the salty taste.

(ii) Sour taste– is produced by acids i.e., which are ionizable and on being ionized they liberate H^+ ion, which give rise to the sour taste.

(iii) Sweet taste– is produced by a large number of compounds, most of which are organic substances. Notable examples are various sugars (glucose, fructose, sucrose etc.) alcohols (ethyl alcohol glycol, glycerol etc) and some complex molecules like Saccharin. Some inorganic substances (e.g. lead acetate) are also known to have sweet taste.

(iv) Most of the bitters are organic compounds and many of them are alkoloids e.g. quinine, morphine, strychnine etc.

Some inorganic compounds of Mg and Ca also are bitter. An example of organic but non-alkaloid bitter is bile-salt.

(v) Metallic taste– is found with certain drugs e.g. Metronidazole causes metallic taste.

(vi) Alkaline taste– is related to the substances which are highly alkaline in nature.

Assesement of Bhoutik composition of Rasas

As mentioned earlier, the Bhoutik composition of Rasas is assessed through inference only. Basing upon the pharmacological actions of a particular Rasa its composition may be predicted. For example

(1) Ushnatwa and Abhishyandatwa of Lavana Rasa will provide us a clue that it contains Agni and Jala bhutas[1].

(2) Urdhwa bhaga hara property of Vamana dravyas will give an inference about Agni, Vayu and Akasa bhutas and Adho bhaga hara property of Virechana dravyas indicate towards Prithvi & Jala bhutas[2]. (However, the author is of the openion that this assessment is not helping to find out the Rasa of drug. Hence is not a suitable example. But it is found that many scholars observe it as an example for assesement of bhoutik composition on the basis of Rasa).

(3) Through Madhura rasa Kapha aggravation is seen which is the result of Jala bhuta. Similarly it subsides Pitta which is Agneya inature. This aspect gives us an inference that Madhura Rasa is made up of Prithvi and Jala.

---

१. स च सन्निवेश: कार्यदर्शनेनोन्नेय: तेन तत्र कार्यं दृश्यते तत्र कल्प्यते यथा- लवणो उष्णात्वा-
दग्निर्विष्यन्दित्वाच्च जलमनुमनुमीयते । (चक्रपाणि- च. सू. २६)

२. तत्राग्नि मारुतात्मका: रसा: प्रायेणोर्ध्वभाज:,
लाघवादुत्प्लवनाच्च वायोरूर्धज्वलनाच्चवह्ने:,
सलिलपृथिव्यात्मकास्तु प्रायेणाधोभाज: पृथिव्या
गुरुत्वान्निगम्नगत्वच्चोदकस्य, व्यामिश्रात्मका:
पुनरुभयता भाज: । (च. सू. २६)

The geometro-chemical aspects of tastes and their potency are proposed by Rajesh Behari Mathur (1962). They are tabulated below:

Group	taste	other effects on the system
C I N	Bitter	Hot, Coloration
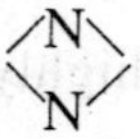 N N	Bitter	Hot
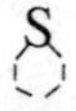 S	Bitter	Cold, Coloration
COOH COOH	Sour	Cold
CHS-COOH	Sour	Hot
N-CH or NH-CH	Pungent	Hot
OH-CH	Sweet	Cold
OH-COOH	Astringent	Cold
NH-OH or NH_2-COOH	Alkaline	
NH_2-COOH	Saltish	
N-CH_3	Bitter, Acrid	Poisonous
CO-NCH_3	Sweet, Acrid	Poisonous
NH-CH_3	Bitter, Acrid and Pungent	Hot, Constriction
- COOH	Acid (Amla)	Contraction & attraction
- OH	Alkaline	Cold, attraction & fixation
CO-OHC or CO-NH	Sweet & alkaline	Cold, astriction i.e., contracting and binding
or Co O	Sweet & a bit acidic	

-CO-	Sweet, bitter	cold and absorptive
	Neo-taste	cold & dry
-CHO	Sweet, Alkaline	cold, reaction & adhesion
$-CH_3O$	Sweet	cold, permeable
$-CH_2O$	Sweet	cold, diuretic
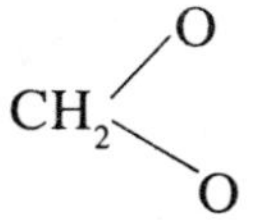	Bitter, Sweet	cold, laxative
$- CH_2Cl$	Bitter, pungent & saltish	Appetiser
$-CH (NH_2) COOH$	Saltish, acidic	Digestive, assimilative and heat producer.

All the configurative Rasas mentioned from essential constitution of the important organic compounds are characterized as:

a. Growth promoting and retarding factors which control growth of the tissues.

b. Dietary factors which give strength to the body.

c. Digestive and combustive factors which digest the food to convert it into energy.

d. Sensorial factors which develop senses and carry sensations to the mind.

e. Anti-disease factors which check diseases. Their actions on the body are due to the energies they hold in their bonds which are released when the bonds are ruptured.

Thus Rasas are 'vital forces' of the body on which the organs depend for their existance, reaction to stimulus and their internal and external actions. Increase and decrease of particular Rasas can even create genetic mutation in the body there by changing its character.

Diagramatic representation of evolution of rasas:

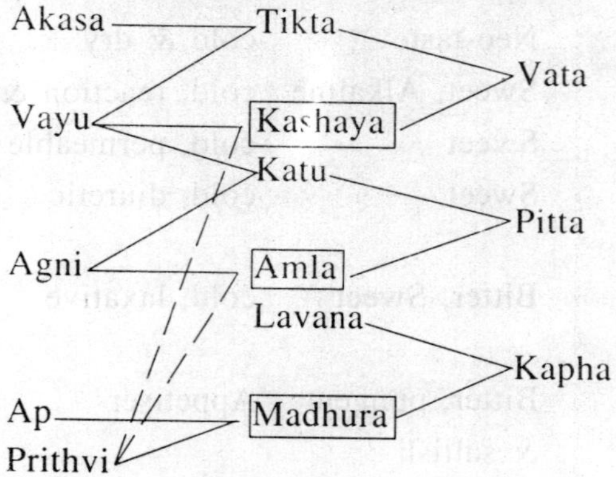

Diagramatic represention or rasas and their bhuta composition:

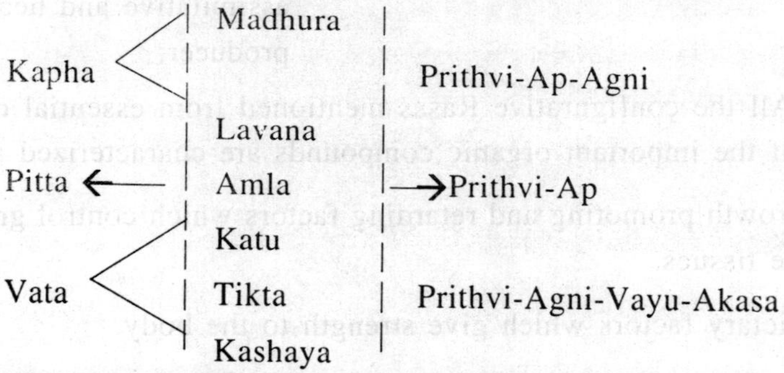

6. Difference between Rasa and Anu Rasa

Every drug will have a primary taste followed by a secodary taste i.e., Pradhana Rasa and Anu Rasa respectively[1].

Charaka quoted that the taste which is immediately expressed when the drug is in dry state, is known as Pradhana Rasa. The taste which is perceived after some time and in the wet state of a dravya is known as Anu Rasa. Vagbhata also expressed the same view[2].

१. (i) व्यक्तः शुष्कस्य चादौ च रसो द्रव्यस्य लक्ष्यते ।
विपर्ययेणानुरसो, रसो नास्तीह सप्तमः ॥ (च. सू.)
(ii) तत्र व्यक्तो रसः स्मृतः; अव्यक्तोऽनुरसः किञ्चिदन्ते व्यक्तोपि चेष्यते । (अ.हृ.सू. १/३-४)
(iii) तत्र व्यक्तो रसः । अनुरसस्तु रसेनाभिभूयत्वादव्यक्तो व्यक्तो वा किञ्चिदन्ते । (अ.सं.सू. १७)
(iv) तत्र व्यक्तो रसः । यस्तु रसनाभिभूतत्वान्न व्यज्यते वा किञ्चिदन्ते सोऽनुरसः । (योगेन्द्रनाथः)
२. (i) तस्मान्नैकरसं द्रव्यं भूतसंघातसंभवात् । (अ.हृ.सू. १)
(ii) सर्वं द्रव्यं पञ्चमहाभूतसमवायसंभवं, तस्मादनेकरसम् । (योगेन्द्रनाथः)

The concept of primary and secondary tastes is found with many drugs in Ayurveda. For example, Aswagandha will have Madhura and Tikta Rasas. Twak will have Madhura and Katu rasas. Basing upon Rasa-Anurasa concept we find several drugs mentioned under more than one Skandha among the six Rasa Skandhas.

RASA	ANURASA
1. Found in the dry state 2. Expressed in the begining 3. Experienced immediately 4. Predominant taste	1. Found in the wet state 2. Expressed in the end 3. Experienced lately 4. Secondary taste

7. Effects of seasons, determination of bhoutik evolution of Rasa

There are six Rutus (six seasons) and accordingly six Rasas also[1]. There is some relavence between these two numbers and their genesis. Indukara high-lighted the relation between seasons, pancha-bhuta composition of rasas and evaluation of Rasas[2].

Formation of Rasas according to season

S.N.	Season	Mahabhuta composition	Produced Rasa
1.	Sisira Ritu	Vayu + Akasa	Tikta
2.	Vasanta Ritu	Vayu + Prithivi	Kashaya
3.	Grishma Rita	Vayu + Agni	Katu
4.	Varsha Ritu	Prithivi + Agni	Amla
5.	Sarat Ritu	Ap + Agni	Lavana
6.	Hemanta Ritu	Prithivi + Jala	Madhura

१. (i) षड्ृतुकत्वाच्च कालस्थोपपन्नो महाभूतानां न्यूनातिरेकविशेषः । (च.सू. २६)
(ii) स षड्ृतुकत्वात् कालस्य महाभूतगुणैरूनातिरिक्तैः संसृष्टो विषम विदग्धः .....विपरिणमते ।
(अ.सं.सू.१८)

२. कथं महाभूतानां ऊनाधिक्यं? उच्यते-कालस्य संवत्सराख्यस्य षड्ऋतुकत्वाद्रसस्यापि षड्भेदत्वम्। तथा च शिशिरे वाय्वाकाशयोराधिक्याद्रसस्य तिक्तता, वसन्ते वायुपृथिव्योः कषायता, ग्रीष्मेऽग्नि वाय्वोः कटुता, वर्षास्वग्नि पृथिव्योरम्लता, शरद्यम्न्युदकयो लवणता, हेमन्ते पृथिव्यृन्दयोर्मधुरतेति प्राधान्यात् व्यपदेशः, तेनान्यत्रऋतुउद्भवानामपि रसानां यथोक्त महाभूतद्वयाधिक्यमेव कारणं विज्ञेयम्।
(इन्दुकरः- अ.सं. सू. १८)

Indukara further classified that certain rasas will form in other seasons also but the formation of rasas in the specified seasons will be the best.

Chakrapani quoted that little var ation in Mahabhutas and seasons is always expected. Therefore some variations may occur in the formation of rasas also. Therefore the above mentioned seasonal effect is explained on the basis of general behaviour.

In this context it is very important to identify the difference between utility of rasas during various seasons and formation of rasas during various seasons. For example, Lavana Rasa forms during Sarat Ritu; but its utility is best during Varsha ritu to tackle aggravated Vata.

8. Causes of sense of taste: *(Rasopalabdhi)*

When a substance is brought into touch with the Rasanendriya or tongue, then the taste will be known[1]. In otherwords taste will be known from the moment of exposure of a substance to organ of taste.

Badhanta Nagarjuna explained that taste can be perceived by means of three methods: They are:

(i) Pratyaksha - through direct means.

(ii) Anumana - through inference.

(iii) Aptopadesa - by the elders sayings[2].

Certain tastes are perceived directly e.g. sweetness of sugar, sourness of mango etc.

Some of the tastes are assessed through inference as the taste is not possible by direct means e.g. sweetness of urine in diabetes after observing ants surrounding the urine of diabetic patient.

Other times, the taste may be assessed on the basis of elders sayings e.g. when ever there is a controversy in concluding the primary and secondary tastes, the Saints/Acharyas words are considered[3].

१. रसो निपाते द्रव्याणाम् । (च.सू. २६)

२. प्रत्यक्षतोऽनुमानादुपदेशतश्च रसानामुपलब्धि: । (र.वै. ३ सू. १०८)

३. आस्वाद्य प्रत्यक्षत उपलभ्यते, अनुमानात् पूर्वोक्त लिङ्गं दृष्ट्वा मधुरोऽयमित्युपलभ्यते । उपदेशात् आगमात् कषायं मधु, मधुरमुदकम् इत्यादि । अथवा आस्वादतो रसानां सामान्यत उपलब्धिर्भवति, अनुमानाल्लिङ्गपूर्वकाद् विशेषोपलब्धिर्भवति, उपदेशत: कर्मणि रसानां प्रवृत्तिरूपलभ्यते । अथवा सर्वमास्वादत एव रसो न गृह्यते, आगमतश्च क्वचित्, क्वचिदनुमानाच्चेति ।(भाष्यं-र.वै.३ सू.१०८)

For the proper reception of this special sense, the Indriya Pancha Panchakas of Rasanendriya mentioned earlier are very essential.

Dr. S.C. Dhyani had evaluated a "Dilution method" for the identification of Rasas. By this method the "taste threshold" of a given Rasa shall be determined.

Method of testing– 5 gm of the powderd drug is mixed with 10 ml of distilled water and stirred till they mix thoroughly. Then it is filtered with the help of a filter paper. Afterwards one drop of the filtered solution is applied over the tongue and distilled water will be added drop by drop till the taste on the tongue disappears. This particular point of disappearance of taste will indicate the 'taste threshold' of the given drug.

To differentiate Pradhana Rasa and Anurasa, the drugs for which taste is to be established are given along with another equally potent drug. there fore Rasa and Anurasa can not be differentiated directly. Then the Rasas present in the mixture are identified with the help of above method seperately. In the end it may be concluded that the Rasa with higher theshold is "Pradhana Rasa" and the one with lower threshold is "Anu Rasa".

Rasas are of several types on the basis of Tara and Tama bheda. To estimate the three grades of taste viz., mild moderate and maximum, the threshold of each Rasa is divided into three equal categories e.g. Madhura, Madhura Tara, Madhura Tama etc.

The observations of Dr. Sivcharan Dhyaniji are as following:

Taste threshold	Degree of taste	Taste threshold	Degree of teste
0-1400 ml	Madhura	0-1133 ml	Katu
1401-2800 ml	Madhura tara	1135-2266 ml	Katu tara
2801-4200 ml	Madhura tama	2267-3400 ml	Katu tama
0-420 ml	Amla	0-3933 ml	Tikta
421-840 ml	Amla tara	3934-7866 ml	Tikta tara
841-1260 ml	Amla tama	7867-11800 ml	Tikta tama
0-260 ml	Lavana	0-1000 ml	Kashaya
261-520 ml	Lavana tara	1001-2000 ml	Kashaya tara
521-780 ml	Lavana tama	2001-3000 ml	Kashaya tama

Dhyaniji is of the openion that the evaluation of Rasas of known and unknown dravyas shall be done with this method. This is felt so because, out of 553 drugs listed out from various Nighantus, the Rasas for only 40 drugs are alike and for 513 drugs different authors mentioned different Rasas. Therefore the validity of Rasas delineated in the ancient texts become questionable. Some method like the above is essential to confirm the Rasa of Ayurvedic herbs etc.

When any food (Ahara) or drug (Oushadha) material is brought into contact with the tongue or taste buds (Jihwa or Rasanendriya) then Rasa jnana (taste sensation) will occur. The orally administered drug will mix with Bodhaka sleshma (Saliva) and Prapaka (first chemical change) will occur. By this certain electromagnetic stimuli are generated and they inturn stimulate the gustatory centers. Depending on their frequency and wavelength, different tastes will be perceived. The concept of Soumya and Agneya Rasas may be well explained on the basis of this principle.

Limitations in determining the rasas by using the orgonoleptic methods: (Sharma P.V. & Bandhopadhyay N.G., 1970).

1. Observation is purely subjective and liable to vary from individual to individual.
2. Perception may vary due to any abnormality or disease in the organ.
3. As solubility of the substance is an essential factor for perception of taste, Rasa of an insoluble drug may not be known.
4. Some substances may not put on the tongue due to ethical or psychological reasons such as urine, faeces etc.
5. Poisonous substances, if put on tongue may prove fatal and as such an unknown drug may not be advised to be put on tongue.

Hence some objective methods should be evolved to know the Rasa of an unknown drug or to re-establish the tastes of classical Ayu. drugs.

The following observation were made by sharma P.V. & Bandyopadhyay (1970) in their study:

S. N.	Madhura Dravyas	Protein	Carbohy-drate
1.	Atibala	+	+
2.	Bala	+	+
3.	Masha	+	+
4.	Yashti Madhu	+	+
5.	Shatavari	+	+
6.	Masha parni	+	+
7.	Mridvika Acidic	+	+
8.	Kharjura	+	+
9.	Kapikachchu	+	+
10.	Gokshura	—	+

S.N.	Amla Dravyas	Reaction
1.	Jambira	Acidic
2.	Dadima	Acidic
3.	Chincha	Acidic
4.	Amalaki	Acidic
5.	Badara	Acidic
6.	Changori	Acidic
7.	Bhumyam-alaki	
8.	Āmra	Acidic
9.	Amlavetasa	Acidic
10.	Amrataka	Acidic

Lavana Dravyas	Na^+	Cl_3^-
Samudra Lavana	+	+
Saindhava Lavana	+	+
Krishna Lavana	+	+

S. N.	Katu Dravyas	Alkaloid	Glyco-side	Essn-oil	Phenol	Coura-min	Sterol
1.	Tulasi	—	+	+	—	—	—
2.	Chitraka	—	+	+	—	—	—
3.	Pippali	+	+	+	—	—	—
4.	Maricha	+	+	—	—	—	—
5.	Ārdraka	+	—	+	—	—	—
6.	Jiraka	+	—	+	+	—	—
7.	Yavani	+	—	+	+	—	—
8.	Sarṣhapa	+	—	+	—	—	—

S. N.	Tikta Dravyas	Alkaloid	Glyco-side	Essn-oil	Phenol	Coura-min	Sterol
1.	Guduchi	+	—	+	—	—	—
2.	Nimba	+	—	—	—	—	—
3.	Katuki	+	—	—	—	—	—

4.	Kirata tikta	+	—	—	—	—	—
5.	Parijata	+	+	—	—	—	—
6.	Karanja	+	—	—	—	—	—
7.	Kutaja	+	—	—	+	—	—
8.	Sapta parna	+	—	+	+	—	—
9.	Vāsa	+	—	+	—	—	—
10.	Kālamegha	+	—	—	—	—	—

S.N.	**Kashaya Dravyas**	**Tannins**
1.	Arjuna	+
2.	Ashoka	+
3.	Dhataki	+
4.	Mayaphala	+
5.	Mocha Rasa	—
6.	Haritaki	+
7.	Khadira	+
8.	Lodhra	+
9.	Udumbara	+
10.	Jambu phala	+

There is little difference between Katu and Tikta dravyas. According to Pancha bhoutik configuration, Vayu is common to both but in addition there is Agni in Katu Rasa and Ākasa in tikta rasa. Owing to this negligible demarcation these two may be confused together in practice.

9. Transformation of Rasas

The Rasa of a dravya may undergo different changes. Badhanta Nagarjuna explained them in the following manner:

(1) Sthana: ***(Storge)***

If a substance is kept at once place for some time, its taste will change. e.g. coocked rice which is Madhura in taste will become Amla (sour) if it is stored for few days.

Similarly, if a substance is kept in a vessel for some time, its taste will change. e.g. curd kept in bronze vessel will become pungent in taste[1].

(2) Samyoga: ***(Mixing)***

If one substance is mixed with another one, the taste will change. e.g. tamarind mixed with lime water becomes sweet[2].

(3) Agni: ***(Coocking)***

Coocking a substance with fire wood on fire will chagne its taste e.g. on coocking tamarind turn to be sweet[3].

(4) Atapa: ***(Sun-light)***

On exposure to sun light the taste will change e.g. the Sourness of Amalaki reduces on drying in sun-light[4].

(5) Bhavana: ***(Soaking)***

If one substance is soaked in another material its taste may change. e.g. by soaking bitter drugs with lime juice the taste will be made as sour[5].

(6) Desa: ***(Place)***

Particular area may bring about some change in the taste of a substance e.g. Bananas will be very sweet in some areas and sour in other areas. Similarly Mangos in certain areas are very sweet compared of the other areas[6].

(7) Kala: ***(Time)***

Time will bring about certain changes in the original taste of a substance e.g. Mango will be astringent when it is tender and becomes very sour later. Finally it will become sweet in taste[7].

---

१. अन्यथात्वगमनं स्थानात् । (र.वै. ३/२०)

२. संयोगत: .... । (र.वै. ३/३०)

३. ....अग्ने: पाकात् । (र.वै. ३/३०)

४. आतपात् । (र.वै. ३/३१)

५. भावनथा । (र.वै. ३/३२)

६. देशकालाभ्याम् । (र.वै. ३/३२)

७. परणिामत: । (र.वै. ३/३३)

(8) Parinama: ***(Change in form)***

Certain changes in the form of a substance will change the taste also e.g. Milk will be sweet to begin with but later turns to be sour when the same becomes curd[1].

(9) Upasarga: ***(Infected)***

When a substance is infected by pests or bugs it will give rise to a new taste. e.g. Suger cane which is infected by pests will yield bitter or sour juice[2].

(10) Vikriya: ***(Peculiar tricks)***

Certain peculiar tricks will also change the original taste of a substance e.g. when palm fruit is coocked and rubbed against floor, it becomes bitter[3].

The above mentioned are some of the factors which are responsible for transformation of one rasa into another rasa. These procedures will be helpful in pharmacy while preparing drugs. They will be more useful to cover the tastes like bitter, pungent and astringent.

10. General Classification of Rasas

Depending upon the general behaviour of Ushna (hot) and Seeta (cold) characters or depending upon their effect on doshas or depending up on their effect on digestive process the Rasas are classified into three main categories. They are:

I. Soumya and Āgneya Rasas[4].

१. उपसर्गत: । (र.वै. ३/३४)

२. विक्रियत: । (र.वै. ३/३५)

३. अग्निषोमियाज्जगतो रसा द्विविधा: - सौम्या आग्नेयाश्च ।
मधुरतिक्तकषाया: सौम्या:, कट्वम्ललवणा आग्नेया: । (सु.सू.४२/७)
*डल्हण:- सौम्याश्चाग्नेयाश्चेति चकारद्वयात् स्नेहरूक्षगुरुत्वलघुत्वैरपि द्वैविध्यं सूचयति ।

४. (i) स्वादुरम्लाऽथ लवण: कटुकस्तिक्त एव च । कषायश्चेति षट्कोऽयं रसानां संग्रह: स्मृत: ॥
स्वाद्वम्ललवणं वायुं, कषायस्वादु तिक्तका:।
जयन्ति पित्तं, श्लेष्माणं कषायकटु तिक्तका: ॥ (च.सू. १/६५-६६)
(कट्वम्ललवणं पित्तं, स्वाद्वम्ललवणा: कफम् । कटुतिक्तकषायाश्च कोपयन्ति समीरणम् ॥)
पाठान्तर:

(ii) तत्र मधुराम्ललवणा वातघ्ना:, मधुरतिक्तकषाया: पित्तघ्ना:,
कटुतिक्तकषाया: श्लेष्मघ्ना: । (सु.सू. ४२/४)

क्रमश: पृष्ठ १११ में..........

II. Dosha Prakopaka and Dosha Sāmaka Rasas[1].

III. Vidahi and Avidahi Rasas.

(I) Soumya Āgneya Rasas

Soumya	**Agneya**
(1) Madhura Rasa	(1) Katu Rasa
(2) Tikta Rasa	(2) Amla Rasa
(3) Kashaya Rasa	(3) Lavana Rasa

(II) Dosha Prakopaka & Samaka Rasa

Prakopaka	**Samaka**
(1) Vata - Katu, Tikta, Kashaya	(1) Vata - Madhura, Amla, Lavana
(2) Pitta- Katu, Amla, Lavana	(2) Pitta - Kashaya, Tikta, Madhura
(3) Kapha - Madhura, Amla, Lavana	(3) Kapha - Katu, Tikta, Kashaya

(III) Vidāhi - Avidāhi Rasas

Vidahi	**Avidahi**
(1) Katurasa	(1) Madhura rasa
(2) Amla rasa	(2) Tikta rasa
(3) Lavana rasa	(3) Kashaya rasa

11. Characteristics, Functions & Properties of Six Rasas:-

Characteristics of Sadrasas and their Etymology

(1) **Madhura Rasa:** The character which tempts an individual to consume the entire material is known as Madhura bhava. It indicates

---

पृष्ठ ११० से क्रमशः.............

(iii) तत्र वायोरात्मैवात्मा, पित्तमाग्नेयं श्लेष्मासौम्यमिति । (सु.सू. ४२/५)

(iv) त एते रसाः स्वयोनिवर्धनाअन्ययोनिप्रशमनाश्च ॥ (सु.सू.४२/६)

तत्राद्या मारुतं घ्नन्ति त्रयस्तिक्तादयः कफम् ।
कषायतिक्तमधुरा पित्तमन्ये तु कुर्वते ॥ (अ.हृ.सू.१/१४-१६) और (अ.सं.सू. १अ.)

(v) रसाः स्वाद्वम्ललवणतिक्तोषणकषायकाः। षड्द्रव्यमाश्रितास्ते तु यथापूर्वं बलावहाः ॥

१. (i) मधु = यावत् पिबाम्यहम् । (वाचस्पत्यम्)

(ii) मधु = मन्यन्ते विशेषेण जानन्ति जना यस्मिन् । (श.क.द्रु.)

(iii) मधु माधुर्य्यं राति इति मधुरः । (अ.को.)

that people ae attracted towards it owing to the sweet nature[1].

(2) **Amla Rasa:** Author's teacher Manikya Sharma (Prof. Govt. Ayu. College, Hyderabad) used to define it as the taste which is responsible for the causation of several diseases[2].

(3) **Lavana Rasa:** The character which is responsible for scraping away the doshas or the character which causes dryness to the tongue[3].

(4) **Katu Rasa:** The character which spreads all over the tongue due to its severity or the character which produces secretions from eyes, mouth, nose etc[4].

(5) **Tikta Rasa:** The character which spreads all over the tongue with in no time[5].

(6) **Kashaya Rasa:** The character which causes discomfort to the throat or which adversely affects the taste reception[6].

The Local Action of Rasas

Etymology of each rasa is indicating towards local effects only. More over Rasa action occurs immediately after exposure to Rasanendriya. Afterwards the action of vipaka and virya begins. There fore the systemic effects mentioned for Rasas are meant for Samana Pratyayarabdha dravyas on the basis of theory of probability. e.g. Milk with Madhura rasa will under go Madhura Vipaka hence its final effect can be assessed by means of Rasa only. But Āmalaki with

---

१. (i) अम्ल:= अम+क्ल । रस भेदे । (श.क.द्रु.)
(ii) अमयते सर्वान् रोगानुत्पाद्यते इत्यम्ल: । (स्व.)

२. 'लू' छेदने । लव-लेशे, विनाशे, छेदने च। लुनाति जिह्वामिति लवण: ।(श.क.द्र. और वाचस्यत्यम्)

३. कटति तीक्ष्णतया रसनां मुखं वा आवृणोति यद्वा कटति वर्षयति चक्षुर्मुखनासादिभ्यो जलं स्रावयतीति । कट वर्षावरणयो: । (श.क.द्रु.)

४. तिक्तं = तेजयतीति तिक्तं । तिज+बाहुलकात् क्त: । (वाचस्पत्यम्)

५. कषति कण्ठम् इति। कष् + आय: । कष वधे हिंसायाम्
कष्यते विस्वाद्यते इति कषाय: । (श.क.द्रु. और वाचस्पत्यम्)

६. (i) तेषां विद्याद्रसं स्वादु यो वक्रमनुलिम्पति । आस्वाद्यमानो देहस्य ह्लादनीऽक्षप्रसादन: ॥
प्रिय: पिपीलिकादीनाम् .... । (अ.हृ.सू. १०/२-३)
(ii) तत्र य: परितोषमुत्पादयति प्रह्लादयति तर्पयति जीवयति मुखोपलेपं जनयति श्लेष्माणं चाभिवर्धयति स मधुर: । (सु.सू. ४२/९)
(iii) तेषां स्वादुरास्वाद्यमानो मुखमुपलिम्पतीन्द्रियाणि प्रसादयति, देहं प्रह्लादयति, षट्पदपिपीलिकादीनामपीष्टतम: । (अ.सं.सू. १८)

Āmla rasa will under go Madhura Vipaka and its final effect (Rasayan) can not be assessed by means of Rasa.

(1) Madhura Rasa

It will coat entire oral cavity with its sweet taste, a feeling of generalized well beingness, pleasure and strength to body organs will be seen. It is more attracted by ants flys etc[1].

(2) Amla Rasa

It washes or clears the oral cavity, it results in pilocrection, tingling sensation of teeth, blinking of eyes due to its sour taste[2].

(3) Lavana Rasa

It spreads all over the oral cavity and causes dryness due to osmosis (Syandana). It also results in burning sensation in the buccal cavity and throat[3].

(4) Katu Rasa

It stimulates the tip of the tongue, causes burning sensation over the tongue and oral cavity, results in watering from eyes, mouth, and nose. It also produces burning in the buccal cavit[4].

---

१. (i) ....अम्लं क्षालयते मुखम् ।
हर्षणो रोमदन्तानायक्षिभ्रुवनिकोचनः ॥ (अ.हृ.सू. १०/३)
(ii) यो दन्तहर्षमुत्पादयति मुखस्रावं जनयति श्रद्धां चोत्पादयति सोऽम्लः । (सु.सू.४२/९)
(iii) अम्लस्तु जिह्वामुद्वेजयत्थुरः कण्ठं विदहति, मुखं स्रावयति, अक्षिभ्रुवं संकोचयति, दशनान् हर्षयति, रोमाणि च । (अ.सं.सू. १८)

२. (i) लवणः स्यन्दयत्यास्यं कपोलगलदाहकृत् । (अ.हृ.सू. १०/४)
(ii) यो भक्तरुचिमुत्पादयति, कफप्रसेकं जनयति मार्दवं चापादयति स लवणः । (सु.सू. ४२/९)
(iii) लवणो मुखं विष्यन्दयति, कण्ठकपोलं विदहति, अन्नं प्ररोचयति । (अ.सं.सू. १८)
(iv) लवणं विष्यन्दयति । (च.सू. २७/४)

३. (i) उद्वेजयति जिह्वाग्रं कुर्वंश्चिमिचिमां कटुः ।
स्रावयत्यक्षिनासास्यं कपोलौ दहतीव च ॥ (अ.हृ.सू. १०/५)
(ii) यो जिह्वाग्रं बाधते उद्वेगं जनयति शिरो गृह्णीते नासिकां च स्रावयति च कटुकः ।(सु.सू.४२/९)
(iii) कटुको भृशमुद्वेजयति जिह्वाग्रं चिमचिमायति कण्ठकपोलं स्रावयति मुखाक्षिनासिकं विदहति देहम् । (अ.सं.सू. १८)

४. (i) तिक्तो विशदयत्यास्यं रसनं प्रतिहन्ति च ॥ (अ.हृ.सू. १०/४)
(ii) यो गले चोषमुत्पादयति मुखवैशद्यं जनयति भक्तरूचिं चापादयति हर्षं च स तिक्तः ।(सु.सू.४२/९)
(iii) तिक्तो विशदयति वदनं, विशोधयति कण्ठं, प्रतिहन्ति रसनाम् । (अ.सं.सू. १८)

(5) Tikta Rasa

It catches the entire oral cavity and disallow other taste reception. It reduces the desire to eat, causes burning in the throat[1].

(6) Kashaya Rasa

It produces a feeling of stiffness of tongue, dry & stiffness in the throat and other channels (Srotas) of the body. It results in catching pain in the heart[2].

Generalized Effects of Rasas

(1) Madhura Rasa[3]

Effect on doshas: Vata-Pitta Samaka; Kapha Vardhaka.

Actions: Dhatu vardhana, Ojo vardhana, Āyushya, Indriya prasadana, Balya, Varnya, Vishahara, Trishna Prasamana, Daha Prasamana, Kesya, Kantya, Jeevaniya, Brimhaniya, Sandhana kara, Stanya Janana etc.

Indication: Vata Rogas, Murcha, Asthi bhagna, Kshata kshina, Rakta-pitta,

---

१. (i) कषायं जडयेज्जिह्वां कण्ठस्रोतोविबन्धकृत् । (अ.हृ.सू. १०/६)
(ii) यो वक्त्रं परिशोषयति जिह्वां स्तम्भयति कण्ठं बध्नाति हृदयं कर्षति पीडयति च स कषाय इति । (सु.सू.४२/९)
(iii) कषायस्तु जडयति जिह्वां, बध्नाति कण्ठं पीडयति हृदयम् । (अ.सं.सू. १८)

२. (i) तत्र मधुरोरसः शरीरसात्म्याद्रसरूधिरमांसमेदोस्थिमज्जौजः शुक्राभिवर्धन आयुष्यः षडिन्द्रियप्रसादनो बलवर्णकरः पित्तविषमारूतघ्नस्तृष्णादाहप्रशमनस्त्वच्यः केश्यः कण्ठयो बल्यः प्रीणनो जीवनस्तर्पणो बृंहणः स्थैर्यकरः क्षीणक्षतसन्धानकरो घ्राणमुखकण्ठौष्ठ जिह्वाप्रह्लादनो दाहमूर्च्छाप्रशमनः षट्पदपिपीलि-कानिमिष्टतमः स्निग्धः शीतो गुरुश्च । (च.सू. २६/४३-१)
(ii) तत्र, मधुरो रसो रसरक्तमांसमेदोऽस्थिमज्जौजः शुक्रस्तन्यवर्धन चक्षुष्यः केश्यो वर्ण्यो बलकृत्सन्धानः शोणितरसप्रसादनो बालवृद्धक्षतक्षीणहितः षट्पदपिपीलिकानामिष्टतमस्तृष्णा-मूर्च्छादाहप्रशमनः षडिन्द्रियप्रसादनः कृमिकफकरश्चेति । (सु.सू. ४२/१०-१)
(iii) .... मधुरोरसः ॥
आजन्मसात्म्यात्कुरूते धातूनां प्रबलं बलम् । प्रशस्तो बृंहणं कण्ठ्यः स्तन्यसन्धानकृद्गुरुः । आयुष्यो जीवनः स्निग्धः पित्तानिलविषापहः ॥ (अ.हृ.सू. १०/६-९)
बालवृद्धक्षतक्षीणवर्णकेशेन्द्रियौजसाम् ।
(iv) तत्र मधुरो रसो जन्मप्रभृति सात्म्यात्सर्वधातुविवर्धन आयुष्यो बालवृद्धक्षतक्षीणबलवर्णेन्द्रियत्वक्केशकण्ठहितः प्रीणनो बृंहणो जीवनस्तर्पणः स्थैर्यसन्धानस्तन्यकरो वातपित्तविषदाहमूर्च्छातृष्णाप्रशमनः स्निग्धः शीतो मृदुर्गुरुश्च । (अ.सं.सू. १८)

(2) Amla Rasa[1]

Effect on doshas: Pitta-Kapha Vardhaka; Vatanulomana.

Actions: Deepana-Pachana, Brimhana, Hridya, Prinana, Koshta Vidahi, Vyavayi.

Indications: Hridroga, Agnimandya, Vāta rogas etc.

(3) Lavana Rasa[2]

Effect on doshas: Vata Samaka; Pitta-Kapha Vardhaka.

Actions: Pachana, Kledana, Deepana, Chedana, Bhedana, Vikasi, Sroto Sodhaka, Sareera mardavakara, Samsodhana, Dhatu Saithilyakara, Ruchya.

Indications: Vata rogas, Agni mandya, Sula, Madhumeha, Swasa etc.

(4) Katu Rasa[3]

Effect on doshas: Kapha Samaka; Vata-pitta Vardhaka.

---

१. (i) अम्लो रसो भक्तं रोचयति, अग्निंदीपयति, देहं बृंहयति ऊर्जयति, मनो बोधयति, वातमनुलोमयति, हृदयं तर्पयति, आस्यमास्रावयति, भुक्तमपकर्षयति क्लेदयति जरयति, प्रीणयति, लघुरुष्णः स्निग्धश्च । (च.सू. २६/४३-२)

(ii) अम्लो जरणः पाचनो दीपनः पवनग्रहणोऽनुलोमनः कोष्ठविदाही बहिःशीतः क्लेदनः प्रायशो हृद्यश्चेति । (सु.सू. ४२/१-२)

(iii) अम्लोऽग्निदीप्तिकृत्स्निग्धो हृद्यः पाचनरोचनः । उष्णवीर्यो हिमस्पर्शः प्रीणनः क्लेदनो लघुः।। करोति कफपित्तास्रं मूढवातानुलोमनः । (अ.हृसू.१०/१०-१२)

(iv) अम्लोऽनिलनिबर्हणोऽनुलोमनः कोष्ठविदाही रक्तपित्तकृदुष्णवीर्यः शीतस्पर्शो बोधयतीन्द्रियाणि रोचनः पाचनो दीपनो बृंहणस्तर्पणः प्रीणनः क्लेदनो व्यवायी लघुः स्निग्धो हृद्यश्च।(अ.सं.सू.१८)

२. (i) लवणो रसः पाचनः क्लेदनो दीपनश्च्यावनश्छेदनो भेदनस्तीक्ष्णः सरो विकास्यधः स्रंस्यवकाशकरो वातहरः स्तम्भबन्धसङ्घातविधमनः सर्वरसप्रत्यनीकभूतः, आस्यामास्रावयति, कफं विष्यन्दयति, मार्गान् विशोधयति, सर्वशरीरावयवान् मृदूकरोति, रोचयत्याहारम् , आहारयोगी, नात्यर्थं गुरुः स्निग्धोष्णश्च । (च.सू. २६/४३-३)

(ii) लवणः संशोधनः पाचनो विश्लेषणः क्लेदनः शैथिल्यकृदुष्णः सर्वरसप्रत्यनीको मार्गविशोधनः सर्वशरीरावयवमार्दवकरश्चेति ।। (सु.सू. ४२/१०-३)

(iii) लवणः स्तम्भसंघात बन्धविध्मापनोऽग्निकृत् ।। स्नेहनः स्वेदनस्तीक्ष्णो रोचनश्छेदभेदकृत् । (अ.हृ.सू. १०/१२-१३)

(iv) लवणः स्तम्भबन्धसंघातविध्मापनः सर्वरसप्रत्यनीको दीपनो रोचनः पाचनः क्लेदनः शोषणः स्नेहनः स्वेदनो भेदनः छेदनः सरो व्यवायी विकासी हरतिपवनं विष्यन्दयति कफं विशोधयति स्रोतांसि नातिगुरुः स्निग्धतीक्ष्णोष्णश्च । (अ.सं.सू. १८)

३. (i) कटुको रसो वक्रं शोधयति, अग्निं दीपयति, भुक्तं शोषयति, घ्राणमास्रावयति, चक्षुर्विरेचयति, स्फुटीकरोतीन्द्रियाणि, अलसकश्वयथूपचयोदर्दाभिष्यन्दस्नेहस्वेदक्लेदमलानुपहन्ति, रोचयत्यशनं,

क्रमशः पृष्ठ ११६ में.............

Action: Mukha Sodhana, Agni deepana, Indriya dourbalya, Kandu hara, Vrana ropona, Krimi hara, Mamsa lakhana, Sroto Vivarana etc.

Indications: Kandu, Vrana, Grahani, Agnimandya, Kapha Vikaras etc.

(5) Tikta Rasa[1]

Effect on doshas: Pitta-Kapha Samaka, Vata Vardhaka.

Actions: Visha hara, Krimihara, Daha prasamana, Kandu hara, Trishna prasamana, Kushtaghna, Lekhana, Stanya Sodhana, dhatu Soshana.

Indications: Amla pitta, Āma vata, Kushta, Krimi Roga, Medo roga etc.

पृष्ठ ११५ से क्रमश:.............

कण्डूर्विनाशयति, व्रणानवसादयति, क्रिमीन् हिनस्ति, मांस विलिखति, शोणितसंघातं भिनन्ति, बन्धांश्छिनन्तिः, मार्गन् विवृणोति, श्लेष्माणं शमयति, लघुरुष्णो रूक्षश्च । (च.सू. २६/४३-४)

(ii) औष्यतैक्ष्ण्यरोक्ष्यलाघववैशद्यगुणलक्षणं पित्तं, तस्य समानयोनि: कटुको रस:, सोऽस्य औष्ण्या-दौष्ण्यं वर्धयति, तैक्ष्ण्यात्तैक्ष्ण्यं, रौक्ष्याद्रौक्ष्यं, लाघवाल्लाघवं वैशद्याद्वैशद्यमिति।(सु.सू. ४२/८-२)

(iii) कटुको दीपन: पाचनो रोचन: शोधन: स्थौल्यालस्यकफकृमिविषकुष्ठकण्डूप्रशमन: सन्धिबन्धविच्छेदनोऽवसादन: स्तन्यशुक्रमेदसामुपहन्ता चेति । (सु.सू. ४२/१०-४)

(iv) कटुर्गलामयोदर्दकुष्ठालसकशोफजित् । व्रणावसादन: स्नेहमेद:क्लेदोपशोषण: ॥
दीपन: पाचनो रूच्य: शोधनोऽत्रस्य शोषण: ।
छनन्ति बन्धान् स्तोतांसि विवृणोति कफापह: ॥ (अ.हृ.सू. १०/१७-१८)

(v) कटुकोऽलसकश्वयथूदर्दस्थौल्याभिष्यन्दकृमिवक्ररोगविषकुष्ठकण्डूप्रशमनो व्रणावसादन: स्नेह-क्लेदशोषणो रोचन: पाचनो दीपनो लेखन: शोधन: शोषयत्यन्नं स्फुटयतीन्द्रियाणि भिनन्ति शोणि-तसंघातं छिनन्ति बन्धान् विवृणोति स्रोतांसि क्षपयति श्लेष्माणं लघुरूक्षतीक्ष्णोष्णश्च।(अ.सं.सू. १८)

१. (i) तिक्तो रस: स्वयमरोचिष्णुरप्यरोचकघ्नो विषघ्न: क्रिमिघ्नो मूर्च्छादाहकण्डू कुष्ठतृष्णाप्रशमन-स्त्वङ्मांसयो: स्थिरीकरणो ज्वरघ्नो दीपन: पाचन: स्तन्यशोधनो लेखन: क्लेदमेदोवसामज्जाल-सीकापूय-स्वेदमूत्रपरीषपित्तश्लेष्मोपशोषणोरूक्ष: शीतोलघुश्च । (च.सू. २६/४३-५)

(ii) तिक्तइछेदनो रोचनो दीपन: शोधन: कण्डूकोठतृष्णामूर्च्छाज्वरप्रशमन: स्तन्यशोधनो विण्मूत्र-क्लेदमेदोवसापूयोपशोषश्चेति । (सु.सू. ४२/१०-५)

(iii) तिक्त: स्वयमरोचिष्णुररूचिं कृमितृड्विषम् ॥ कष्ठमूर्च्छाज्वरोत्क्लेशदाहपित्तकफान् जयेत् ।
क्लेदमेदोवसामज्जशकृन्मूत्रोपशोषण: ॥
लघुर्मेध्यो हिमो रूक्ष: स्तन्यकण्ठविशोधन: । (अ.हृ.सू.१०/१४-१६)

(iv) तिक्त: स्वयमरोचिष्णुररूचिविषकृमिमूर्च्छोत्क्लेदज्वरदाहतृट्कुष्ठकण्डूहर: क्लेदमेदोवसामज्ज-विण्मूत्रपित्त-श्लेष्मणोपशोषणो दीपन: पाचनो लेखन: स्तन्यकण्ठशोधनो मेध्यो नातिरूक्ष: शीतो लघुश्च। (अ.सं.सू. १८)

(6) Kashaya Rasa[1]

Effect on doshas: Pitta-Kapha hara; Vata vardhaka.

Actions: Samsamana, Sangrahi, Sandhana kara, Ropana, Soshana, Sthambhana, Rakta prasamana, Lekhana, Twachya, Āma sandharana, Vishtambhi, Jwarahara, Chedana etc.

Indications: Atisara, Grahani, Twak vikara, Medoroga etc.

12. Arrangement of gunas (qualities) of Rasas as per the Degree of Activity

Broadly all the constituents of dravya including Rasa are considered as gunas only. However the Rasas will also possess some individual qualities. Though these qualities are there in the form of the characters of the given dravya, when specifically described they are considered as Rasa gunas. The following tables denote the qualities of respective Rasas and their degree of activity viz., mild, medium and best.

Table showing qualities of Rasa[2]**:**

Rasa (Taste)	**Guna (Properties)**
Madhura	Snigdha, Seeta, Guru.
Amla	Snigdha, Ushna, Laghu.
Lavana	Snigdha, Ushna, Guru.
Katu	Ruksha, Ushna, Laghu.
Tikta	Ruksha, Seeta, Laghu.
Kashaya	Ruksha, Seeta, Guru.

१. (i) कषायो रसः संशमानः, संग्राही, सन्धानकरः, पीडनो, रोपणः, शोषणः, स्तम्भनः, श्लेष्मरक्तपित्त-प्रशमनः, शरीरक्लेदस्योपयोक्ता रूक्षः शीतोऽलघुश्च । (च.सू. २६/४३-६)

(ii) तत्र शैत्यरौक्ष्यलाघववैशद्यवैष्टम्भ्यमुणलक्षणो वायुः, तस्य समानयोनिः कषायो रसः, सोऽस्य शैत्याच्छैत्यं वर्धयति, रौक्ष्याद्रौक्ष्यं, लाघवाल्लाघवं, वैशद्याद्वैशद्यं, वैष्टम्भाद्वैष्टम्भ्यमिति । (सु.सू. ४२/८-१)

(iii) कषायः संग्राहको रोपणः स्तम्भनः शोधनो लेखनः शोषणः पीडनः क्लेदोपशोषणश्चेति । (सु.सू. ४२/१०-६)

(iv) कषायः पित्तकफहा गुरुरस्रविशोधनः । पीडनो रोपणः शीतः क्लेदमेदोविशोषणः ॥
आमसंस्तम्भनो ग्राही रूक्षोऽति त्वक्सादनः । (अ.हृ.सू. १०/२०-२१)

(v) काषायो बलासं सपित्तं सरक्तं निहन्त्याशु बध्नाति वर्चोऽतिरूक्षः । गुरुस्त्वक्सवर्णत्वकृत्क्लेदशोषी हिमः प्रीणनो रोपाणो लेखनश्च ॥ (अ.सं.सू. १८)

क्रमशः पृष्ठ११८ में........

Table showing degree of activity of Rasa qualities[1]:

S.N.	Guna (quality)	Uttama (best)	Madhyama (moderate)	Avara (mild)
1.	RUKSHA	Kashaya	Katu	Tikta
2.	SNIGDHA	Madhura	Amla	Lavana
3.	USHNA	Lavana	Amla	Katu
4.	SEETA	Kashaya	Madhura	Tikta
5.	GURU	Madhura	Kashaya	Lavana
6.	LAGHU	Tikta	Katu	Amla

* Katu-Tikta-Kashaya Rasas may act as Baddha Vinmutra because of their Rukshatwa.

** Lavana-Amla-Madhura Rasas may increase urination and faces quanity because of Guru and Seeta gunas.

The individual qualities of each rasa therefore result in particular pharmacological property.

13. Combination and Permutations of Rasas:-

The basic six tastes will have several combinations and permutations and are 63 types[2]. They are:

पृष्ठ ११७ से क्रमशः.........

२.(i) तत्र मधुराम्ललवणाः स्निग्धा गुरवश्च; कटुतिक्तकषाया रूक्षा लघवश्च; सौम्याः शीताः, आग्नेया उष्णाः॥ (सु.सू. ४२/७)

(ii) माधुर्यस्नेहगौरवशैत्यपिच्छिलगुणलक्षणः श्लेष्मा; तस्य समानयोनिर्मधुरो रसः, सोऽस्य माधुर्यान्माधुर्यं वर्धयति, स्नेहात् स्नेहं, गौरवाद्गौरवं, शैत्याच्छैत्यं, पैच्छिल्यात् पैच्छिल्यमिति ॥(सु. सू. ४२/८)

(iii) तस्य पुनर्योनिः कटुको रसः, स श्लेष्मणः प्रत्यनीकत्वात् कटुकत्वान्माधुर्यमभिवर्धयति,रौक्ष्यात् स्नेहं, लाघवाद्गौरवम् औष्ण्याच्छैत्यं वैशद्यात् पैच्छिल्यमिति ।तदेतन्निदर्शनमात्रमुक्तं भवति । (सु.सू.४२/८)

(iv) जग्धाः षडधिगच्छन्ति बलिनो वश्यतां रसाः । यथा प्रकुपिता दोषा वशं यान्ति बलीयसः॥ (सु.सू. ४२/१३)

१. रसाः कट्वम्ललवणा वीर्योष्ण यथोन्तरम् ॥ तिक्तः कषायो मधुरस्तद्वदेव च शीतलाः ।
तिक्तः कटुः कषायश्च रूक्षा बद्धमलस्तथा । पट्वम्लमधुराः स्निग्धाः सृष्टविण्मूत्रमारूताः ।
पयेः कषायस्तस्माच्च मधुरः परमं गुरुः ॥
लघुरम्लः कटुस्तस्मादपि च तिक्तकः । (अ.हृ. सू. १०/३६-३९)

२.(i) भेदश्चैषां त्रिषष्ठिविकल्पो द्रव्यदेशकालप्रभावात् । (च.सू. २६)

(ii) त्रिषष्ठिस्यात्वसंख्येया रसानुरस कल्पनात् । (च. सू. २६)

(iii)तत्रैतेषां रसानां संयोगास्त्रिषष्टिर्भवन्ति । तद्यथा-पञ्चदशद्विकाः विंशतिस्त्रिकाः, पञ्चदश चतुष्काः, षट् पञ्चकाः, एकशः षड्साः, एक षट्क इति ॥ (सु.सू. ४२/१२)

(iv)संयोगः सप्तपञ्चाशत्कल्पना तु त्रिषष्ठिधा ॥
रसानां योगिकत्वेन यथास्थूलं विभज्यते । (अ.हृ.सू. १०/३९-४०)

Eka Rasa (one taste)	-	6
Dwi Rasa (two tastes)	-	15
Tri Rasa (three tastes)	-	20
Chatushka (four tastes)	-	15
Pancha Rasa (five tastes)	-	6
Sad Rasa (six tastes)	-	1
Total:		63

Examples for each combination:

Eka Rasa

1. Madhura	-	Sarkara
2. Amla	-	Jambira
3. Lavana	-	Samudra Lavana
4. Katu	-	Maricha
5. Tikta	-	Katuki
6. Kashaya	-	Amrasthi Lodhra

Dwi Rasa:

7. Madhur-amla	-	Badara
8. Madhura Lavana	-	Ushtra Kshura
9. Madhura Katu	-	Sunaka Mamsa
10. Madhura Tikta	-	Sarja Rasa
11. Madhura Kashaya	-	Tila Taila
12. Amla Lavana	-	Kshara Mrittika
13. Amla Katu	-	Chukra
14. Amla Tikta	-	Sura
15. Amla Kash-aya	-	Suka mamsa
16. Lavana Katu	-	Sarja Kshara
17. Lavana tikta	-	Naga (lead)
18. Lavana Kashaya	-	Samudra Phena
19. Katu Tikta	-	Pushkara mula
20. Katu Kasha aya	-	Katphala
21. Tikta Kashaya	-	

Tri Rasa:

22. Madhuramala Lavana	-	Hastima-msa
23. Madhuramla Katu	-	Salya mams
24. Madhuramla Tikta	-	Godhuma
25. Madhuramla Kashaya	-	Takra
26. Madhurala-vana Katu	-	Kapota Mamsa
27. Madhura lavana Tikta	-	
28. Madhura Kashaya	-	Guda+ Kamala kanda
29. Madhura, Katuka Kashaya	-	Honey
30. Madhura, Katu Tikta	-	Eranda taila
31. Madhura, Tikta Kashaya	-	Guduchi
32. Amla, Lavana Katu	-	Silajatu
33. Amla, Lavana Tikta	-	Hasti mutra

34. Amla, Lavana - Kashaya
35. Amla, Katu - Tikta
36. Amla, Katu, Kashaya - Amlavetase
37. Amla, Tikta - Kashaya
38. Lavana, Katu - Tikta
39. Lavana, Katu - Kashaya
40. Lavana, Tikta - Kashaya - Samudraphena
41. Katu, Tikta - Kashaya - Aguru

Chatushka:

42. Madhura, Amla - Lavana, Katu - Gomutra Silajatu
43. Madhura, Amla - Lavana, Tikta - Gomutra
44. Madhura, Amla - Lavana, Kashaya - Sandhava yukta Takram
45. Madhura, Amla - Katu, Tikta - Lasuna yukta Sura
46. Madhura, Amla - Katu, Kashaya
47. Madhura, Amla Tikta, Kashaya
48. Madhura, Lavana Tikta, Katu - Vārtaka
49. Madhura, Lavana Katu, Kashaya
50. Madhura, Katu - Tikta, Kashaya - Guggulu, Tila
51. Madhura, Lavana - Tikta, Kashaya
52. Amla, Lavana Katu, Tikta
53. Amla, Lavana, Katu Kashaya
54. Amla, Lavana Tikta, Kashaya
55. Amla, Katu Tikta, Kashaya
56. Lavana, Katu - Tikta, Kashaya - Bāla Mulaka

Pancha Rasa:

57. Madhura, Amla, Lavana Katu, Tikta
58. Madhura, Amla, Lavana Tikta, Kashaya
59. Madhura, Amla Lavana Katu, Kashya
60. Madhura, Amla - Katu, Tikta, Kashya - Haritaki
61. Madhura, Lavana - Katu, Tikta, Kashaya - Rasona
62. Amla, Lavana - Katu, Tikta, Kashaya - Bhallataka

Shadrasa:

63. Madhura, Amla - Lavana, Katu Tikta, Kashaya - Ena Mamsa

14. Exceptions in the general laws of Rasa activity

Charaka mentioned about certian drugs with Rasa viruddha virya i.e. which exhibit some peculiarity compared to other general rasas.

They are[1]:

Madura, Kashaya, Tikta Rasas - Brihat Pancha mula - Ushna virya

Madhura, Kashaya, Tikta Rasas - Ānupa Mamsa - Ushna virya

Lavana Rasa	-	Saindhav lavan	-	Seeta virya
Amla Rasa	-	Āmalaki	-	Seeta virya
Tikta Rasa	-	Arka, Agaru & Guduchi	-	Ushna virya

While commenting on this Chakra pani gave few more examples[2]:

1. Madhura Rasa	-	Tanduliyaka	-	Avrishya
2. Kashaya, Katu, Tikta & Madhura Rasa	-	Tila	-	Pitta-kapha Vardhaka
3. Katu, Tikta Rasa	-	Vārtaka	-	Vāta hara

There exceptions are considered as Vikriti Vishama samaveta or Vichitra pratyayarabdhata.

15. Knowledge of samana, kopana of doshas and dushyas by the Rasa

The effect of Rasas on doshas is already mentioned under Rasa classification. The effect of Rasas on doshas and dushyas is tabulated below:

S.N.	Rasa	Effect on Prakopaka	Tri-doshas Samaka	Effect on Dhatus
1.	Madhura	Kapha Vardhaka	Vata-Pitta Samaka	Dhatu vriddhi

---

१. मधुरं किञ्चिदुष्णं स्यात् कषायं तिक्तमेव च । अर्कागुरुगुडूचीनां तिक्तानापुष्णमुच्यते ॥
तस्माद्रसोपर्देशेन न सर्वं द्रव्यमादिशेत् । दृष्टं तुल्यरसेऽप्येवं द्रव्ये द्रव्ये गुणान्तरम् ॥
यथा महत्पञ्चमूलं यथाऽब्जानूपमामिषम् ॥ लवणं सैन्धवं नोष्णमम्लमालकं तथा । (च.सू. २६)

२. तत्र रसस्य विकृतिसमवायो यथा- मधुरे तण्डुलीयके मधुरो हि प्रकृत्यास्नेहवृष्यात्वादिकरः, तण्डुलीयके तु विकृतिविषमसमवेतत्वेनतन्नकरोति विषमसमवेतास्तु तिले कषायकटुतिक्तमधुराः; यदि हिमे रसाः समया मात्रया समवेताः स्युस्ततस्तिलोऽपि पित्तश्लेष्महरस्त्रिदोषहरो वा स्यात् पित्तकफकरस्त्वयं तेनात्ररसानां क्वचित् कर्त्तुत्वमकर्त्तुत्वं च क्वचिदिति वैषम्यमुन्नीयते । नानात्मकानामित्यादि हेतुत्रयं तु विकृतिसमवायविषमसमवायोरेवोपलश्यकं । यत्र वार्ताकं कटुतिक्तत्वेन वातकरत्वं प्राप्तमपि च विकृतिविषमसमवायात्तन्न भवति, तत्राचार्येण वार्ताकं वतघ्नं इत्युक्तमेव । (चक्रपाणि-च.वि. १अ.)

2.	Amla	Kaph-pitta Vriddhi	Vata Samak	Hridya (Rasa dhatu)
3.	Lavana	Kapha-Pitta Vriddhi	Vata Samaka	Sukra Kshaya
4.	Katu	Pitta-Vata Prakopa	Kapha Samaka	Dhatu Kshaya
5.	Tikta	Vata Prakopa	Kapha-Pitta Samaka	Dhatu Kshaya
6.	Kashya	Vata prakopa	Kapha-pitta Samak	Dhatu Kshaya

It is claimed that Madhura Rasa (sweet) will nourish all the tissues because glucose is stored in the muscles as glycogen and circulating all over the body as glucose in the blood. The cerebral cortex contain maximum quantity of glucose and its depletion results in death during hypoglycaemic attacks.

Similarly Amla Rasa (Sourness) is claimed to be Hridya (good for heart). It is known that vit-c is helpful in preventing atherosclerotic changes and thus help the heart and cvs.

The other effects of the rasas are described in the respective contexts.

16. The order in usage of Rasas in Oushadha & Āhara:-

Rasa usage as oushadha ***(Medicine)***

Kashyapa mentioned about the utilization of Rasas in various disease states. For example:

(1) In Kapha disorders- Katu, tikta & kashaya Rasas shall be used gradually in the same order. By using Katu rasa in the beging both Pichchila and Gurutwa qualities of Kapha will be subsided. It is followed by administration of Tikta rasa which reduces sweetness of mouth caused by Kapha and therefore helps in reduction of Kapha. Finally Kashaya rasa is given to remove the Sneha (oily mature) of Kapha. In this manner three rasas chronologically will help in subsiding Kapha diseases.

(2) In pitta disorders– Tikta, Madhura & Kashaya Rasas shall be used gradually in the same order. By using Tikta rasa in the begining

Āma pachana is possible. Afterwards Madhura rasa will subside the Pitta by its Guru, Snigdha and Seeta Gunas. In the end Kashaya rasa is administered to exhaust the liquidity of pitta by means of Ruksha guna.

(3) In Vata disorders– Lavana, Amla & Madhura rasas shall be used chronologically. By using Lavana rasa in the begining Vibandhitwa, Seetalatwa and Laghutwa of Vata are subsided through Kleda, Ushna and Guru gunas respectively. There after amla rasa is used to cause Sroto vikāra (Vasodilatation) and brings about Anuloma gati to vata by means ofGuru, Pichchila and Snigdha gunas.

Rasa usage as Āhara *(food)*

Suśruta advocated three phases for using the rasas in diet. Food must be started with Madhura rasa followed by Amla and Lavana Rasas[1].

Prathama Avastha (first phase)	-	Madhura Rasa
Madhyama Avastha (middle phase)	-	Amla & Lavana rasas
Antima Avastha (last phase)	-	Tikta, Katu & Kashaya rasas

However, Bhavamishra is in favour of administering Madhura rasa in the end. He is of the openion the Madhura rasa will tackle the ill effects of Lavana, Amla, Katurasas, Ushna & Vidahi aspects of food items. Hence shall be taken at the end of principal meal[2].

Bhavamishra also quoted that salt and ginzer must be taken before meals to increase appetite and to clear the oropharynx[3].

Above paras prove that both drug and diet are used on the basis of rasas. This knowledge is very essential since treatment according to Ayurveda do possess Āhara, Vihāra and Oushadha.

17. Diseases borne due to excessive usage of certain Rasas:–

(1) Madhura Rasa

Sthoulya (obesity), Mardava (laxity), Ālasya (lazyness), Govrava (heaviness), Aruchi (tastelessness), Agni Mandya (loss of appetite),

---

१. पूर्वं मधुरमश्नीयान्मध्येऽम्ल लवणौ रसो । पश्चाच्छेषान् रसान् वैद्यो भोजनेष्ववचारयेत् ॥ (सु.सू. ४६)

२. लवणाम्ल कटूष्णानि विदाहीन्यत्ति यानि तु । तद्दोषं हर्त्तुमाहारं मधुरेण समापयेत् ॥ (भा.प्र.)

३. भोजनाग्रे सदा पथ्यं लवणार्द्रकभक्षणम् । अग्निसंदीपनं रूच्यं जिह्वा कण्ठ विशोधनम् ॥ (भा. प्र.)

Ati Swapna (more sleeping), Asya & Kanta Mamsa Vriddhi (excessive formation of muscle tissue of buccal region and throat), Swasa (breathlessness), Kasa (cough), Pratisyaya (common cold), Alasaka, Seeta jwara, Ānaha, Āsya Madhurya, Chardi (vomiting), Sanjna Nasa (loss of conciousness), Swara bhanga, Gala ganda & Ganda mala (lymphedino pathy), Sleepada (elephantiasis), Sopha (swelling), Vasti roga, Dhamani lepa, Netra rogas etc; Kapha vikaras will occur[1].

(2) Amla Rasa

Danta harsha (tingling sensation of teeth), Trishna (thirst), Roma harsha (epilation), Pitta vriddhi, Rakta vikaras, Mamsa vidaha, Sarira saithilya (weakness), Sotha in weak persons, Hridaya daha, Kanta daha (burning in the throat), burning all over the body etc., Pitta vikaras will occur[2].

१.(i) स एवंगुणोऽप्येक एकार्थमुपयुज्यमानः स्थौल्यं मार्दवमालस्याभिवृद्धिं श्वासकासप्रतिश्यायालसकशीतज्वरानाहास्यमाधुर्यवमथुसंज्ञास्वरप्रणाशगलगण्डगण्डमालाश्लीपदगलशोफबस्तिधमनीगलोपलेपाक्ष्यामयाभिष्यन्दानित्येवं प्रभृतीन् कफजान् विकारानुपजनयति । (च.सू. २६/४३-१)

(ii) स एवं गुणोऽप्येक एवात्यर्थमासेव्यमानः कासश्वासालसकवमथुवदनमाधुर्यस्वरोपघातकृमिगलगण्डानापादयति तथाऽर्बुदश्लीपदबस्तिगुदोपलेपाभिष्यन्दप्रभृतीञ्जनयति । (सु.सू. ४२/१०-१)

(iii) कुरुतेऽन्युपयोगेन स मेदः श्लेष्माजान् गदान् ।
स्थौल्याग्निसादसन्न्यासप्रमेहगण्डार्बुदादिकान् ॥ (अ.हृ.सू. १०/६-९)

(iv) एवं गुणोऽपि स सदाऽत्युपयुज्यमानः स्थौल्याग्निसादगुरुताऽलसकातिनिद्राः । श्वासप्रमेहगलरोगविसंज्ञता ऽऽस्यमाधुर्यलोचनगदार्बुदगण्डमालाः ॥ छर्दुदर्दमूर्द्धरूक्कासपीनस क्रिमीन् ।
श्लीपदजलोदरष्ठी-वनानि चावहेत् ॥ (अ.सं.सू. १८)

२.(i) स एवं गुणोऽप्येकं एवात्यर्थमुपयुज्यमानो दन्तान् हर्षयति, तर्षयति, संमीलयत्यक्षीणी, संवेजयति लोमानि, कफं विलापयति, पित्तमभिवर्धयति, रक्तं दूषयति, मांसं विदहति, कायं शिथिलीकरोति, क्षीणक्षतकृशदुर्बलानां श्वयथुमापादयति, अपि च क्षताभिहतदुष्टदग्धभग्नशूनप्रच्युतावमूत्रितसर्पितमर्दितच्छिन्नभिन्नविश्लिष्टोद्विद्धोत्पिष्टादीनि पाचयत्याग्नेय-स्वभावात्, परिदहति कण्ठमुखे हृदयं च । (च.सू. २६/४३-२)

(ii) स एवं गुणोऽप्येक एवात्यर्थमुपसेव्यमानो दन्तहर्षनयनसंमीलनरोमसवेजन कफविलयन शरीरशैथिल्यान्यापादयति, तथा क्षताभिहतदग्धदष्टभग्नरूग्णशूनप्रच्युतावमूत्रितविसर्पतच्छिन्नभिन्नविद्धोत्पिष्टादीनि पाचयन्याग्नेयस्वभावात् परिदहति कण्ठमुगोहृदयं चेति ॥ (सु.सू. ४२/१-२)

(iii) सोऽत्यभ्यस्तस्तनोः कुर्याच्छैथिलयं तिमिरं भ्रमम् ॥
कण्डुपाण्डुत्ववीसर्पशोफविस्फोटतृट्ज्वरान् । (अ.हृ.सू. १०/११-१२)

(iv) जनयति शिथिलत्वं सेवितः सोऽति देहे कफविलयनकण्डूपाण्डुतारूग्विघातान् ।
क्षतविहितविसर्पं रक्तपित्तं पिपासां श्वयथुमपि कृशानां तैजसत्वाद्भ्रमं च ॥ (अ.सं.सू. १८)

(3) Lavana Rasa

Pitta Vriddhi, Rakta Vikara, Trishna; Murcha (syncope), Santapa (raise in temperature), Mamsa kotha (necrosis), Kushta (skin diseases), Sotha (oedema), Danta chalana (loose teeth), Napumsakatwa (male infertility/impotency), Vali (wrinkling of skin), Palita (grey hair), Khalitya (baldness), Raktapitta (haemorrhage), Amlapitta (hyperacidity), Visarpa (herpes), Vata Rakta (Gout), Vicharchika (eczema) etc., will occur[1].

(4) Katu Rasa

Napumsakatwa, Murcha, Glani, Krisatwa (weight loss), Bhrama (giddiness), Daha (burning), Trishna, Kampa, Sarvanga sula, Vata rogas etc. will occur[2].

१.(i) स एवंगुणोऽप्येकं एवात्यर्थमुपयुज्यमानः पित्तं कोपयति, रक्तं वर्धयति, तर्षयति, मूर्च्छयति, तापयति, दारयति, कुल्णाति मांसानि, प्रगालयति कुष्ठानि, विषं वर्धयति, शोफान् स्फोटयति, दन्तांश्च्यावयति, पुंस्त्वमुपहन्ति,इन्द्रियाण्युपरुणद्धि, वलीपलितखालित्यमापादयति, अपि च लोहितपित्तमाम्लपित्त वीसर्पवातरक्तविचर्चिकेन्द्रलुप्तप्रभृतीन्विकारानुपजनयति ।(च.सू. २६/४३-३)

(ii) स एवं गुणोऽप्येक एवात्यर्थमासेवमानो गात्रकण्डूकण्ठशोफवैवर्ण्यपुंस्त्वोपघातेन्द्रियोपताप-मुखाक्षिपाक रक्तपित्तवातशोणिताम्लीकाप्रभृतीनापादयति ॥ (सु.सू. ४२/१०-३)

(iii) सोऽतियुक्तोऽस्रपवनं खलतिं पलितं वलिम् ॥
तृट्कुष्ठविषवीसर्पान् जनयेत्क्षपयेद्बलम् । (अ.हृ. सू. १०/१३-१४)

(iv) खलतिपलिततृष्णातापमूर्च्छाविसर्पश्वयथुकिटिभकोठा क्षेपरोधास्रपित्तम् । क्षतविषमन्दबुद्धिं वातरक्तं करोति क्षपयति बलमोजः सोऽति वा सेवनेन ॥ (अ.सं.सू. १८)

२.(i) स एवं गुणोऽप्येक एवात्यर्थमुपसेव्यमानो भ्रममदगलताल्वोष्ठशोषदाहसंताप बलविघातकम्पतो-दभेदकृत् करचरणपार्श्वपृष्ठप्रभृतीषु च वा शूलानापादयति ॥ (सु.सू. ४२/१०-४)

(ii) स एवंगुणोऽप्येक एवात्यर्थमुपयुज्यमानो विपाकप्रभावात् पुंस्त्वमुपहन्ति; रसवीर्यप्रभावान्मोहयन्ति, ग्लापयति, सादयति, कर्शयति, मूर्च्छयति, नमयति, तमयति, भ्रमयति, कण्ठं परिदहति, शरीरता-पमुपजनयति, बलं क्षिणोति, तृष्णां जनयति; अपि च वाय्वग्निगुणबाहुल्याद्भ्रमदवथुकम्पतोद-भेदैश्चरणभुजपार्श्वपृष्ठप्रभृतिषु मारुतजान् विकारानुपजनयति ॥ (च.सू. २६/४३-४)

(iii) कुरुते सोऽतियोगेन तृष्णां शुक्रबलक्षयम् ।
मूर्च्छामाकुञ्चनं कम्पं कटिपृष्ठादिषुव्यथाम् ॥ (अ.हृ.सू. १०/१९)

(iv) कुरूतेऽतिनिषेवितः स तृष्णामदमूर्च्छादवमोहदेहसादान् ।
बलशुक्रगलोपशोषकम्पभ्रमतापग्लपनातिकर्शनानि ॥
करचरणपार्श्वपृष्ठप्रभृतिष्वनिलस्य कोपमनितीव्रम् ।
संकोच-तोद-भेदैर्वाय्वग्नि गुणाधिकत्वेन ॥ (अ.सं.सू. १८)

(5) Tikta Rasa

Rukshatwa, Visha lakshanas, Dhatu kshaya (wasting), Ojo kshaya, Sroto kharatwa (atherogenesis), Glani, Moha, Bhrama, Mukha Sosha (dryness of mouth), Sarira Sosha (dehydration), Dourbalya (weakness) etc., will occur[1].

(6) Kashaya Rasa

Mukha Sosha (dryness of mouth), Hridaya Peeda (catching pain in the heart), Adhmana (bloating), Vak graha (aphasia), Sroto rodha, bluish discoloration, impotency, impaired digestion, obstruction to urine, constipation, Krisatwa (weight loss), Pakshaghata (hemiplegia), Ardita (facial paralysis), Apatanaka (conculsive disorders), Vata rogas etc., will occur[2].

Above paras indicate in detaile about the importance of proper utilization of the Rasas. When used in balanced quantities they provide health and excessive usage will result in diseases[3]. Charaka

---

१.(i) स एवंगुणोऽप्येक एवात्यर्थमुपयुज्यमानो रौक्ष्यात्खरविषस्वभावाच्च रसरूधिरमांसमेदोऽस्थिमज्जाशुक्राण्युच्छोषयति, स्रोतसां खरत्वमुत्पादयति, बलमादत्ते, कर्शयति, ग्लपयति, मोहयति, भ्रमयति, वदनमुपशोषयति, अपरांश्च वातविकारानुपजनयति ॥ (च.सू.२६/४३-५)

(ii) स एवं गुणोऽप्येक एवात्यर्थमुपसेव्यमानो गात्रमन्यास्तम्भाक्षेपकार्दित शिरःशूलभ्रमतोदभेदच्छेदास्यवैर-स्यान्यापादयति ॥ (सु.सू. ४२/१०-५)

(iii) धातुक्षयानिलव्याधीनतियोगात्करोति सः ॥ (अ.हृ. सू. १०/१६)

(iv) धातुबलक्षयमूर्च्छाग्लानिभ्रमवातरोगपरूषत्वम् । खरविशदरौक्ष्यभावैः सोऽतिसमासेवितः कुर्यात् ॥ (अ.सं.सू.१८)

२.(i) स एवंगुणोऽप्येक एवात्यर्थमुपयुज्यमान आस्यं शोषयति, हृदयं पीडयति, उदरमाध्मापयति, वाचं निगृह्णाति, स्रोतांस्यवबध्नाति, श्यावत्वमापादयति, पुंस्त्वमुपहन्ति, विष्टभ्य जरां गच्छति, वातमूत्रपुरीषरेतांस्यवगृह्णाति, कर्शयति, ग्लपयति, तर्षयति, स्तम्भयति, खरविशदरूक्षत्वात् पक्षवधग्रहापतानकार्दितप्रभृतींश्चं वातविकारानुपजनयति ॥ (च.सू. २६/४३-६)

(ii) स एवंगुणोऽप्येक एवात्यर्थमुपसेव्यमानो हृत्पीडास्यशोषोदराध्मानवाक्यग्रहमन्यास्तम्भगात्रस्फुरणचुमचुमायनाकुञ्चनाक्षेपणप्रभृतीञ्जनयति । (सु.सू.४२/१०-६)

(iii) करोति शीलितः सोऽति विष्टम्भाध्मान हृद्रुजः ॥
तृट्कार्श्यपौरूषभ्रंशस्तोतोरोधमलग्रहान् । (अ.हृ.सू. १०/२१-२२)

(iv) अन्यभ्यासात्सोऽपि शुक्रोपरोधं तृष्णाध्मानस्तम्भविष्टम्भ कार्श्यम् । स्रोतोबन्धं वातविण्मूत्रसङ्गं पक्षाघाताक्षेपकादींश्च कुर्यात् ॥ (अ.सं.सू. १८)

३. सर्वरसाभ्यासो बलकराणाम्, एकरसाभ्यासो दौर्बल्यकराणाम् । (च.सू. २५/४०)

* चक्रपाणिः- एकरसाभ्यासः कर्शनानामिति अपवादं वर्जयित्वा, तेन घृताभ्यासो रसायनानामिति न विरूध्यते ।

mentioned that Eka Rasabhyasa (consuming only one Rasa excessively) is condemnable. He considered Sarva Rasabhyasa (balanced diet with all Rasas) as ideal[1].

18. Superiority of Rasa

In the context of dravya its superiority and importance were discussed. Similarly on the basis of Adhikarana Siddhanta now, the importance of Rasa is highlighted here. Sushrita proposed four points while Badanta Nagarjuna proposed eight points.

Suśruta's view

(1) Āgama ***(classics):*** In the ancient treatises both foods and drugs are described on the basis of Rasas e.g. Madhura skandha dravyas, Tikta skandha dravyas etc[2].

(2) Upadesa ***(elderly advises):*** Through classical texts our elders have well documented the utility of herbs on the basis of their Rasas only. e.g. Madhura, Amla, Lavana rasas will act as Vāta Sāmaka etc[3].

(3) Anumana ***(inference):*** An inference is made about the action of a particular dravya on the basis of its Rasa only. e.g. Lavana rasa is Sukra hara, Amla rasa is Hridya etc[4].

(4) Rishi Vachana ***(sayings of saints):*** Ancient Acharyas specifically mentioned certain drugs with particular rasa for a particular purpose e.g. Ghrita possessing Madhura ras is used for Jivaniya Karma; asking for Madhura dravyas to perform Yajna (ritual)[5].

Badhanta Nagarjunaś view

(1) Adhikara ***(base for treatment):*** Treatment is based upon Rasas

---

१. इत्येवमेते षड्रसा: पृथकत्वे नैकत्वेन वा मात्रश: सम्यगुपयुज्यमाना उपकाराय भवन्त्यध्यात्मलोकस्य, अपकारकरा: पुनरतोऽन्यथा भवन्त्युपयुज्यमाना:, तान् विद्वानुपकारार्थमेव मात्रश: सम्यगुपयोजयेदित्ति । (च.सू. २६/४४)

२. आगमात् , आगमो हि शास्त्रमुच्यते; शास्त्रे हि रसा अधिकृता:,
यथा- रसायत्त आहार इति, तस्मिंस्तु प्राणा: । (सु.सू. ४०/४)

३. उपदेशाच्च, उपदिश्यन्ते हि रसा:, यथा: मधुराम्ललवणावातं शमयन्ति । (सु.सू. ४०/४)

४. अनुमानाच्च- रसेन ह्यनुमीयन्ते द्रव्यं, यथा- मधुरमिति । (सु.सू. ४०/४)

५. ऋषिवचनाच्च- ऋषिवचनं वेदो यथा- किंचिदिज्यार्थं मधुरमाहरेदिति तस्माद्रसा: प्रधानं; रसेषु गुणसंज्ञा । (सु.सू.४०/४)

only e.g. Pachana with Katu Rasa; Balya with Madhura Rasa etc.[1]

(2) Upadesa: See above[2].

(3) Anumana: See above[3].

(4) Āgama: See above[4].

(5) Upasamhara ***(for collective use):*** When certain drugs are to be picked up collectively, then they are described on the basis of Rasa only e.g. when Vidarigandhadi gana is to be compared with another group, it is compared with Madhura Skandha on the basis of Madhura Rasa[5].

(6) Vyapatti Nimittata ***(vitiation dependent):*** Vitiation of Rasa may result in vitiation of dravya and vipaka also e.g. if Madhura Rasa of milk is disturbed then milk will spoil and its vipaka is also changed[6].

(7) Apadesa ***(frequent usage):*** Rasa is frequently used to explain different aspects of life e.g. Madhura Gana (melodious song), Madhura Vani (sweet voice), Katu Swabhava (angry nature) etc[7].

(8) Aneka Vishayatwa ***(multiplicity of issues):*** On the basis of tastes the drugs are innumerable[8].

---

१. रसानधिकारात् । (र.वै. १सू. १११)

* भाष्यं:-केचिद् रसान प्रधानान् ब्रुवतेऽधिकारात् । ते ह्यधिकृताश्चिकित्साणामिति । कथं षट्स्वेव युक्तं वमनं, षट्सु युक्तं विरेचनम् । षट्सुचास्थापनं युक्तं, षट्सु संशमनं हितम् ॥

२. उपदेशात् । (र.वै.१ सू. ११४)

३. अनुमानात् । (र.वै.१सू. ११५)

४. आगमाच्च । (र.वै.१सू.१२०)

५. तेनोपसंहारात् । (र.वै.१सू.११२)

* भाष्यं:- यथाविदारिगन्धादीन् द्रव्यगणान् एकत्वा यानि यान्येवंप्रकाराणि मधुरस्कन्धपरिसंख्येयानि भवन्ति ।

६. तद्व्यापत्तौ शेषव्यापत्तेः । (र.वै.१सू.११३)

* भाष्यं:- रसव्यापत्तिनिमित्तं शोषाणां द्रव्यादीनां व्यापत्तेः- यथाक्षीरस्य रसे दुष्टे क्षीरं न गृह्यते, तद्विपाकादयश्च विपन्ना इति ।

७. अपदेशात् । (र.वै.१सू.११५)

* भाष्यं:- अपदेशो नाम अन्येनान्योऽयोऽपदिश्यते उपमारूपेण......प्रधानेन.....मधुरं गान्धर्वं, मधुरवाणी, कटुकः फणीति ।

८. नानाविषयत्वात् । (र.वै.१सू. ११७)

Further References on Rasa

1. Agashe B.K.; "Experimental measurement of Tikta Rasa". Dept. of D.G., Tilak Ayu Mahavidyalaya, Pune. 1993-94 (M.D. Thesis)
2. Changede J.V.; "Experimental measurement of Madhura Rasa". Dept. of D.G., Tilak Agu Mahavidyalaya, Pune. 1993-94 (M.D. Thesis).
3. Dhyani S.C.; "Determination of taste and taste threshold of drugs". Dept. of D.G., IPGTRA, G.A.U., Jamnagar. (Ph.D Thesis).
4. Hiremath V.N.; "Determination of Alteration in taste threshold of single drug powder storage (A study on preservation)". Dept. of D.G., IPGTRA, G.A.U., Jamnagar. (M.D. Thesis).
5. Khander (Mrs.) M.B.; "Experimental measurement of Madhura Rasa". Dept. of D.G., Tilak Ayu. Mahavidyalaya, Pune, 1995-96. (M.D. Thesis).
6. Khemani Naresh; "Effect of storage on taste threshold of crude drugs", Dept. of D.G., IPGTRA, G.A.U., Jamnagar (M.D. Thesis).
7. Kshirsagar M.S.; "Experimental measurement of Amla Rasa". Dept. of D.G., Tilak Ayu. Mahavidyalaya, Pune, 1993-94. (M.D. Thesis).
8. Murkute (Ms.) M.B.; "Experimental measurement of Katu Rasa". Dept. of D.G., Tilak Ayu. Mahavidyalaya, Pune. 1993-94. (M.D. Thesis).
9. Murthy D.S.; "Rasonipate Dravyanam". Dept. of D.G., IPGTRA, G.A.U., Jamnagar. 1997. (M.D. Thesis). 1974
10. Parasai M.R.; "Rasa Vijnaa". Dept. of D.G., IPGTRA, G.A.U., Jamnagar. 1958. (M.D. Thesis).
11. Parmar Sudhaben; "Shadrason Ke Gunon Ka Bhoutika Star Par Nirdharana". Dept. of D.G., IPGTRA, G.A.U., Jamnagar. 1981. (M.D Thesis).
12. Puranik (Ms.) D.B.; "Experimental measurement of kashaya Rasa". Dept. of D.G., Tilak Ayu. Mahavidyalaya, Pune. 1994-95. (M.D. Thesis).
13. Salave (Mrs.) S.V.; "Experimental measurement of Madhur-tikta". Dept. of D.G., Tilak Ayu. Mahavidyalaya, Pune. 1995-96. (M.D. Thesis).
14. Sheela Keralem; "Study on Tikta Rasa with special reference to its Jwaraghna property". Dept. of D.G., Govt. Ayu. College, Trivendrum. 1990. (M.D. Thesis).
15. Vaishnav P.V.; "Determination of Rasas and their Degrees in the Drugs". Dept. of D.G., IPGTRA, G.A.U. Jamnagar. 1977. (M.D. Thesis).
16. Rajesh Behari Mathur; "Rasas-their origin & action". Nagarjuna Vol. V, No. 11 July 1962.
17. Sharma P.V. & Bandyopadhyay N.G.; "Objective Method for Determination of Rasa". Nagarjuna, May 1970.
18. Pandit Y.R.; "Concept of Rasa and its actions". Nagarjuna. Vol. V, No.7, March 1962, pp. 569-583.

Chapter-VI
Concept of Vipaka

1. Etymology of Vipaka

The end product of a Dravya which is the out come of digestion/ metabolism is know as Vipaka. It is believed that Vipaka is the bio-transformative phase of Rasa[1].

Gangadhara also defined it as the final transformative state of Rasa of the given dravya[2].

Sivadas sen mention vipaka as a state which is different from Avastha paka. This definition appears to be more important in the context of Dravya guna since the food metabolism and drug metabolism are different in many aspects[3].

2. Characteristics of Vipaka

Charaka and Suśruta did not make serious attempt to define Vipaka prescisely. It is vagbhata who exclusively defined it as "the factor which is the final out come of the bio transformation of Rasa through the action of Jāṭarāgni (degestive enzymes)[4].

Badhanta Nagarjuna mentioned this transformation (Parinama) as the characteristic feature of Vipaka[5].

3. Analysis and Determination of Vipaka

It is a well known fact that either the food or the drug material we consume, will undergo some changes inside the GIT. It is

---

१. विशिष्टः जरणनिष्ठाकाले रसविशेषस्य पाकः प्रादुर्भावः विपाकः । (प्रशस्तपाद)

२. पाकः पचनं द्रव्याणां स्वरूपरसयोः परावृत्तिः । सा च स्वरूपान्तरत्वेन रसान्तरत्वेन च परिणतिः, तस्याविशेषो विपाकः । (गंगाधरः)

३. अवस्थापाकापेक्षया विशिष्टः पाकः विपाकः । (शिवदासः)

४. जाठरेणाग्निना योगाद्यदुदेति रसान्तरम् । रसानां परिणामान्ते स विपाक इति स्मृतः ॥ (अ.हृ.सू. ९)

* अरूणदत्तः- रसानां परिणामान्ते जरणनिष्ठाकाले, यद् रसान्तरं रसविशेषः उदेति उत्पद्यते स विपाकः ।

५. परिणामलक्षणो विपाकः । (र.वै.१.सू. १७०)

* भाष्यंः- परिणामोऽर्थान्तरभावः, जोतिरित्यर्थः । एवं विदाहानामपि पाकावयवत्वं युज्यते ।

Chakrapani who proposed the concept of Avasthapaka and Nishta paka in the context of digestion (Vide: ch.chi. 15 chapter)[1].

Charaka described that generally all the food materials will under go three phases of digestion in the Maha srotas (GIT and other Organs). They are:

(i) Madhura paka (Prapaka), (ii) Amla paka & (iii) Katu paka. In this context one should clearly identify the difference between Avastha paka and Prapaka. Chakrapani specifically used the term Prapaka for Madhura Avastha paka but not for Avastha paka. However scholars like Dr. C. Dwarakanath and others have considered Prapaka term as synonymous to Avastha paka.

Dr. C. Dwarakanath considers liver (Yakrit) as the site of Bhutagni paka which can be comparable to micro enzymic activity in drug metabolism.

Āhara (food & drugs) will under go two phases of transformation inside the body. They are:

(1) Avastha paka (Digestion)– initial phase.

(2) Nishta paka (Metabolism)– final phase.

Suśruta quoted that the dravyas which are made up of Panchabhutas will under go the paka with the helf of respective Agni and enchance the concerned characteristics inside the body.

From these references it appears that Charaka mainly concentrated on digestion while Sushrita emphasized metabolism.

(1) Avastha Paka

When the food comes into contact with Jāṭarāgni (digestive enymes), then the process of Avasthapaka (digestion) begins with Madhura paka or Prapaka (the sweet phase) in the Āmasaya (oral

---

१. अन्नस्य भुक्तमात्रस्य षड्रसस्य प्रपाकतः । मधुराद्यात् कफोभावात् फेनभूत उदीर्यते ॥
परं तु पच्यमानस्य विदग्धस्याम्लभावतः । आशयात् च्यवमानस्य पित्तमच्चमुदीर्यते ॥
पक्वाशयं तु प्राप्तस्थ शोष्यमाणस्य वह्निना। परिपिण्डितपक्वस्य वायुः स्यात् कटुभावतः ॥ (च.चि. १५)
* चक्रपाणिः- भुक्तमात्रस्येति भुक्तानन्तरमेव ।.........षड्रसस्थापि प्रथमं मधुरता निरूक्ताभवतीति दर्शयति । प्रपाकत इति प्रथम पाकतः; प्रपाक आदिकर्मणि । मधुरश्चासौ आद्यश्चेति मधुराद्यः ....।

cavity to first part of duodenum). Later food is ejected into Pachyamanasaya (second part of duodenum to ileum), where it undergoes Amla paka (the acid phase). Finally the food reaches the Pakwasaya (caecum to rectum) where the process of digestion ends with Katu vipaka (alkaline phase)[1].

The comparative study of these three stages from modern physiology will provide the exact picture.

(i) The food first under goes digestion in saliva chiefly under the influence of salivary amylase (ptylin). Usually ptylin acts on boiled starch. Hence coocked food (Ānna) is considered for Avastha paka. Ptylin converts starch up to the maltose. The main action ptylin takes place in the stomach before the HCl concentration becomes high. On an average it continues for 30-40 min. Digestion of proteins and fats is not possible in saliva or before gastric juice involment. Upto this stage the process of digestion was denoted as Prapaka or Madhura paka in Ayurveda.

(ii) Gastric juice does not possess any carbohydrate splitting enzyme, but gastric HCl can carry on some hydrolysis of sucrose. Protein and fat digestion begins in gastric juice and completes with the action of succus entericus. Gastric juice contains proteolytic enzyme pepsin which digests them upto peptones. Gastric lipase breaks neutral fat into 1mol. of glycerol and 3 mol. of fatty acids. This occurs in Pachyamanasaya according to Ayurveda.

Next, the action of Achcha pitta (pancreato-biliary secretions) begins:

(a) Pancreatic amylase acts on starch and dextrin. Maltase acts on maltose.

(b) Pancreatic trypsin converts protein into peptones and amino acids. 50-60% of protein digestion is over in pancreatic juice. Here tryptic digestion ends and erepsin action begins.

(c) Fat digestion mainly occurs in duodenum by pancrcatic lipase (steapsin). Emulsification of fat takes place by bile salts, fatty acids,

१. पञ्चभूतात्मके देहे आहारः पाञ्चभौतिकः । विपक्वः पञ्चधा सम्यग्गुणान् स्तानभिवर्धयेत् ॥ (सु.सू. ४६)

cholesterol, monoglycerides, lysolecithins and proteins. Bile salts make the fats water-soluble. Fat digestion is nearly completed in pancrcatic juice. Fat is converted into glycerol and fatty acids.

Till this state, the process of digestion is considered as Amla avastha paka in Ayurveda.

(iii) Succus entericus contain amylase and maltose which helps in the conversion of carbohydrates into glycose. The other disaccharides taken in food are hydrolysed by lactase and sucrase (investase) present in this juice.

Digestion of protein in intestinal juice depends upon tryptic activity. Erepsin consists of a mixture of enzymes viz., aminopeptidases and dipeptidases which act in alkaline medium. They convert lower peptides completely into amino acids.

Lipase in succus entericus is insignificant since fat digestion will be almost over in pancreatic juice.

Apart from these digestive changes the digested food loose most of the water content once stool formation is over in large intestines. This final form is slightly alkaline in reaction. This third phase is mentioned as Katu Avastha paka in Ayurveda.

2. Nishta Paka

After the food is subjected to Jataragni paka and Bhutagni paka, the nutrients absorbed along with the chyle from the small intestine (Adho-āmāsaya) will have a further transformation known as 'Nishta Pāka'.

Karma nishta is the conclusive action of a dravya. Chakrapani explain Nishta paka or Vipaka as Karma Parisamapti i.e., conclusion of action in its entirety. Even though various Rasas undergo transformative changes, the contribution made by their special functions due to further transformative changes in known as vipaka or Nishta paka. The final action will increase the symptoms of Kapha, Sukra etc[1].

---

१. अवस्थापाकात् कफपित्तयोर्वृद्धिः तथा निष्ठापाकाच्च मलरूपतया उत्पादः । (च.द.)

The concept of Nishta paka vis-a-vis post-digestive changes which occurs in Adho amasaya after absorption under the influence of Bhutagni paka and Dhatvagni paka etc. This process is denoted as metabolism. Modern physiology belives that- 'All metabolic reactions are connected in a single integrated whole in which individual links can replace one another' (Byllow K.M., 1958).

During Nishta paka the pancha Bhuta Amsas of a dravya will be converted into its basic components like prithvi, ap, tejas, vayu & Akasa. The Sthayi dhatu poshana will be done by this Vipaka[1].

The 'Madhura Nishta paka' results in the final formation of glucose and its conversion into glycogen for the utility of tissues. Metabolic end-products characterized as 'Amla Nishta paka' and 'Katu Nishta paka' may be the outcome of cellular respiration. The term Amla Vipaka may refer to intermediate metabolites (keto acids) as the laetic acid and pyruvic acids which are the 3-carbon compounds. These are *laghu* in nature when compared to amino acids, glucose, glyceral and fatty acids and *gunu*, as compared to the end-products of cellular respiration which are characterized as Katu Vipaka.

Thus, the terms Amla and Katu vipakas, in the context of Nishta paka, may refer to the basic molecular structure of the given substance.

The following are the differences between Avasthapāka and Nishta paka:

AVASṬHĀ PĀKA	NIṢHṬĀ PĀKA
1. It is an initial transformative phase	1. It is the final transformative phase
2. It is assessed by direct or visible process	2. It is assessed through inference

१. (i) कर्मनिष्ठया इति कर्मणो निष्ठा निष्पत्तिः; कर्मनिष्ठया क्रियापरिसमाप्तिः ।
(चक्रपाणि-च.सू. २६/६६)

(ii) रसोपयोगे सति योन्त्याहारपरिणामकृतः कर्मविशेषः कफशुक्राभिवृद्ध्यादिलक्षणः,तेन विपाको निश्चीयते ।

3. Normal doshas are produced	3. Doshas in the form of excreta are produced
4. Effect Asthayi dhatus (Poshya dhatus)	4. Effects the sthayi dhatus (Poshaka dhatus)

Chakrapani further substantiate his view that during Dhatu paka process Rasa dhatu produces Kapha as its mala and Rakta dhatu produces Pitta as mala. On the other hand druing the Ahāra pachana process through Jataragni Prakrita Kapha, Pitta and Vāta are produced in the Avastha paka.

The Avastha pāka and Nishta pāka of Ayurvedic herbal drugs must be studied carefully with this concept.

The above paras have proved beyond doubt that Avastha paka and Nishta paka are mainly described in relation to food metabolism in Ayurveda. It is essential to review the definition of digestion and metabolism in relation to Avastha and Nishta pāka.

Digestion— It is the process of bio-chemical transformation of complex and larger food particles in the gut enzymatically into a simple form suitable for absorption and assimilation, the complex and higher molecules being unsuitable for absorption.

Metabolism— Metabolism of a food substance is a series of specific bio-chemical reactions occuring within the living organism from the time of its incorporation into the cell or tissue till its exeretion, of which some are concerned with tissue synthesis and others with tissue break-down what are termed as anabolism and catabolism respectively.

Though natural products are used as medicine in Ayurveda, drug metabolism of these harbs etc., shall be considered differently since some of the digestive and metabolic states differ from that of food substances. For example, Swarasa, Kalka, Churna etc., preparation may not have any starch reaciton with saliva as they are not boiled. But kashaya, lehya etc., will undergo the salivery digestion also.

On the other hand the secondary metabolites of the plants i.e., active principles etc., will under go certain chemical changes inside the body under the influence of liver and tissue micro-enzymes resulting in respective pharmacological actions. The drug effects produced through the process of metabolization shall only be considered as vipaka. The unmetabolized active principle of drug responsible for pharmacological action may be considered as virya. e.g. the third phase of effects of morphine are seen after conjugation (i.e., after vipaka) while first two phases of its effects are due to virya (unmetabolized active ingredient).

The concept of Vipaka in Ayurveda will cover the drug metabolism or pharmacokinetics dealt in modern pharmacology. Depending upon this view the fate of an herbal drug administered orally may be exlained in this way:

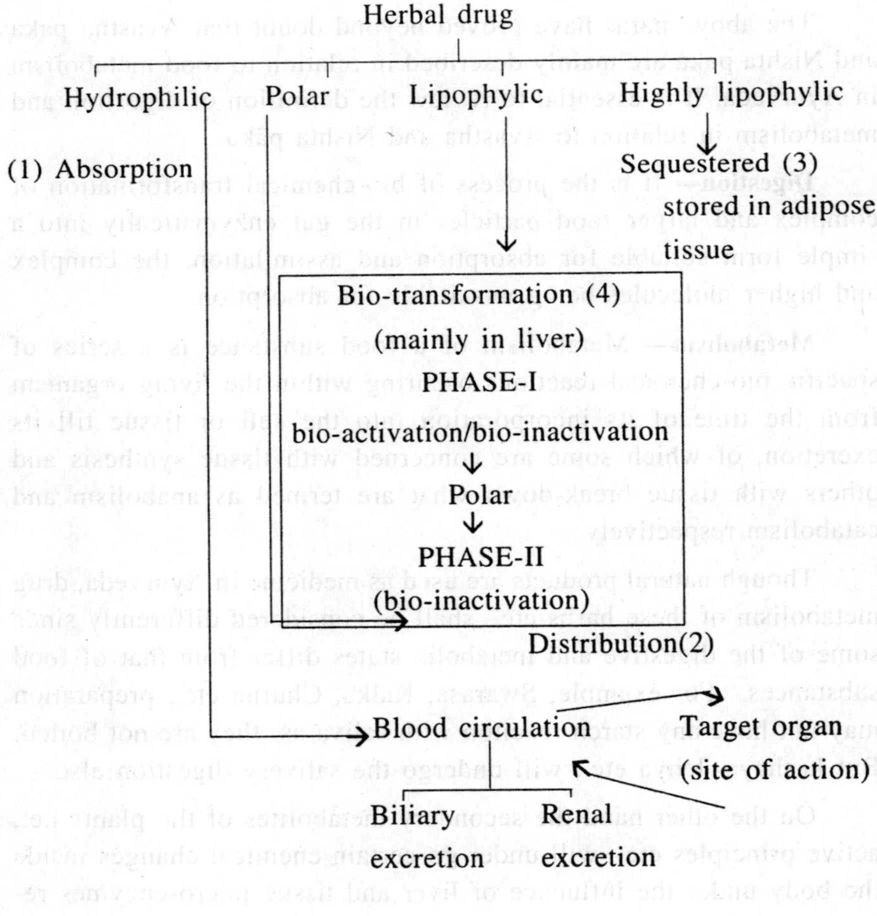

The above diagram represents the macro or micro molecules of the herbal drugs stored in various tissues of the plants. These chemical constituents will be arranged in four categories viz., hydrophilic, polar, lipophylic and highly lipophylic.

(i) Hydrophilic— They enter blood stream immediately after absorption and reach the site of action or target organ. The end products are eliminated through bile and urine.

(ii) Polor— They will readily enter into the body fluids and under go second phase of biotransformation and finally attain bio-inactivation. This process is also completed quickly compared to lipophylic compounds.

(iii) Lipophylic— They undergo first phase of biotransformation initially and become activated or inactivated. If activated the polar compenents are formed which will further undergo second phase of bio-transformation to become inactive.

(iv) Highly lipohylic— They are sequestered and stored in the adipose tissue.

From these findings it may be tentatively concluded that the drug action of hydrophilic and polar components may be similar to that of Virya, while lipophylic components acting on end organ is due to vipaka. The former one does not require complete bio-transformation while the later one does require.

Polar compounds bye-passing phase-I metabolism demonstrate the concept of Vyavayi, Vikasi, Asukari etc., gunas. The main difference between Vipaka and Virya will be that "Vipaka acts throug '*distribution*' while, Virya acts through *absorption*."

The two phases of metabolism may be represented as:

Phase I- Functionalization reaction

Phase II- Synthetic or conjugating reaction.

Phase	Biotransformation pathways		Subcellular localization
Phase-I	Oxidation	- Hydroxylation	- Microsome, Nuclear membrane
		- Epoxidation	- Microsome (ER)
		- Dealkylation	-
		- Dehalogenation	- -
		- Alcohol	- Cytosol
		- Amino oxidases etc	- Mitochondria
	Reduction	- Azo reduction	- Microsome
		- Nitro reduction	- Microsome, cytosol
		- Aldehyde reduction	- Cytosol
	Hydrolysis	- De-esterification	- Microsome
		- Deamination	
Phase-II	Conjugation	- Glucuronidation	- Microsome
		- Sulfonation	- Cytosol
		- Acetylation etc.	
	Miscellaneous	- Ring Scission	- Not known
		- Molecular scission	
		- Cyclization	

Thus the pathway by which drugs and foreign compounds are chemically altered in side the body is known as 'metabolism' or 'process of detoxication'.

During their journy inside the body the compounds may be excreted partially unchanged or may be converted into other forms. The toxic compounds thus formed will be converted into relatively non-polar lipophilic compounds which are very difficult for excretion. But the more polar hydrophilic compounds are excreted within a short period of time.

If the lipid soluble non-polar compounds are not metàbolized as polar water soluble compounds, then they tend to remain in the blood and tissues and will produce the pharmacological effects for an indefinite time.

On the other hand certain compounds are insoluble in the body fluids and are resistant to the chemical/enzymatic reactions in the GIT. Therefore they are eliminated through stools and do not exhibit any biological action e.g. mineral oil, barium sulphate.

Some compounds which are freely soluble in body fluids and resistant to chemical changes are relatively non-toxic and rapidly excreted e.g. aromatic and aliphatic compounds.

The following aspects of drug metabolims are essential for every drug:

(a) Rates and Site of absorption of both the drug and its metabolite.

(b) Plasma and tissue levels.

(c) Plasma protein binding.

(d) Rate of metabolism and half-life of the drug in blood and tissues.

(e) Rates and routes of excretion.

Sites of drug metabolism

Liver is the primary site of drug metabolism and metabolism of all substances which enter blood circulation via the GIT (through portal circulation). The oxygenated blood perfuses through liver cells where nutrients are removed or stored.

Drugs are metabolized into water soluble derivatives and returned to circulation for excretion by the kidneys. Bile also acts as one of the means of excretion of metabolic products through faeces.

Metabolism of drugs and foreign substances in the liver is carried out by a number of specific and non-specific enzymes. Generally, drug metabolism may involve the following types of bio-transformations.

(i) a single step conversion of biologically active compound to an inactive compound which is excreted;

(ii) a two step conversion, in which there is first inactivation followed by conjugation with glucuronic acid;

(iii) a two step process in which an inactive compound is converted to a biologically active compound followed by inactivation and excretion;

(iv) a two step process in which there is first a change in activity of an active compound followed by inactivation.

Types of Metabolic Conversions

(a) Oxidation— It is normally the first step involved in the drug metabolism unless the drug compound possess functional groups like -OH, -SH, $-NH_2$, $-CO_2H$ which are capable of conjugation. A complex of non-specific microsomal enzymes present in the liver catalyse metabolic oxidation of a large variety of compounds both endogenous substances like steroid hormones and exogenous substances like drugs and pollutants. The most important enzyme involved in this type of oxidation is cytochrome p-450.

(b) Reduction— Metabolic reductions are carried out by enzyme systems which make use of NADPH as a hydrogen donar.

(c) Hydrolysis— Esterases such as pseudocholine esterase present in plasma will catalyse the hydrolysis reactions of drug substances.

(d) Conjugation Reaction— In the case of drugs and other molecules containing groups like -OH, -SH, $-NH_2$ or $-CO_2H$ conjugation with glucuronic acid, sulphate, amino acids and peptides in the major pathway for metabolic elimination. However, in the absence of such reactive groups, oxidation, reduction, hydrolysis etc., proceeds the conjugation reaction.

These aspects confirm that the phenomenon through which a drug molecule gets converted into different form is termed as 'biotransformation' or metabolism. Most of the metabolized end products are usually more polar in character than the parent drug molecule. This increased polarity renders the metabolite less absorbable through the renal tubules and also makes it transient in the body. There will be a disparity due to the genetic differences among different races.

4. Different types of Vipaka

There are different views and theories over the number of vipakas also.

(1) Shadvidha Vipaka Vāda (concept of six vipakas)

(i) Niyata or Yatha Rasa Vipaka Vāda- definite Vipaka concept.

(ii) Aniyata Vipaka Vāda- indefinite vipaka concept.

(2) Pancha vidha Vipaka vāda (concept of five vipakas)

(3) Trividha Vipaka vāda (concept of three vipakas)

(4) Dvividha Vipaka vāda (concept of two vipakas)

(1) Shadvidha Vipaka Vāda

(i) Yatha Rasa Vipaka Vāda– This concept proposes that each Rasa will under go its individual vipaka and results in six vipakas respectively e.g. Madhura rasa gives rise to Madhura vipaka; Amla rasa leads to Amla vipaka etc[1]. However, many Acharyas did not agree with this concept owing to several exceptions to this genal belief that each Rasa will have its own vipaka e.g. Vrihi (Rice) is Madhura (sweet) in taste but it undergoes Amla vipaka, similarly Āmalaki is Amla (sour) in taste and under goes Madhura vipaka.

Badanta Nagarjuna strongly opposed this concept by stating that Rasa and Vipaka are expressed at different times and they also act upon the body at different times. Even their perception is different and effects are also different. Therefore Vipaka need not depend upon Rasa alone.

But, both Suśruta and Nagarjuna have quoted about Shadvidha vipaka vada by mentioning it as the view of other Acharyas. According the following are the vipakas based upon six tastes:

(a) Madhura Rasa - Madhura Vipaka

(b) Amla Rasa - Amla Vipaka

(c) Lavana Rasa - Lavana Vipaka

---

१. (i) तत्राहुरन्ये- प्रतिरसं पाक इति । मधुरो मधुरस्याम्लोऽम्लस्यैवं सर्वेषामिति । दृष्टान्तं चोपदिशन्ति- यथा शालियवमद्गादयः प्रकीर्णाः स्वभावमुत्तरकालेऽपि न परित्यजन्ति तद्वदिति ॥ (सु.सू. ४०)

(ii) यथारसं विपाकमेके ब्रुवते । (र.वै.४ सू. ३१)

(iii) किचं प्रतिरसं रससदृशः पाकस्तथा बलवत्पराधीनता च पाकस्य रसद्वारा प्रतिपाद्यमाकार्येणैव लभ्येत, तेनैतत् पक्षद्वयमपि न निष्ठापाके चिन्तनीयं, रसस्वरूपनिरूपणेनैवोक्तार्थत्वात् । (शिवदासः)

(iv) प्रायशो ग्रहणात् क्वचिन्नैवंविधोऽपि । यथा शुण्ठीपिप्पल्यादीनां कटूनां मधुरो विपाकः, कषायस्य कुलत्थस्याम्लः, कषाया हरीतकी अम्लमामलकं च मधुरं पच्यते, मधुरो ....हश्चाम्लं, तथाविधं तैलं पुनः कटुकम् । (योगेन्द्रनाथः)

(v) यथारसं जगुः पाकान् षट् केचित्तदसांप्रतम् । यद् स्वादुव्रीहिरम्लत्वं न चाम्लमपि दाडिमम् ॥ याति तैलं च कटुतां कटुकापि न पिप्पली । यथा रसत्वे पाकानां न स्यादेवं विपर्ययः ।(अ.सं.सू. १७)

(d) Katu Rasa - Katu Vipaka

(e) Tikta Rasa - Tikta Vipaka

(f) Kashaya Rasa - Kashaya Vipaka

My beloved teacher Dr. K. Nisteswar revealed during some discussion that he came across Tikta vipaka of certain dravyas in Bhava prakasa. That means some of the acharyas have followed this concept also.

Suśruta provided an example to substantiate this view- "the plants like Sali (rice),Yava (barley), Mudga (moong dal) etc. will produce the same plants through their seeds respectively but not other plants. Similarly one rasa can under go its respective vipaka but not any other vipaka".

(ii) Aniyata Vipaka Vada

The believers of this view are of the openion that the Vipaka is finalized by the dominant Rasa only. The Rasa which is predominant in a particular dravya will nullify the effect of other rasas and emerge itself as the vipaka in the end. Therefore vipaka can not be assumed on the basis of the original rasa of a dravya. e.g. Aswagandha is Tikta rasa but Katu vipaka; Pippali is Katu rasa but Madhura vipaka[1].

Many scholers do not accept this theory because indefinite approch has no value in scientific medicine.

(2) Pancha Vidha vipaka Vada

Suśruta mentioned about the five Vipakas on the basis of Panchabhutas e.g.: Akasa dravya under goes Akasa bhutagni pāka, vayu dravya under goes vayu bhutagni pāka etc[2].

१.(i) केचित् पुनरबलवन्तो बलवतां वशमायान्ति । तस्मादनवस्थित: पाक इति । (सु.सू ४०)

(ii) अन्ये तु ब्रुवते- रसा द्विविधा बलवन्तोऽबलवन्तश्च; बलवत्त्वं च व्यक्तत्वेन मात्राबाहुल्येन वा, अबलवत्त्वं पुनरेतद्विपर्ययेण; तत्राल्पतयाऽबलवन्तो रसा बलवतां वशमायान्तीति, तेन निष्ठापाके बलवता रसेन दुर्बलरसाभिभावान्न रसप्रतिनियमेन मधुरस्य मधुर एव पाकोऽम्लस्य चाम्ल एवेत्यादि; प्रतिनियमाभावाच्चानवस्थित: पाक इति । अनियतत्वपक्षेऽपि षट्कत्वमेव, कदाचित् कस्यचित् संभवात् इति । उक्तं च- बहवोऽभिभवन्त्यल्पान् बहिर्मिश्रीकृता रसा: । तेन निश्चितमेवैके पाकमाहुर्मनीषिण: । (शिवदास:)

२.(i) इत्यनेन पञ्चधा पाकोऽभिहित: । (चक्रपाणि- सु.सू. ४६)

(ii) इत्यनेन पञ्चधाऽपि विपाकस्तेनैवोक्त: । (शिवदास:)

The five vipakas are :		
	(i) Parthiva vipaka	Guru vipaka
	(ii) Āpya vipaka	
	(iii) Taijasa vipaka	Laghu vipaka
	(iv) Vayavya vipaka	
	(v) Nabhasa vipaka	

Actually these five vipakas will come under two vipakas only viz., Guru and laghu vipakas.

(3) Trividha Vipaka Vada

This is the widely accepted concept of Vipaka. It is mainly emphasized and proposed by Charaka, Vagbhata, Parasara etc[1]. The six rasas will under go three vipakas as denoted here:

(i) Madhura vipaka	-	Madhura & Lavana Rasas
(ii) Amla vipaka	-	Amla Rasa
(iii) Katu vipaka	-	Katu, Tikta & Kashaya Rasas

In Ashtanga Sangraha we find a question of Parāsara where in he questioned that "if Tikta and Kashaya rasas will under go Katu vipaka, how they will act as Pitta samaka (pitta subsiding factors)" There fore he accepted three vipakas with a little modification:

(i) Madhura vipaka	-	Madhura,Lavana,Tikta Kashaya Rasa
(ii) Amla vipaka	-	Amla Rasa
(iii) Katu vipaka	-	Katu Rasa

This Trividha vipaka concept is other wise known as 'Rasa vipaka vada' as it is purely based upon the Rasas.

---

१. (i) त्रिधा विपाको द्रव्यस्य स्वाद्वम्ल कटुकात्मक: ॥ (अ.हृ.सू. १/१७)

(ii) कटुतिक्तकषायांणा विपाक: प्रायश: कटु: ।
अम्लेऽम्लं पच्यते, स्वदुर्मधुरं लवणस्तथा ॥ (च.सू. २६)

(iii) पाकास्त्रयो रसानामम्लोऽम्लं पच्यते कटु: कटुकम् ।
चत्वारोऽन्ये मधुरं संसृष्टं रसास्तु संसृष्टम् । कटुतिक्तकषायाणां कटुको येषां विपाक इति ।
पक्षस्तेषां पित्तविघाते तिक्तकषायौ कथं भवत: ॥ (अ.सं.सू. १७)

(iv) इमे मधुराम्लकटुरूपेण रसानां त्रयो विपाकश्च स परिणामा: रसाख्ये आद्यधातौ गुणा भवन्ति, न तु पाकारम्भचरमपर्यन्तं पच्यमाने षड्रसद्रव्ये प्रथममध्यमचरमावस्थासु मधुराम्लकटुरूपा: । (गङ्गाधर:)

Yogendranath sen proposed it as "Tridosha vipaka vada" since the drugs which are under going these three vipakas will either increase or decrease of Tridoshas[1].

They are:

Madhura vipaka	-	Kapha vardhaka
Amla vipaka	-	Pitta vardhaka
Katu vipaka	-	Vata vardhaka

Sivadas sen described that Kapha and Kapha-Vata leads to Madhura vipaka; Kapha-Pitta leads to Amla vipaka and Vata, Pitta & Vata-pitta leads to Katu vipaka. However many do not agree with this view because rasa can only be transformed into Vipaka and therefore their effects on dosha will be seen. But dosha alone can not determine vipaka.

(4) Dwividha Vipaka Vada

Suśruta mentioned Vipaka as mainly two types viz., (i) Madhura vipaka and (ii) Katu vipaka. These two are respectively known as Guru vipaka and Laghu vipaka on the basis of their predominant guna (property)[2].

Badhanta Nagarjuna proposed the concept that qualities like Seeta, Snigdha, Guru, Pichchila etc., are responsible factors for Vipaka[3]. He also concluded that the transformation of food or drug material will end with genesis of either Guru guna or Laghu guna. Hence vipakas are two only viz., Gunu vipaka and Laghu vipaka[4]. He

---

१. (i) वस्तुतस्तु दोषाणां त्रैविध्याद्विपाकस्यापि तदनुगुणतया त्रैविध्यमेवोचितम् । (योगेन्द्रनाथ

(ii) अन्ये तु वातादिभ्यो दोषेभ्य एव त्रीन् पाकानिच्छन्ति- कफात् वातकफाच्च मधुरः, कफपित्तादम्लः, वातात् पित्तात् वातपित्ताच्च कटुक इति । तदुक्तं- कफात् वातकफात् स्वादुरम्लः पित्तकफोद्भवः । दोषैस्त्रयोऽनिलात् पित्तात् वातपित्तात् कटुर्मतः । (शिवदासः)

२. आगमस्त्वाह- द्विविध एव पाको मधुरः कटुकश्च, तयोर्मधुराख्यो गुरुः, कटुकाख्यो लघुरिति । तत्र पृथिव्यप्तेजोवाय्वाकाशानां द्वैविध्यं भवति तद्गुणसाधर्म्याद् गुरुता, लघुता च, पृथिव्यापश्च गुर्व्यः शेषाणि लघूनि, तस्माद् द्विविध एव विपाक इति ॥ (सु.सू. ४०/)

३. गुणाः विपाकयोः कारणम्, शीतस्निग्धगुरूपिच्छिला गुरूविपाकस्य, लघुरूक्षविशदतीक्ष्णा लघुवि-पाकस्येति । (र.वै. १ सू. १२३)

४. द्वौ, द्वैविध्यदर्शनात् परिणामस्य । गुणकारणत्वाद् गुणद्वैविध्याच्च । (र.वै.१सू. ५०-५१)

*भाष्यं:- यथा खदिरसारादीनि चिरादग्निसंयोगे परिणामं गच्छन्ति, पललादीन्यचिरादिति ।

condemned the concept of three vipakas and stated that Vipaka of a dravya is two types- "Chira kālika" (digestion taking more time) and "Achira kālika" (digestion completed in no time).

According to this view the six Rasas will under go only two vipakas in the following manner–

(i) Madhura vipaka – Madhura, Amla, Lavana Rasas

(ii) Katu vipaka – Katu, Tikta, Kashaya Rasas

Nagarjunas view is expressed in the following way:

(a) Guru Vipaka- Seeta, Snigdha, Guru, Pichila gunas.

(b) Laghu vipaka- Laghu, Ruksha, Visada, Tikshna gunas.

Trividha Vipaka Vāda vis-a-vis Dwividha Vipaka Vada

Suśruta mentioned that the Trividha Vipaka vāda is incorrect because Amla vipaka can neither exist by means of qualities of bhutas nor mentioned in the classical texts. On the other hand Pitta will have Katu rasa and Amla rasa in normal state (Prakrita Avastha) and vitiated state (Vidagdha Avastha). Here the Amla state is only temporary and vitiate phase. If vitiate state is also considered, then one must accept the Lavana vipaka. It is because vitiated Kapha attains Lavana Rasa. Hence vipakas are considered as two[1].

The Madhura vipaka will act as Vata and Pitta samaka while Katu vipaka subsides Kapha. In this way all the doshas are covered by two Vipakas.

Yogendranath sen elaborated his views on this concept and proposed that- Charaka accepted Amla, Katu rasas for normal Pitta while Suśruta accepted only katu rasa. According to Sushrita Amlatwa is attributed to Pitta in vitiate state only[2].

---

१. केचित् त्रिविधमिच्छन्ति- मधुरम्, अम्लं, कटुकं चेति । तत्तु न सम्यक्,
भूतगुणादागमाच्चाम्लो विपाको नास्ति, पित्तं हि विदग्धमम्लतामुपैत्याग्नेयत्वात् ।
यद्येवं लवणोऽप्यन्य:पाको भविष्यति, श्लेष्माहि विदग्धो लवणतामुपैति। (सु.सू. ४०)

२ .अम्लपाकस्याभ्युपगमयोर्बीजं तु चरके पित्तं प्रकृत्याऽम्लं कटु च, सुश्रुते तु कटुरसं,
यत् पुनरम्लत्त्वं तदस्य विदग्धस्यैवेति सुश्रुतेन पित्तस्य प्राकृतस्याम्लत्वानङ्गीकारात्,
सुतरामम्लपाकोऽपि नाङ्गीक्रियते, निष्प्रयोजनत्वात्, इह पुनरम्लपाक: सप्रयोजन एव । (योगेन्द्रनाथ:)

There was a debate even on the qualities of Vipakas:

Vipaka	Charaka	Yogendranath, Chakrapani Sivadas sen	Gangadhara Yadavji Trikamji P.V. Sharma
Madhura vipaka	Guru	Guru	Guru
Amla vipaka	Laghu	Guru	Laghu
Katu vipaka	Laghu	Laghu	Laghu

Trividha Vipaka vada is mainly based upon Tridoshas while Dwi Vidha Vipaka vada is mainly based upon Pancha bhutas[1&2].

Badhanta Nagarjuna also condemned the concept of three Vipakas. He delineated three reasons in support of his view[3]:

(i) Kālatah: Some substance will be digested very lately and some will be digested immediately. Therefore Vipaka is two types viz., Chira kalika (Guru) and Achira kalika (Laghu).

(ii) Guṇatah: On the basis of qualities Vipaka can be only two varieties viz., Guru & Laghu Vipakas.

(iii) Rasatah: The transformation of Rasas will occur in two forms viz., Katu-Tikta-Kashaya Rasas—Laghu Vipaka and Madhura-Amla-Lavana Rasas—Guru Vipaka.

Yogendranath claborately discussed on Amla vipaka. Usually prithvi bhuta is responsible for Guru Vipaka and Agni bhuta is responsible for Laghu Vipaka. Thence it is difficult to decide the Amla Vipaka since Amla is the combination of Prithvi and Agni bhutas. He

---

१. (i) कालतो गुणतो रसतश्चानुपपत्तिः त्रित्वस्य । (र.वै.१ सू. ५०)
* भाष्यं:- कालतस्त्रित्वं नोपपद्यते चिराचिरकालव्यतिरिक्तस्वभावात् ।
गुणतश्च त्रित्वं नोपपद्यते, गुरूभूतजनिता, लघुभूत जनिता इति गुणद्वैविध्यादिति ।
रसतश्च त्रित्वस्यानुपपत्तिः, कटुतिक्तकषायास्तु लघवः, गुरवः परे इति द्विविधः- भेदावरोधात् इति ।
(ii) मधुरो गुरूत्वात् लघुत्वाच्च कटुकः (र.वै.१सू.५२)

२. पृथिव्यम्बुगुणभूयिष्ठतया स्निग्धानां मधुराम्ललवणानां त्रयाणां मधुरो विपाकः
वायुगुणातिरेकाद्रूक्षाणां कटुतिक्तकषायाणां त्रयाणां कटुकः । (योगेन्द्रनाथ)

३. तेषां गुरुः स्यान्मधुरः कटुकाम्लवतोऽन्यथा । (च.सू.)

quotes that Charaka accepted Pitta as Amla as well as Katu in normal state. But Suśruta accepts only Kaut for Pitta in the normal state. On this issue both the Acharyes differed and there from Trividha and Dwividha Vipaka concepts are proposed respectively.

Some scholars will consider Amla Vipaka as a part and parcel of Madhura (Guru) Vipaka and some include it under Katu (Laghu) Vipaka. Even Charaka described Madhura as Guru Vipaka and Amla and Katu as Laghu Kipakas in one context.

Before more description is made on Vipaka, it is essential to finalize the concept of Vipaka. It appears that the concept of Vipaka as mentioned by Charaka (i.e. Trividha vipaka vada) is mainly aimed at Āhara (food). At the same time Suśruta's concept of Dwividha Vipaka vada reflects the drug metabolism. On review of literature the author could not trace out even a single oushadha dravya undergoing Amla vipaka. (Vide- classification of drugs on the basis of Vipaka in III chapter). So it will be quite appropriate to conclude that Trividha and Dwividha Vipaka concepts will be reflecting the food and drug metabolism respectively in Ayurveda.

The reason for not mentioning these two aspects seperately and directly is that Ayurveda mainly uses natural products/herbs in the therapeutics. Thus drug metabolism as described in modern pharmacology is not directly applicable in every aspect of Vipaka concept. However herbs are used as Āhara (food) as well as Oushadha (drug). For example, Pushkara mula (Inula racemosa) which contains inulin as primary metabolite is used in diet while the secondary metabolites flavonoids are used in medicine.

From these discussions, a common conclusion may be drawn that the concept of Dwividha Vipaka is more suitable in the context of Dravya guna vijnana with special reference to herbs.

5. Properties and functions of Vipaka

Vipaka of a drug will effect the doshas, dhatus and malas also. Charaka very lucidly described the qualities and actions of three

Vipakas. They are tabulated below[1]:

S. N.	Types of Vipaka	Properties	Effect on Doshas	Effect on Dhatus	Effect on Malas
1.	Madhura	Snigdha, Guru	enhances Kapha, decre-ases Vata-Pitta	improve dhatus, Sukrala	increases the quan-tity of stools & urine
2.	Amla	Snigdha, Laghu	enhances Pitta subsides Vata	Sukra hara	-do-
3.	Katu	Ruksha, Laghu	enhances Vata, subsides Kapha	Sukra hara	decrease the quantity of stools & urine

Similarly Suśruta and Badhanta Nagarjuna have explained the qualities and effects of Guru and Laghu vipakas. But, they did not mention about the effect on Sukra dhatu by the two vipakas. Their properties are tabulated[2].

S. N.	Type of Vipaka	Bhuta Predo-minance	Effect on Doshas	Effect on Malas
1.	Guru (Madhura)	Prithvi & Ap	Kapha Vardhaka & Vata-pitta hara	Srishta vit-Mutra-(increase in quan-tity of stools & urine
2.	Laghu (Katu)	Vayu, Agni & Akasa	Kapha hara & Vata-pitta vardhaka	Baddha Vit-Mutra (decrease in quan-tity of stools & urine)

---

१. मधुरो लवणाम्लौ च स्निग्धभावात् त्रयो रसाः । वातमूत्रपुरीषाणां प्रायो मोक्षो सुखा मताः ॥
शुक्रहा बद्धविण्मूत्रो विपाको वातलः कटुः । मधुरः सृष्टविण्मूत्रः विपाकः कफशुक्रलः ॥
पित्तकृत् सृष्टविण्मूत्रः पाकोऽम्लः शुक्रनाशनः । तेषां गुरुः स्यान्मधुरः कटुकाम्लावतोऽन्यथा ॥
कटुतिक्तकषायास्तु रूक्षभावात् त्रयो रसाः । दुःखाय मोक्षे दृश्यन्ते वातविण्मूत्ररेतसाम् ॥ (च.सू. २५)

२. गुरुलघुविपाकावुक्तगुणौ । गुरुपाको वातपित्तघ्नः लघुपाकः श्लेष्मघ्नः ।
गुरुपाकः सृष्टविण्मूत्रतया कफोत्क्लेशेन च, लघुर्बद्धविण्मूत्रतया
मारुतकोपनेन च ॥ (सु.सू. ४१)

In this context it was clarified that the Guru and Laghu Vipakas need not be dosha vardhaka and dosha samaka respectively in all cases[1].

Vagbhata considers that Vipaka exhibits its effects similar to those of Rasas e.g. Madhura Rasa properties and actions can be seen with Madhura Vipaka etc[2].

Before the effects of Vipaka are concluded, it is important to know about the degree of variation (Tara-Tama bheda) of Vipaka. According to Charaka there are three degrees of variation for Vipaka[3].

(i) Uttama (superior)

(ii) Madhyama (average)

(iii) Avara/Alpa (inferior)

Gangadhara also mentioned that Gunas like Snigdha, Ruksha etc., will decide the degree of variation of Vipaka.

S.No.	Vipaka	Superior	Average	Inferior
1.	Madhura	Madhura	Amla	Lavana
2.	Katu	Kashaya	Katu	Tikta

6. Means to assess Vipaka

Vipaka is assessed finally after the complete metabolization of the drug and through the final effect of the drug. That means the end phase of biotransformation resulting in ultimate therapeutic effect is the soure to assess Vipaka (Vipaka Upalabdhi Hetu).

Vipaka can not be percieved directly. It can be assessed with the help of inference (and logic). Chakra pani is of the openion that Vipaka shall be assessed even in the absence of Pratyakshatwa (absence of visible proof).

---

१. वर्धनक्षपणप्रशमप्रकोपेषु तयोरनियम: । (र.वै. १ सू. ५३)

* भाष्यं:- यथा-लघुविपाकमुदकं श्लेष्माणं वर्धयति, लघुविपाकं मधु श्लेष्माणं हरतीति ।
तस्मादयमेव गुरुविपाको वर्धन एव, लघुविपाक: शमन एव इति॰ नियमो नास्ति ।

२. रसैरसौ तुल्यफल: । (अ.सं.सू. १७)

३. (i) विपाकलक्षणस्याल्पमध्यभूयिष्ठतां प्रति ।
द्रव्याणां गुणवैशेष्यात्तत्र तत्रोपलक्षयेत् ॥ (च.सू. २६)

(ii) द्रव्यगुणविशेषेण चास्याल्प मध्यभूयस्त्वमुपलक्षयेत् । (अ.सं. सू. १७)

Yogendranath sen also accepted the same view and stated that Vipaka can be determined by means of final therapeutic effect. For example, the effect of food or drug can be finalized by its effect on dosha-dhatu-malas in the form of increase or decrease in their activity.

Sivadas sen further quoted some exceptions and described that Vipaka can not be assessed basing upon Rasa or Virya alone. Some times it must be assessed with out their help also. e.g. Vrishyatwa of Pippali indicate that it under goes Madhura Vipaka; Srishta Vinmutra of Saindhava lavana indicate its Madhura Vipaka etc.

Experimental Model to assess Vipaka[1]

The author proposes an animal model for the assessement or determination of Vipaka of unknown drugs. It will also help to rcassess the Vipaka of classical drugs.

The main parameters shall be (i) measurement of faeces and urine quantities (to assess Badha or Srishta Vinmutra) and (ii) mating behaviour and testicular biopsy of the animals selected for study.

The proposed model consists of two groups of animals (10 each). Preferably albino rats or rabitts may be picked up. One group will be given the drug and the other group is kept as control group. the study should be conducted in the metabolic cages by segregating each animal in individual cages. The quantity of faeces and urine shall be measured everyday for one week or 10 days. The mating behaviour of the animal may also be documented simultaneously or seperately. Afterwards the animal may be sacrificed to study the testicular histology. All these aspects may be compared with the control group.

---

१. (i) विपाक: कर्मनिष्ठया । (च. सू. २६)

(ii) विपाको नित्यपरोक्ष: तत्कार्येणानुमीयते । (चक्रपाणि)

(iii) विपाक: कर्मण: आहारपरिणामकृतस्य निष्ठा निष्पत्ति: दोषशुक्रवृद्धिक्षयलक्षणा, तया उपलभ्यते । (योगेनद्रनाथ:)

(iv) अथं च विपाकाधेयो रसो न रसेन्द्रियग्राह्य:, किन्तु तत्तत्कार्येणैवोन्नीयते- यथा कटुरसाया उष्णवीर्याया अपि शुण्ठ्या वृष्यत्वेन मधुर: पाकोऽनुमीयते, तथा लवणस्य सृष्टविण्मूत्रत्वेन मधुर: पाक उन्नीयते, तथा तिक्तकषाययोर्बद्धविण्मूत्रतया कटुपाक उन्नीयते । (गङ्गाधर:)

(v) (विद्यात्) विपाकं द्रव्याणां कर्मण: परिनिष्ठया । (अ.सं.सू.१७)

* इन्दुकर:- विपाक विशेषं तु कर्मण: तत्कृतस्य परिनिष्ठया निष्पत्ते: दोषवृद्धिक्षय विशेषेण विद्यात् ।

The drugs which increased the quantity of urine, faeces and spermetogenesis is may be labled as Madhura Vipaka and vice verse may be labed as Katu Vipaka.

[The author requests the knowledgeable section of readers to pick-up this model and study the Vipaka of Ayurvedic herbs].

7. Difference between Rasa and Vipaka

It is already discussed that Vipaka is the final out come of Rasa transformation inside the body. Thence a question may arise that-when Vipaka is dependent of rasa what is the necessity to explain both the entities seperately? We find the following points which differentiate both of them[1].

(i) dissimilar characters or properties.

(ii) difference in the time taken for their actions.

(iii) difference in their therapeutic effects.

(iv) dissimilarity in their perception.

Rasa	Vipaka
1. It is known by means of Rasanendriya (tongue)	1. It is known by means of its final effect on the body.
2. Quick and local effects are seen.	2. Delayed and systemic effects are seen.
3. It can be directly detectable	3. It will be detected by inference.

P.V. Sharmaji is of the openion that Rasa mainly effects the mind (Manas) and Vipaka mainly effects the body (sareera). This view may not stand food for logic and scientific discussion since Medhya drugs which are used in psychiatric conditions are acting both on mind and body e.g., Guchi with Madhura paka and Manduka parni with Tikta Rasa are both acting as Medhya Rasayanas. Both the drugs are acting upon psyche and soma.

---

१. भिन्नलक्षणत्वात्; आस्वादग्राह्यो रसः, परिणामलक्षणो विपाक इति । विपाकस्य मधुररता कथमास्वाद्यते? यद्यास्वाद्येत, रसलक्षणत्वात् रस एवेति विपाकाभावः । यदि नास्वाद्येत, कथं भवता मधुरं पच्यते इत्युपलब्धमित्युक्तं भवति। (भाष्यं- र.वै.४ सू. ३१)

Dr. K. Nisteswar in his text on Dravya guna differed with P.V. Sharmaji's view. He also disagreed with the concept of local action and systemic action of Rasa and Vipaka respectively. But the author is of the openion that Rasa usually reflects the local effects of a drug than the systemic effects. Field of action of Rasa is limited to Rasanendriya (tongue) only. However, if the drug is once administered to a man it crosses the field of tongue and under goes the conversion into Virya and Vipaka. Thence some of the system effects are attributed to Rasa.

8. Superiority of Vipaka

Among the constituents of a dravya, it is Vipaka that is responsible for various pharmacological actions. This again depends upon proper or improper transformation. If a drug is properly metabolized it produces good effects and improperly metaboliozed drug is responsible for ill effects (or side-effects). These two properties are denoted as 'Samyak Vipaka' and 'Mithya Vipaka' by Sushrita.

Some scholars may consider the former as Samana pratyarabdhatwa and the later as Vichitra pratyayarabdhatwa. For example, Chitraka which under goes Katu Vipaka according to its Rasa, Guna & Vipaka will be responsible for Baddha vit-mutra (constipating and anti-diuretic properties). While, Pippali which under goes Madhura Vipaka irrespective of its Rasa, Guna & Virya will act as Sukra Vardhana (spermatogenic[1]).

---

१. (i) विपाकस्य प्राधान्यं प्रत्यके ब्रुवते । (र.वै. १ सू. १४१)

(ii) नेत्याहुरन्ये, विपाकः प्रधानमिति । कस्मात् ? सम्यङ् मिथ्याविपाकत्वात् ; इह सर्वद्रव्याण्यभ्यवहृतानि सम्यङ् मिथ्याविपक्कानि गुणं दोषं वा जनयन्ति । (सु.सू. ४०)

* चक्रपाणिः- सम्यक् विपक्कानि गुणं, मिथ्याविपक्वानि दोषं जनयन्ति सम्यक्पाकः समेनाग्निना, मिथ्यापाकस्तु हीनातिपाकरूपो यथाक्रमं मन्देन तीक्ष्णेन वाऽग्निना क्रियते ।.......किंवा सम्यक् पाको द्रव्यानुगुणः पाकः यथा चित्रकः........मिथ्यापाको तद्द्रव्यगुणविसदृशः पाकः यथा पिप्पल्यः । तेन..........यथोक्तं गुणं दोषं वा करोति ।

** हारणचन्द्रः- अत्र द्रव्यगुणानुरूपोनिष्ठापाकः सम्यग्निपाक उच्यते, तद्विपरीतस्तु मिथ्याविपाकः। तयोराद्यः कटुकश्चित्रकः पाकेऽपि कटुक इन्यादौ, द्वितीयस्तु कटुका पिप्पली पाके मधुरा इत्येवमादौ बुभुत्सितत्यः । गुणं दोषं वा इति वा शब्दश्चार्थे, सम्यग्विपक्वानि मिथ्याविपक्वानि वा गुणं दोषं च जनयन्ति, मिथ्याविपक्वा पिप्पली य शुक्रवर्धनादिरूपं गुण प्राक्स्वेदजननादिरूपं दोषं च जनयति । यद्वा अग्निसाम्यात्र हीनं नापि चाधिकं निष्ठापाकः । तत्र सम्यग्विपाके यथोक्ता गुणाः मिथ्याविपाके चामादिदोषाः संभवन्तीत्यायुर्वेदविदो भाषन्ते ।

The superiority of Vipaka is explained on the basis of four points by Bandhanta Nagarjuna. They are:

(1) Nimittatwa: ***(responsible factor)***

Stimulation or supression of the doshas is under the control of Vipaka. Hence its is important[1].

(2) Dhatupadehat: ***(tissue construction)***

Tissue construction or building up various tissues of the body is possible through digestion/metabolism. Therefore Vipaka is important[2].

(3) Vipakākshepatwa: ***(dependency for theraputic effects)***

All the food and drug materials will depend upon proper and improper Vipaka to exhibit either good effects or ill effects. Hence Vipaka is important[3].

(4) Sastra Pramanya: ***(emphasis by classics)***

Classical texts/treatises quote Vipaka as an important entity of dravya. Hence it is superior[4].

❋

Further Readings on Vipaka

1. Dave Navin H.; "Vipako Karma Nishtaya: Ek Prayogik Adhyayan". Dept. of D.G., IPGTR, G.A.U., Jamnagar, 1978. (M.D Thesis).
2. Vohara V.M.; "Vipaka Vijnana", Dept. of D.G., IPGTR, G.A.U. Jamnagar, 1958. (M.D Thesis).

---

१. तन्निमित्तत्वात् प्रशमनवर्धनयोः । (र.वै. १ सू. १४२)

२. धातुपदेहात् । (र.वै. १ सू. १४३)

३. (i) विपाकाक्षेपत्वादितरेषां, प्रायशोविपाकसादगुण्ये च गुणवतामप्यदोषात् । (र.वै.१ सू. १४५)
(ii) विपाकवैगुण्ये गुणवतामपि दोषात् । (र.वै. १ सू. १४५)

४. शास्त्रप्रामाण्यात् । (र.वै. १ सू. १४६)

Chapter-VII
Concept of Virya

1. Etymology of Virya

Virya term is derived from the Sanskrit root 'Vir' meaning that which is powerful or potent (Vikranta).

Acharya P.V. Sharmaji quoted Virya as the factor which is capable of or which responsible for producing drug action[1].

Its equivilant is 'Potency' in modern pharmacology. Potency is the word derived from Latin term *Potentia* meaning that strength of a medicine or strenght or force or power.

2. Characteristics and Nature of Virya

Veerya is characterized by the drug action. Because all types of drug actions are under the control of virya only[2].

Vriddha Vagbhata considered the most potent qualities of a drug as Virya. Other ordinary qualities can not be treated as Virya[3].

Charaka presicely quoted Virya as the factor which will perform the pharmacological action. This is the main characteristic of Virya[4].

Yadvji Trikamji Acharya accepted Virya as the "active principle" of a dravya. Acharya Priya vrata sharmaji considered active principle as Virya adhishtana.

Actually Vagbhata mentioned four points in support of his Virya vāda[5].

---

१. (i) 'वीर विक्रान्तौ' । (द्र.मै.सि.)
   (ii) वीरयते विक्रान्त: कर्मसमर्थो भवति अनेन इति वीर्यम् । (द्र.गु.वि.)

२. वीर्यं तु क्रियते येन या क्रिया । ना वीर्यं कुरूते किञ्चित् सर्वा वीर्य कृता क्रिया: ॥ (च.सू. २६)

३. गुर्वाद्या वीर्यमुच्यन्ते शक्तिमन्तोऽन्यथा गुणा: । पर सामर्थ्य हीनत्वात् गुणा एवेतरे गुणा: ॥ (अ.सं.सू. १७)

४. येन कुर्वन्ति तत् वीर्यम् । (च.सू. २६)

५. वीर्यं शक्ति:, सा च पृथिव्यादीनां भूतानां य: सारभागस्तदतिशयरूपा बोध्या ।
   सा च द्विविधा चिन्त्याचिन्त्य क्रिया हेतुत्वेन...... परमार्थत: शक्तिरेव वीर्यं सा पुनर्बलवत् क्रिया निर्वर्तन क्षमा रसादिनाऽयोन्निरूपाधिरिति तस्या: शीतोष्णादयो गुणा: उपाधित्वेनाङ्गीकृता: ।(शिवदास:)

(i) **Samagra guna Saratwa**— (most potent qualities) There are eight potent qualities which are known as Viryas.

(ii) **Saktyat Karshata**— (powerful action): They provide more powerful actions than Rasa etc.

(iii) **Vyavahāra Mukhyatwa**— (important in utility) They have more important in utility compared to other qualities.

(iv) **Bāhulyata**— (abundency) They are much abundent in dravya compared to other qualities.

Chakrapani in one context quoted Virya as two types viz, Sahaja (Natural) and Kritrima (Artificial). Though there are no classical examples for them the individual Viryas of Guduchi and Guduchi Sattwa; Palasa and Palasa kshara etc., may be the suitable examples.

Virya has been assessed and studies from various angles in the modern times. Some of the findings are as following

(1) Action of Ushna & Seeta virya drugs on skeletal muscle

Total 24 drugs of 12 each belonging to Ushna and Seeta viryas have been selected at random. Their aqueous extracts (10% water infusion) were tested for their activity against contractions of frog skeletal muscle (Frog Rectus Abdominis) by using Burn model (1954).

Two similar dose response curves with Acetylecholine were taken (1r, 2r doses) before and after injecting i ml of 10% solution of the trial drug.

The drugs Kutaja (Seeta virya) and Ati visha (Ushna virya) have shown complete blockade of (100% inhibition) Ash induced contraction. Jatiphala and Pushkara mula have shown maximum potentiation (73.3% & 70.5%). Useera and Maha Bala from Seeta virya group potentiated them.

However, statistical analysis showed insignificant inhibition of both the viryas. There fore the skeletal muscle experiment does not reveal any specificity about the nature of Ushna and Seeta Virya drugs (Nisteswar K. et. al.).

(2) Effect of Ushna & Seeta Virya drugs on frog heart muscle

The aqueous extracts of 16 Ushna and 16 Seeta Virya drugs were screened on 32 healthy frog hearts. Conventional method for this experiment was followed as suggested by Burn (1952). The effect of Ushna and Seeta Virya drugs in different doses (0.2ml and 0.4ml) was assessed on the basis of heart rate (Chronotropic activity) and amplitude (Inotropic activity of isolated frog heart during and after perfusion).

Both groups have exhibited positive as well as negative inotropic and chronotropic activities. However, large number of drugs have shown positive chronotropic activity from Seeta Virya groups at 0.2 ml dose as compared to Ushna Virya group. Where as large number of Ushna Virya drugs exhibited negative inotropic activity at the dose level of 0.2 ml and 0.4 ml in comparision with Seeta Virya group.

Seeta Virya group has shown significant decrease of amplitude ($P < 0.05$) at the dose of 0.4 ml while Ushna Virya drugs have shown significant depressant action at 0.2 ml and 0.4 ml doses ($P < 0.01$).

It is evident that more depressant effect on amplitude was exercised by Ushna Virya group in comparision with Seeta Virya group. Both Seeta and Ushna Virya drugs have shown insignificant decrease of heart rate.

Comparision of Seeta and Ushna Virya drugs specifically mentioned to have some effects on heart (Hridaya) like Vāsa, Bhavya, Gokshura, Apamarga, Bakuchi and Jātiphala does not very much from the above. Hence the action of Ushna and Seeta Virya drugs can not be associated with positive and negative chronotropic and Ionotropic effect since both the groups have not shown a specific action on frog heart rate and amplitude (Nisteswar K. et al.).

(3) Effect of Seeta and Ushna Virya drugs on B.M.R.

Two Seeta Virya drugs namely Yashtimadhu and Shatavari, and two Ushna Virya drugs namely Chitraka and Jatiphala have been taken for this study. In healthy volunteers initially B.M.R. was recorded with Mc Kisson Metaboler. Then the drug was administered three times for only one day (Chitraka and Jatiphala 2 gm each and Yashtimadhu and Shatavari 5 gm each).

Each drug was studied in six healthy volunteers for each group. the administration of Seeta virya drugs increased the B.M.R. A significant increase ($P < 0.05$) has been observed with Yashti, while increase in B.M.R. with Shatavari is not very significant.

The action of Ushna Virya drugs is quite opposite i.e., they bring about a decrease in B.M.R. after administration. Both Chitraka and Jatiphala have shown a very significant action ($P < 0.05$).

Therefore Seeta and Ushna Viryas, which represents the Saumyatwa and Agneyatwa of a drug or food, may be responsible for synthesizing or metabolizing the Dhatus due to their Santarpaka or Apataspaka actions. (Nisteswar K et al.).

(4) Study of Virya vis-a-vis 'pH' value of Drugs

Total 25 Ushna and 25 Seeta Virya drugs have been screened for 'PH' value in cold water and hot water with PH water. 10 gms of each drug was soaked in 100 ml of distilled water and kept for one hour. After one hour the 'pH' of the sample was tested. Then the sample was kept on water both for 30 minutes and again 'pH' was recorded.

In the end all the screened drugs have shown acidic reaction. From Ushna Virya group, drugs like Sirisha, Sunthi, Talisa patra, Syonaka and Guduchi have shown weak acidic reaction while Vāsa, Useera and Rakta Chandana have shown weak acidic reaction from Seeta virya group. Haritaki and Āmalaki from Ushna and Seeta Virya groups respectively have exhibited strong acidic reactions. The decrease in 'pH' values in hot water was observed with most of the drugs.

It is evident from the present study that Ushna and Seeta Virya drugs have not exhibited specific difference in 'pH' values (Nisteswar K and Dhayani S.C.).

(5) Viryam tu Karma Nishtaya

Dr. K. Nisteswar proposed this denovo concept. He is of the openion that "Rasa, Guna, Virya, Vipaka and Prabhava, reside in the dravya and exercise their own action. Rasa of substances are considered to be extremely susceptable to changes during the process of Kāyāgni pāka. Vipaka described interms of Rasa is the out come of highly specialized reactions implied in Kayagnipaka. The end products of these Rasas are described as Visishta Rasa and the action performed by these Rasas is related to their gunas. Out of 20 gunas described by Acharyas of Ayurveda, considerable significance has been attached to the eight gunas as they are deemed to be effective in the performance of actions. Though Acharyas have mentioned that the gunas attributed to dravya only and by Sahacharya (co-existance) it appears that they are Gunas of Rasa, they described the action of Rasa and Vipaka in terms of Gunas. The two principles viz., Virya (potent gunas) and Prabhava (inexplicable in nature) only should be considered as the principles of durg action. Virya of a dravya should be assessed by Nishta karma (Viryam tu Karmanishtaya) on dosha, dhatu and malas.

The above studies will delineate the regarding analytical study of Virya from various aspects. However virya may not be assessed through Nishta Karma. Some of the studies proved that the effect of Seeta and Ushna Virya dravyas could not prove significant different on skeletal and heart muscles. Only B.M.R. studies have shown some encouraging results in support of Seeta and Ushna virya concept.

The exothermic and endothermic reactions in vitro with Ushna and Seeta virya drugs have been reported (Shukla D.K. et al., 1979). This may be one of the correct approaches towards the assessement of Virya.

According to Dwarakanath (1954) Ushna Virya represents kinetic energy derived from food substances in bio-chemical reactions, while Seeta Virya represents potential energy stored in different tissues either as a part of their structure or as a reserve fuel depot.

If virya can be responsible for the final effect of the durg then the effect of Ushna and Seeta Virya drugs on skeletal and heart muscle must be specific and significant.

After having these discussion, the author would like to conclude that Virya means the pharmacologically active ingredient of the drug.

It will show the effect at the site of action and as long as the peak plasma levels are maintained. It will be more appropriate to equate it with 'potency' of a drug.

Estimation of virya: (Sukla D., 1978)

		Ushna virya		**Seeta virya**
1. Reaction with distilled water	-	Exothermic	-	Endothermic
2. Reaction with artificial gastric juice	-	Exothermic	-	Endothermic
3. Appetite	-	Increases	-	Decreases
4. Sleep	-	Decreases	-	Increases
5. Blood pressure	-	Increases	-	Decreases
6. Stools	-	Hard	-	Soft
7. Urine	-	Decreases	-	Increases
8. B.M.R.	-	Increases	-	Decreases

It may be concluded that Rasa Jnana occurs through Nipata; Vipaka Jnana occurs through final action (Nishta karma) and Virya denotes both these actions. Gunas may be explained along with Rasas and Virya may be explained along with Vipaka. The relation between guna and virya will be the same as that is between Rasa and vipaka.

3. Analysis of Virya and different Concept of Virya

Virya concept is on of the frequently debated aspects of Ayurveda. Some times these are controversial approaches regarding virya. Therefore the author wants to discuss the Virya concept of different Acharyas of Ayurveda from ancient times to modern times. The author feel fortunate to have repeated discussions on Virya with his most respected teacher Dr. Nisteswar. Lecturer, Govt. Ayurvedic College, Vijayawada who is the only person in the comtemporary Ayurvedic scholars who had maximum publications and studies on Virya. All those aspects will be discussed with reasoning here.

Commenting on Charaka's view on Virya (i.e., Virya is the character responsible for drug action), Chakarapani proposed that Veerya means a Sakti (power or potency) but not Guna (quality).

Suśruta and Vagbhata have considered Virya as the most potent quality. This view reflects the over the concept of Charaka and Chakrapāni.

Badhanta Nagarjuna mentioned Karma as the characteristic feature of Virya.

Sivadas sen accepted Virya as Sakti and considered it as the essence of Parchabhutas. According to him Virya is two types viz. Chintya and Achintya. Though virya is a type of potency it will possess certain qualities like Seeta, Ushna etc[1].

4. Number of Viryas

The author noticed variability among the scholars of modern times regarding Virya classification. Different openions have been expressed by different scholars.

For example:

(i) Yadavji Trikamji Acharya's view:

- Virya
  - Sakti Virya vāda (Bahu vidha Virya vāda)
  - Pāribhashika Virya vāda (Guna Virya vāda)
    - Ashtavidha Virya vāda
    - Dwi vidha Virya vāda

* Note— He seperately mentioned Nagarjuna's concept on Virya apart from the above classification.

(ii) Acharya Priyavrata Sharma's veiw:

- Virya
  - Guna Virya vāda
    - Sakti matra Virya vāda [Charaka]
    - Paribhashika Virya vāda [Suśruta & Vagbhata]
  - Karma Virya vāda
  - Dravya Virya vāda
    - Chintya (Virya)
    - Achintya (Prabhava)

---

१. समग्रगुणसारेषु शक्त्युत्कर्षविवर्तिषु व्यवहाराय मुख्यत्वात्
बह्वग्रग्रहणादपि अतश्च विपरीतत्वात् संभवत्यपि नैव सा ॥ (अ.हृ.सू. ९)

(iii) Dr. Sivcharan Dhyaniji's view:

Infact it is Sri Dhyaniji who correctly identified different classifications of Virya.

Virya

Sakti Virya vada	Guna Virya vada	Karma Virya vada
(Chintya Virya)	(Paribhashika Virya vada)	

Finally, the auther is to conclude that there are three classifications available in the classics in relation to Virya number.

(1) Sakti Virya vāda (Dravya virya vāda)

(2) Pāribhashika Virya vāda (Guna virya vāda)

(3) Karma Virya vāda

(1) Sakti Virya Vāda

All the drug actions are believed to be the out come of Sakti (power and potency) of a dravya. This school of thought is otherwise known as Bahu-Virya Vāda (concept of multiple viryas).

Charaka accepted Shakti as virya. He believes that the constituents of dravya (i.e., Rasa, Vipaka etc.), will exhibit their therapeutic effects by means of Shakti alone[1].

Vriddha Vagbhata identified 'Sakti matra Virya vāda' as classical. Both Indukara and Hemadri have considered Virya as innumerable[2].

Chakrapani prescicely described that Virya is nothing but Sakti (potency) of a draya through which the drug action is possible[3].

Sivadas sen mentioned Virya as the ultimate factor representing the Pancha bhutas in the form of Shakti. This Shakti may be Chintya or Achintya. The former will be considered as Virya and the later as Prabhava.

---

१. ना वीर्यं कुरुते किञ्चित् सर्वा वीर्य कृता क्रियाः । (च.सू. २६)

२. गुर्वाद्याः वीर्यमुच्यन्ते शक्तिमन्तोऽन्यथा गुणाः ।
परसामर्थ्यहीनत्वात् गुणा एवेतरे गुणाः ॥ (अ.सं.सू. १७)

३. अयं च वीर्यशब्दः पारिभाषिकवीर्यवचनो न भवति, किन्तु शक्तिमात्रवचनः, तेन प्रभावरसादयः सर्व एव स्वकार्यं कुर्वन्तः शक्तिपर्यायरूपवीर्यवाच्या इति ज्ञेयाः । (चक्रपाणि-च.सू. २६)

This theory is otherwise called as 'Dravya Virya vāda also' under this view Virya is not classified into specific number[1].

(2) Pāribhastika Virya Vāda

The most potent qualities among Gurvadi gunas shall be considered as Viryas. This school of thought is also known as 'Guna Virya vāda'. Suśruta and Laghu Vagbhata proposed this view.

Vriddha Vagbhata denoted Guna Virya vāda as Loukikam[2]. The Guna Virya vāda is in turn sub-divided into two theories viz.,

(i) Dwividha Virya vāda (2 viryas concept)

(ii) Ashtavidha Virya vāda (8 viryas concept)

(i) Dwividha Virya vāda– The followers of this view propose that all the dravyas are made up of Panchabhutas and they are in turn classified as Agni (heat) and Soma (cold). Thence the Viryas are also two types viz., Ushna (hot) and Seeta (cold) respectively. This view is strongiy supported by Sushrita and Vagbhata[3].

(ii) Ashta vidha Virya vāda– This school of thought is mainly accepted by Charak. But Sushita and Vagbhata have also mentioned it but not emphasized over it. According to this Guru, Laghu, Seeta, Ushna, Snigdha, Ruksha, Mridu, Tikshna are proposed as eight viryas[4]. Sushrita considered Visada and Pichchila in place of Guru and Laghu.

---

१. शक्तिमात्रं तु वीर्यं स्यादिति केचिद् बुधा विदु: । तन्मते द्रव्यरसयो: पाकस्य च गुणस्य च ॥
मृद्वादे; स्वक्रियोत्पादे शक्तिवीर्यमिति स्थिति: ॥ (द्र.गु.वि.)

२. गुर्वादीनां वीर्यसंज्ञा विशिष्टनाम्नायविहिताऽपि लौकिकीति समुद्भाव्यते । (अ.सं.सू. १७)

३. (i) ....केचिद् (वीर्यं) द्विविधमास्थिता: । शीतोष्णमिति......। (च.सू. २६)
(ii) उष्णशीतगुणोत्कर्षात्तत्र वीर्यं द्विधा स्मृतम् ॥ (अ.हृ.सू.१और अ.सं.सू.१)
(iii) तच्च वीर्यं द्विविधं-उष्णं, शीतं च, अग्निषोमीयत्वाज्जगत: । (सु.सू.४०)
(iv) उष्णं शीतं द्विधैवान्ये वीर्यमाचक्षतेऽपि च ॥
नानात्मकमपि द्रव्यमग्नीषोमौ महाबलौ । (अ.हृ.सू.९)

४. (i) मृदु-तीक्ष्ण-गुरू-लघु-स्निग्ध-रूक्ष-उष्ण-शीतलम् ।
वीर्यं अष्टविधं.. ॥ (च.सू.२६)
(ii) केचिदष्टविधमाहु:-शीतं, उष्णं, स्निग्धं, रूक्षं, विशदं, पिच्छिलं, मृदु, तीक्ष्णं चेति ।
एतानि खलु वीर्याणि स्वबलगुणोत्कर्षाद्रसमभिभूयात्मकर्म कुर्वन्ति । (सु.सू.४०)
(iii) वीर्यं पुनर्वदन्त्येके गुरू-स्निग्धं-हिमं-मृदु ।
लघु-रूक्ष-उष्ण-तीक्ष्णं च तदेवं मतमष्टधा ॥ (अ.हृ.सू.९)

But the commentator on Suśruta Samhita accepted Guru and Laghus only as Virya instead of Visada & Pichchila.

(3) Karma Vriya Vāda

This concept is intitially propsed by Badhanta Nagarjuna and later supported by Bhavamishra and Nimi. Nagarjuna quoted that Karma is the characteristic feature of Virya[1].

He further added that dravya do not perform any function in the absence of Virya even though Rasa and Guna are present. Even Mantras (hymns) perform some Karmas without the help of Rasa and Guna. He described that Neela, Neela tara, Neela tama are different stages of a matter where in 'Neelatwa' is the common factor. Similarly, Gunas will always remain as Gunas and can never act as Viryas. Therefore Virya should be defined on the basis of Karma only.

Bhavamishra quotes special action of a Dravya as Virya e.g. Yashtimadhu which is Madhura Rasa, Snigdha & Seeta Guna acts as Sandhana kara while Ksheera with similar qualities acts as Sramsana. It denotes Achintya Virya concept[2].

Nimi mentioned about 15 types of Karmanya Gunas or Viryas on the basis of Bhautika Sanghatana:

1.	Adhobhaga hara	-	Ap+Prithvi
2.	Urdhwa bhaga hara	-	Agni + Vayu
3.	Ubhaya bhaga hara	-	Prithvi + Agni+Vayu
4.	Sangrahi	-	Prithi + Vayu
5.	Samsamana	-	Vayu + Ap + Prithvi
6.	Deepana	-	Prithvi + Vayu
7.	Jivaniya	-	Prithvi + Ap
8.	Praṇaghna	-	Vayu + Agni
9.	Mādana	-	
10.	Seetikaraṇa	-	Ap

१. कर्मलक्षणं वीर्यम् । (र.वै.सू. १/१६९)

२. मधुररसं स्निग्धं शीतं च यष्टिमधुकं संदधाति, क्षीरं च तादृगेव स्रंसयतीति विशेष: । अस्य कर्मविशेषस्य दर्शनादेतस्माद् रसगुणाख्यात् कारणमन्यद् विद्यते । अस्य विशेषस्य साधकं तद् वीर्यमिति जानीया इति । (भा.प्र)

11.	Sothakara	-	Prithvi + Ap
12.	Sothaghna	-	Akasa + Vayu
13.	Pāchana	-	Agni
14.	Dāraṇa	-	Vayu + Agni
15.	Rōpaṇa	-	Prithvi + Ap

(5) Pancha bhoutikatwa of Virya

Suśruta mentioned about the composition of panchabhutas in Virya[1].

1.	Teekshna and Ushna	-	Agni bhuta
2.	Gura and Seeta	-	Jala bhuta
3.	Snigdha	-	Jala bhuta
4.	Mridu	-	Jala & Ākasa bhutas
5.	Ruksha	-	Vayu bhuta
6.	Laghu	-	Agni, Ākasa & Vayu bhutas.

He further described two types of Viryas in the following manner:

(i) Pichchila Virya - Jala bhuta

(ii) Visada Virya - Prithvi & Vayu bhuta

(6) Functions of Virya

Various effects and functions of eight Viryas are tabulated below-

S.N.	Virya	Effect on doshas	Systemic effects
1.	Ushna[2]	Vāta hara, Kapha hara, and Pitta vardhaka	Deepana, Pachana, Dāha Janana, Murchana, Swedana, Vamana, Virechana, Vilayana,

---

१. अम्बुभूमिजमधोभागं तेजोवायुजमूर्ध्वगम् । तथैवोभयतोभागं मह्यग्न्यनिलजं मतम् ॥
संग्राहिकं विजानीयात् पृथिव्यनिलसंभवम् । वायुसोममहीजातं तथा संशमनं विदुः ॥
पृथिव्यनिलबाहुल्याद्दीपनं परिचक्ष्महे । पृथिव्यपां गुणैरुक्तं जीवनीयमिति स्थितिः ॥
वाय्वनलस्वभावाच्च प्राघ्नं मदनं मतम् । प्राणघ्नं तीव्रभावात्तु दोषधातुप्रकोपनम् ॥
मदनं चलधातुत्वाद् दोषकोपनमेव तु । अपां गुणबहुत्वात्तु शीतीकरणमिष्यते ॥ (निमिः)

२. (i) तीक्ष्णोष्णावाग्नेयौ, गुरुशीताम्बुगुणभूयिष्ठौ अम्बुगुणभूयिष्ठः स्नेहः, तोयाकाशभूयिष्ठं मृदुत्वं, वायुगणभूयिष्ठं रौक्ष्यम्, अग्न्याकाशसमीरणभूयिष्ठं लघुत्वम् ॥ (सु.सू. ४१)
(ii) शीतपिच्छिलाम्बुगणभूयिष्ठौ, क्षितिसमीरणभूयिष्ठं वैशद्यम् । (सू.सू.)

			Bhrama, Trishna, Janana, Āsu paka, Avrishya.
2.	Seeta[1]	Pitta hara Vata-kapha vardhaka	Prahladana, Vishyandana, Sthirikarana, Prasadana, Kledana, Jivaniya, Sthambhana, Rakta prasadana, Balyam.
3.	Snighda[2]	Vāta hara, Kapha vardhaka	Snehana,Brimhana, Santar-pana,Vajikarana, Vayah-sthapana.
4.	Ruksha[3]	Vata vardhaka Kapha-pitta hara	Sangrahana, Peedana, Virukshana, Ropana.
5.	Guru[4]	Kapha vardhaka Vata hara	Upalepana, Brimhana, Balya
6.	Laghu[5]	Kapha hara Vata vardhaka	Lekhana, Langhana, Dhatu kshaya
7.	Mridu[6]	Pitta hara	Rakta prasadana, Mamsa prasadana
8.	Tikshna[7]	Kapha hara	Sangrahi, Āchushana, Avadarana, Sravaṇa

---

१.(i) तत्र कर्माण्यप्युष्णस्य दहनपाचनमूर्च्छनस्वेदनवमनविरेचनानि......उष्णस्निग्धौ वातघ्नौ ।(सु.सू.४१)
(ii) तत्रोष्णं.......विलयनानिलकफशमनानि कोरति । (अ.सं.सू. १७)
(iii) तत्रोष्णं भ्रमतृड्ग्लानिस्वेददाहाशुपाकिता: । शमं च वातकफयो: करोति । (अ.हृ.सू. ९)
(iv) उष्णं कफवातहरं पित्तकरं लघु अवृष्यं च ॥ (द्रव्यगुणसंग्रह:)
२.(i) शीतस्य प्रह्लादन-विष्यन्दन-स्थिरीकरण-प्रसादन-क्लेदन-जीवनानि । (सु.सू. ४१)
(ii) शीतं ह्लादनस्तम्भनजीवनरक्तपित्तप्रसादनादीनि । (अ.सं.सू. १७)
(iii) शीतं कफमारुतकृद्वीर्यं गुरू पित्तनाशनं बल्यम् । (द्रव्यगुणसंग्रह:)
३.(i) स्निग्धस्य स्नेहन-बृंहण-सन्तर्पण-वाजीकरण-वय:स्थापनानि । (सु.सू. ४१)
(ii) उष्णास्निग्धौ वातघ्नौ । (सु.सू. ४१)
४.(i) रूक्षस्य अनिलवृद्धि-संग्रहण-पीडन-विरूक्षणोपरोपणानि । (सु.सू. ४१)
(ii) तीक्ष्णरूक्षविशदा: श्लेष्मघ्ना: । (सु.सू. ४१)
५. लघुतीक्ष्णरूक्षा: श्लेष्मघ्ना: । (सु.सू. ४१)
६.(i) शीतमृदुपिच्छिला: पित्तघ्ना: । (सु.सू. ४१)
(ii) मृदो रक्तमांसप्रसादनसुस्पर्शनानि । (सु.सू. ४१)
७.(i) लघुतीक्ष्णरूक्षा: श्लेष्मघ्ना: । (सु.सू. ४१)
(ii) तीक्ष्णस्य संग्रहाचूषणावदारणस्रावणानि । (सु.सू. ४१)

9.	Visada[1]	Kapha hara	Kledachushana, Virukshana, Uparohana
10.	Pichchila[2]	Kapha vardhaka	Upalepana, Purana, Brimhana, Samsleshara, Vajikarana.

7. Causes of Virya Perception (Veeray Upalabdhi)

Virya can be perceived either by Nipata (by means of external contact with the body) or Adhirasa (by means of internal contact i.e., with site of action). While explaining this Chakrapani quoted that certain drugs may act by means of Nipata-Azdhivasa also[3].

S.N.	Example	Virya	Site of aciton	Type of observation
i.	Ānupa mamsa	Ushna Virya	Adhivāsa	through inference (Anumana Pramana)
ii.	Maricha	Tikshna Virya	Nipata	through direct per ception (Pratyaksha Pramana)
iii.	Maricha	UshnaVirya	Nipata + Adhivasa	Pratyaksha + Anumana

Chakrapani quoted few more examples on peception of Virya.

(a) Seeta Virya of Saindhava lavana and Ushna Virya of Ānupa mamsa may be percieved indirectly i.e., through inference.

(b) Teekshna Virya of Rajika (mustard) is directly pervieved through Ghrana (nose).

(c) Pichchila, Visada, Snigdha, Ruksha etc, are percieved by means of Chakshu & Sparsa (visual & sensory organs).

---

१. (i) तीक्ष्णरूक्षविशदा: श्लेष्मघ्ना: । (सू.सू. ४१)
(ii) विशदस्य क्लेदाचूषणविरूक्षणोपरोहणानि । (सु.सू. ४१)

२. पिच्छिलस्योपलेपनपूरणबृंहणसंश्लेषणवाजीकरणानि । (सु.सू. ४१)

३. वीर्यं यावदधीवासान्निपाताच्चोपलभ्यते ॥ (च.सू. २६)

* चक्रपाणि:- किञ्चिद् वीर्यमधीवासादुपलभ्यते, यथा आनूपमांसादेरुष्णत्वं, किञ्चिच्च,, निपातादेव लभ्यते यथा मरीचादीनां तीक्ष्णत्वादि, किञ्चिन्न निपाताधीवासाभ्यां यथा मरीचादीनामेव । एतेन रस: प्रत्यक्षेर्णेव; विपाकस्तु नित्यपरोक्ष: तत्कार्येणानुमीयते, वीर्यं तु किञ्चिदनुमानेन; यथा सैन्धवमतं शैत्यं, आनूपमांसगतमौष्यं वा, किञ्चिच्च वीर्यं प्रत्यक्षेणैव, यथा राजाकागतं तैक्ष्ण्यं, घ्राणेन, पिच्छिल-विशदस्निग्धरूक्षादय: चक्षुस्पर्शनाभ्यां निश्चीयन्त इति वाक्यार्थ: ।

Sushrita elaborately discussed regarding the type of perception of different viryas.

They are:

Mridu, Seeta & Ushna Viryas	-	Sparsa grahya (known by touch)
Pichchala & Visada Viryas	-	Chakshu & Sparsa grahya (known by vision and touch)
Snigdha & Ruksha Viryas	-	Chakshu grahya (known by vision)
Tikshna Virya	-	Mukha duhkhotpādana (known through its severity or pungency on taste)[1].

8. General Principles and Exceptions of Virya *(Virya Nirdharana)*

As already discussed it is possible to assess or confirm the Gunas of certain dravyas on the basis of their Rasas. Generally Madhura Rasa and Vipaka dravyas are expected to be Seeta Virya in nature; Amla Rasa and Vipaka Dravyas are expected to be Ushna Virya in nature etc. Some of the examples are as following[2].

1. Shatavari	-	Madhura Rasa	-	Madhura Vipaka	-	Seeta Virya
2. Chitraka	-	Katu Rasa	-	Katu Vipaka	-	Ushna Virya
3. Kanjika	-	Amla Rasa	-	Amla Vipaka	-	Ushna Virya

These are all the examples of Samana pratyayarabdha dravyas or Prakriti sama Samaveta dravyas.

On the other hand there are a group of drugs which will not yield Virya in accordance with Rasa etc. These unpredictable Viryas are known as Āchintya Viryas or Prabhava. Charaka quoted the following exceptions to the general rules[3].

१. तेषां मृदुशीतोष्णाः स्पर्शग्राह्याः, पिच्छिलविशदौ चक्षुःस्पर्शाभ्यां, स्निग्धरूक्षौ चक्षुषा, तीक्ष्णो मुखे दुःखोत्पादनेन । (सु.सू. ४१)

२. शीतं वीर्येण यद्द्रव्यं मधुरं रसपाकयोः । तयोरम्लं यदुष्णं च यद्द्रव्यं कटुकं तयोः ॥
तेषां रसोपदेशेन निर्देश्यो गुणसंग्रहः । वीर्यतोऽविपरीतानां पाकतश्चोपदेक्ष्यते ॥
यथा पयो यथा सर्पिर्यथा च चव्यचित्रकौ । (च.सू. २६)

३. मधुरं किञ्चिदुष्णं स्यात् कषायं तिक्तमेव च । यथा महत्पञ्चमूलं यथाऽब्जानूपमामिषम् ॥
लवणं सैन्धवंनोष्णमामलकं तथा । अर्कागुरूगुडूचीनां तिक्तानामुष्णमुच्यते ॥
..........कषायः स्तम्भनः शीतः सोऽभयायातमोऽन्यथा । (च.सू. २६)

Dravya	Rasa	Virya
Ānupa mamsa	Madhura	Ushna
Āmalaka	Aml.ı	Seeta
Saindhava lavana	Lavana	Anushna
Guduchi	Tikta	Ushna
Maha Panchamula	Kashaya, Tikta	Ushna
Haritaki	Kashaya	Ushna

Sushrita quoted following exceptions:

1. Brihat Panchamula	- Kashaya Tikta Rasa	- Vata hara	- Ushna Virya
2. Kulatha	- Kashaya Rasa	- Vata hara	- Snigdha Virya
3. Palandu	- Katu Rasa	- Vata hara	- Snigdha Virya
4. Ikshu Rasa	- Madhura Rasa	- Vata kara	- Seeta Virya
5. Pippali	- Katu Rasa	- Pitta hara	- Mridu & Seeta Virya
6. Āmalaki	- Amla Rasa	- Pitta hara	- Mridu & Seeta Virya
7. Sandhava lavana	- Lavana Rasa	- Pitta hara	- Mridu & Seeta Virya
8. Kākamachi	- Tikta Rasa	- Pitta kara	- Ushna Virya
9. Matsya	- Madhura Rasa	- Pitta kara	- Ushna Virya
10. Mulaka	- Katu Rasa	- Kapha kara	- Snigdha Virya
11. Kapitta	- Amla Rasa	- Kapha hara	- Ruksha Virya
12. Madhu	- Madhura Rasa	- Kapha hara	- Ruksha Virya

9. Superiority of Virya

While mentioning about the superiority of Virya, Suśruta explained that various actions of a Dravya viz., Urdhwabhagahara, Adhobhagahara, Samsodhana, Samsamana, Samgrahika, Agnideepana, Peedana, Lekhana, Brimhana, Rasayana, Vajikarana, Swayathu kara,

Vilayana, Dahana, Dārana, Mādana, Pranaghna, Vishaprasamana etc., are under the control of Virya. Hence Virya is superior[1].

He also quoted that virya will over come the effect of Rasa and exhibit its own effect[2]. For example, Vata hara Rasas do not perform the same function when they are in association with Ruksha. Laghu, Seeta gunas.

The following four aspects are proposed in support to the superiority of Virya by the Acharyas:[3]

(1) Virya Prādhānikatwa

It is considered to be the most important factor among the constituents of Dravya[4].

(2) Karma Kāraṇa

The Karma (action) is dependent on Virya mainly. Sushrita said that Virya is responsible for different actions of the drug[5].

(3) Rasābhibhavam

Virya will supersede the Rasa etc., and exhibit its own effects. Sushrita consider the effects of Virya are due to Balotkarsha (most potent quality)[6].

(4) Aptopadesa

All the classics and Acharyas emphasize Virya and its effects. Hence Virya is superior[7].

❋

---

१. वीर्यं प्रधानमिति । कस्मात्- तद्वशेनौषधकर्मनिष्पत्तेः इहौषधकर्माण्यूर्ध्वाधोभागोभयभाग-संशोधनसंशमनसांग्राहिकाग्निदीपन-पीडनलेखनबृंहणरसायनवाजीकरणश्वयथुकरविलयन-दहनदारणमादन प्राणघ्न विषप्रश-मनादीनि वीर्यप्राधान्याद् भवन्ति । (सु.सू. ४०)

२. एतानि खलु वीर्याणि स्वबलगुणोत्कर्षाद् रसमभिभूयात्मकर्म कुर्वन्ति । (सु.सू. ४०)

३. रसनाग्राह्यो रसः, शेषे गुणाः कायाग्निपाकजो विशिष्ठो रसो विपाकः तत्रैवोत्पन्नो गुणो वीर्यम् । (हेमाद्रिः)

४. वीर्यप्राधान्याद् द्रव्याणाम् । (र.वै. १/१३०)

५. तेन कर्मकरणात् । (र.वै. १/१३१)

६. तुल्यरसगुणेषु विशेषात् । (र.वै. १/१३६)

* भाष्यंः- वीर्यतः कार्यसामर्थ्यं भिषजो विदुः ।

७. आगमाच्च । (र.वै. १/१४०)

Further Readings on Virya

1. Devdas K.V., "An appraisal of the concept of Seetoshna veerya vigyana". D.G. Dept. I.P.G.T.R.A., G.A.U., Jamnagar.
2. Nisteswar K., "A comprehensive study of Veerya". D.G., Dept. I.P.G.T.R.A., G.A.U., Jamnagar. 1980 (M.D. Thesis).
3. Nisteswar K and Dhyai S.C.; "A critical study of virya vis-a-vis drug action". Paper submitted to Hari on Āshram Gold medal competition, 1979.
4. Nisteswar K. et al., "Action of Ushna and Seeta veerya drugs on skeletal muscle (frog rectus abdominis)". Sachitra Ayurveda sept. 80. vol. 33, No. 3.
5. Nisteswar K. et al., "Effect of Seeta and Ushna veerya drugs on Basal Metabolic Rate". Jrl of Res in Ayu. & Siddha. Vol. II, No. 4, 1980.
6. Nisteswar K. et al.; "Effect of Ushna and Seeta virya drugs on heart muscle an in vitro study". Jnl of the NIMA, Feb. 1986.
7. Nisteswar K. & Dhyani S.C.; "Rationale Behind Ashtavidha Virya Vāda." Nagarjuna May 1981. Vol. XXIV No. 9 pp. 192-194.
8. Nisteswar K.; "Role of virya in pharmacokinetics". Paper presented at I.A.H.P.S., Seminar, Calcutta, 1979.
9. Nisteswar K. & Dhyani S.C.; "Study of virya vis-a-vis 'PH' value of Drugs". Nagarjuna Oct. 1982. vol. XXVI No. 2 pp. 24-25.
10. Nisteswar K & Shyani S.C.; "Therapeutic values of Ashta viryas in different Kariya kalas". Nagarjuna, March 1981, Vol. XXIV, No. 7 pp. 152-153.
11. Nisteswar K.; "Viryam Tu Karmanishtaya- An assessement of Virya". Ayu. June 1986.
12. Nisteswar K.; "Viryam Tu Karmanishtaya- a de novo concept of drug action". 1986.
13. Sharma P.V. et al., "An objective method for the determination of virya". Jrl. of Res. in I.M. & H., Vol. II No. 2

14. Sukla Devendra; " Veeryam Yavat Adhivasat Nipatatcha Upalabhyate". D.G. Dept. IPGTRA, G.A.U., Jamnagar 1978 (M.D. Thesis).

15. Sukla D. & Dhyani S.C.; "Dravya evam virya ka prayogika Mulyankan". Paper presented at the seminar on Ayurvedic Drug Research. Nov. 1978, G.A.U., Jamnagar.

16. Vajpai V.S.; " Veerya Vijnanam", D.G. Dept., IPGTR, G.A.U., Jamnagar 1961 (M.D. Thesis).

Chapter - VIII
Concept of Prabhava

1. Etymology of Prabhava

The property which is responsible for a special or peculiar action of a Dravya is known as Prabhava[1].

The term Prabhava has been used by several Acharyas under different contexts and different meanings to denote the "non-specific effects" of a drug.

Prabhava can be considered under different synonyms like: Sakti, Vichitra Pratyayarabdhatwa, Vikriti Vishama Samaveta, Achintya Virya or Achintya, Anavadharaniya, Swabhava etc.

2. Characeristics of Prabhava

It is the property which is characterized by specific actions of substances which can not be explained in terms of the pharmacological actions of various constituents of dravya when they are considered invividually in relation to each other[2].

Chakrapani considered Prabhava as Achintya (unpredictable) since its effect is not comparable to the effects expected generally from the constituents of a Dravya. He also quoted Virya as Chintya and Achintya. The 'Achintya Virya' is considered as Prabhava.

Thus, probhave may also be defined as the special property which produces actions which are different from and contrary to those

---

१. (i) प्रकृष्ट: भाव: प्रभाव: । (स्व.)
(ii) प्रभवति सामर्थ्यविशिष्ठं भवति द्रव्यमनेनेति प्रभाव: । (द्र.गु.वि.)

२. रसवीर्यविपाकानां सामान्यं यत्र लक्ष्यते ।
विशिष्ठ: (विशेष:) कर्मणां चैव प्रभावस्तस्य स स्मृत: ॥ (च.सू. २६)
*चक्रपाणि:- सामान्यमिति तुल्यता । विशेष: कर्मणामिति दन्त्याद्याश्रयाणां विरेचनत्वादीनां सामान्यं लक्ष्यत इत्यनेन रसादिकार्यत्वेन यन्नावधारयितुं शक्यते कार्यं तत् प्रभावकृतमिति सूचयति, अत एवोक्तं- प्रभावोऽचिन्त्य उच्यते; रस-वीर्य-विपाक कार्यतयाऽचिन्त्य इति ।

attributed to Rasa, Gun, Virya and Vipaka[1,2,3].

Badhanta Nagarjuna described Prabhava as 'Anavadharaniya' in the chapter on Virya[4].

The following are the examples of Prabhava as mentioned by Charaka[5]:

(1) Danti (Baliosperumn montanum)- Katu Rasa, Ushna Virya, Katu Vipaka- Virechana.

Chitraka (Plambago zeylanica) -- --- -- Sangrahi

(2) Sthavara Visha (vegetable poisons) acting as antidotes to Jangama Visha (animal poisons).

(3) Ubhaya bhaga hara (emetic as well purgative) property.

(4) Mani dharana (wearing precious stones) in various diseases.

Vagbhata also mentioned several examples for Prabhava or Achintya karma[6,7].

(i) Danti and Chitrak are samana pratyayarabdha dravyas but the former is purgative while the later is not.

---

१. रसादि साम्ये यत्कर्मविशिष्टं तत्प्रभावजम् । (अ.सं.सू. १७)
२. रसगुणभूतसमुदायाश्रय एषानवधारण: । (अ.हृ.सू. ९)
तथा रसभूतसमुदायानामन्येषामन्यथावीर्यत्वात् ॥ (र.वै. ४/२८)
३. सर्वातिशायी द्रव्यस्वभाव: प्रभाव: । (अ.सं.सू. १७)
४. रसवीर्यविपाकादिगुणातिशयवानलम् । द्रव्यस्वभावो निर्दिष्ट: य: प्रभाव: स कीर्तित: ।
(अरुणदत्त:- अ.हृ.सू. ९)
५. कटुक: कटुक: पाके वीर्योष्णश्चित्रको मत: । तद्वद्दन्ती प्रभावात्तु विरेचयति मानवम् ॥
विषं विषघ्नमुक्तं यत् प्रभावस्तत्र कारणम् । ऊर्ध्वानुलोमिकं यच्च तत् प्रभावप्रभावितम् ॥
मणीनां धारणीयानां कर्म यद्विविधात्मकम् । तत् प्रभावकृतं येषां प्रभावोऽचिन्त्य उच्यते ॥(च.सू. २६)
६. दन्ती रसाद्यैस्तुल्यापि चित्रकस्य विरेचनी । मधुकस्य च मृद्वीका घृतं क्षीरस्य दीपनम् ॥
कटुपाकरसस्निग्धगुरूत्वै: कफवातजित् । लशुनो यापक...न्ना तु तैरेव यद्गुणै: ॥
मिथो विरूद्धा वातादीन् लोहिताद्या जयन्ति यत् । कुर्वन्ति यवकाद्याश्च तत् प्रभावविजृम्भितम् ॥
शिरिषादि विषं हन्ति स्वप्राद्यं तद्विवृद्धये । मणिमन्त्रौषधीनां च यत् कर्म विविधात्मकम् ॥
शल्याहरण-पुंजन्म- रक्षायुर्धी-वशादिकम् । दर्शनाद्यैरपि विषं यन्नियच्छति चागद: ॥
विरेचयति यद् वृष्यमाशु शुक्रं करोति च । ऊर्ध्वाधोभागिकं यच्च द्रव्यं यच्छमनादि च ॥
मात्रादि प्राप्य तत्तच्च यत् प्रपञ्चेन वर्णितम् । तच्च प्रभावजं सर्वमतोऽचिन्त्य: स उच्यते ॥
(अ.सं.सू. १७)
७. दन्ती रसाद्यैस्तुल्यापि चित्रकस्य विरेचनी ॥ मधुकस्य च मृद्वीका, घृतं क्षीरस्य दीपनम् । (अ.हृ.सू. ९)

(ii) Yashtimadhu and Draksha (liquorice and grapes) are also Samana pratyayarabdha dravyas but the former is Virechanopaga (synergetic action) while the later is Virechaka (direct action).

(iii) Ksheera and Ghrita (milk and ghee) are Samana pratyayarabdha dravyas but the forme reduces appetite (Agnimandya kara) while the later is appetizer (Agni vardhaka).

(iv) Lasuna (garlic) possess Katu Rasa, Snigdha-Guru Gunas and Katu Vipaka (i.e. vichitra pratyayarabdha). However it acts as Kapha-vata hara (reduces Kapha & Vata) instead of increasing them.

(v) Rakta sali and Yavaka have similar properties but the former is dosha hara while the later is dosha vardhaka.

(vi) Sirisha etc., act as antidotes (Visha hara) and sleep (Swapna), fatty foods etc., aggravate the effects of poisons.

(vii) Salya Āharana (removal of foreign body by using magnet etc), Pumsavana (deciding the male or female birth), Raksha vidhi (asepsis and antesepesis), Ayushya (increasing the longivity), Medhya (brain tonics), Vasikarana (hipnotism), Mani dharana (wearing precious stones) etc., are all described as Prabhava examples.

(viii) Sometimes exposing the individual suffering from poisoning to antidote (Agada darsana) may yield good results.

(ix) Vrishya dravyas (aphrodisiacs) acting as Sukra rechaka (enhancing ejaculation).

(x) Madana phala (Randia dumetorum) and Haritaki (Terminalia chebula) acting as emetic and laxative respectively.

(xi) The dose dependent variation in therapeutic effects of a drug.

Sushrita did not mention about Prabhava directly. However he indicated Prabhava through the concept of "Achintya Veerya". He is of the openion that the Prabhava janya karma is un-predictable (Achintya) and un-questionable (Amimamsya). One has to follow the classical texts in their understanding. For example: we can not make the Ambashtadi gana to act as purgative in any form. Hence Prabhava in ultimate[1].

Some of the scholars have questioned the validity of Prabhava examples like Danti and Chitraka. We find the name Chitraka under Bhedaniya dasaimani of Charaka Samhita (Sutra sthan 4th chapter). Therefore a doubt is expressed by many that both Danti (Chitra) and Chitrak are bhedaniya i.e.; purgatives and are not suitable examples for Prabhava. Here it is very important to realise that Chitra-Chitraka mentioned in Bhedaniya dasaimani are Danti-Dravanti but not Danti-Chitramula. Charaka mentioned Panchangula term only twice in Charka Samhita. Both the instances chakrapani quoted it as another variety of Eranda. Moreover in the context of Sāka varga (vegetables) in Sutra sthan 27th chapter, Charaka mentioned two types of Eranda viz., Urubuka (Eranda) and Panchangula (Chitra Eranda). The author is of the openion that Panchangula must be Rakta Eranda which may be Jatropha gossipyfolia. Gobalivarda Nyaya of Tarka Sastra shall be applied in this context to differentiate the term Chitraka in two instances. Arunadatta mentioned Chitraka as the synonym of Rakta Eranda while commenting on Ashtanga Hridaya. Similarly, Yashtimatdhu acts as prodrug and analogue in Virechanopaga and Virechaka dravyas.

Coming to the discussion on Rasadi samyatwa which is missing with Manidharana, Vasikarana etc., it is essential to understand that Virya is acting on Nipata or Adhivasa or Nipata as well as Adhivasa. Eg: Bhallataka when applied externally produces blisters because of its Ushna Virya. Same Ushna Veerya subsides the Kapha and also results in Rasayana property when Bhallataka is used internally. The former utility is the example of NIPATA and the later utility is the example of ADHIVASA. The invisible effects which are the out come of Nipata might have been quoted as Achintya Virya or Prabhava. If that is not the case where is the effect of Rasa and Vipaka when a drug is used as external application?

---

१. अमीमांस्यान्यचिन्त्यानि प्रसिद्धानि स्वभावतः । आगमेनोपयोज्यानि भेषजानि विचक्षणः ॥
प्रत्यक्षलक्षणफलाः प्रसिद्धाश्च स्वभावतः । नौषधीर्हेतुभिर्विद्वान् परीक्षेत कदाचन ॥
सहस्रेणापि हेतूनां नाम्बष्ठादिर्विरिच्यते । तस्मात्तिष्ठेत्तु मतिमानागमे न तु हेतुषु ॥(सु.सू.४०)

To denote the exceptions to the internal usage of Prabhava dravyas certain other examples like Manidharana, Agada darsana etc., are described in the treatises.

However, the author is of the strong openion that many of the Prabhavajanya Karmas which are quoted to be Achintyas shall be explicable today with the advent of scientific technology. Therefore the emphasis to Prabhava should be reduced than the earlier days. The following are the substantiating factors to the authors view:

a. Mani dharana: diamond which is a C_5 isotope emits certain radiations which may help in various disease con ditions including cancer.

b. Pumsavana: and Virechana human foetus is bisexual till 2-3 months of intra-uterine life. Though sex is genetically predetermined, a substance called 'differentiator' is finally deciding the sex of the human foetus before 3rd month.

c. Virechanopaga: These are Prodrugs and analogues. *Prodrugs* are used to improve pharmacological or biological properties. *Analogues* are used to increase potency and to achieve specificity of action.

d. Ubhayabhaga: hara The dosage of Virechana dravyas and Vamana dravyas is different. Therefore their actions, emesis and purgation are dose dependent.

Inspite of all these facts still there are many pharmacological properties mentioned in modern pharmacology which result in the non-specific activity of the drugs. Usually it is believed that drugs with similar chemical structure will have similar pharmacological actions. But it is not possible to predict their activity on the basis of chemical structure alone. Some times drugs with similar chemical structure may have entirely different actions. e.g.; Morphine and Papavarine are structurally similar but their pharmacological action is different. The former is narcotic and CNS depressant while the later is non-narcotic and muscle relaxant. There are certain drugs like pheno barbitone, chloral hydrate, Paraldehyde etc., which are structurally different but they all are CNS depressants.

In pharmacology the drug activity can be classified as (a) structurally non-specific or (b) structurally specific.

Structurally non-specific activity is dependent on physical properties like solubility, partition coefficients and vapour pressure and not on the presence or absence of some chemical group. Substances such as alkanes, alkenes, alkynes, alcohols, amides, ethers, ketones and chlorinated hydrocarbons exhibit narcotic activity and potency of each substance is related to its partition coefficient. Structurally non-specific action results from accumulation of a drug in some vital part of a cell with lipid characteristics.

On the otherhand structurally specific activity is dependent upon factors such as the presence or absence of certain functional groups, intramolecular distance and shape of the molecule.

Activity is not easily co-related with any physical property and small changes in structure often lead to changes in activity. Structurally specific activity is dependent upon interaction of the drug with a cellular receptor.

3. Functions of Prabhava

According to Charaka drug action is possible by means of three aspects viz.[1],

(i) Dravya Prabhava— drug action independent of the constituents (i.e., Achintyatwa).

(ii) Guna Prabhava—drug action depending up on the constituents (i.e., Chintyatwa).

(iii) Dravya-Guna Prabhava—drug action depending up the Dravya as well as Guna.

Some of the functions of Prabhava with relavent examples are disccussed in the previous pages[2]. The following actions/functions may be exhibited through Prabhava:

१. द्रव्याणि कार्मुकाणि भवन्ति-द्रव्य प्रभावात्, गुणप्रभावात् ,द्रव्यगुणप्रभावाच्च । (च.सू. २६)
२. रसं विपाकस्तौ वीर्यं प्रभावस्तान् व्यपोहति । बलसाम्ये रसादीनामिति नैसर्गिकं बलम् ॥ (च.सू. २६)

(1) Agadiya Karma (Antidotal activity) e.g. Sirisha

(2) Virechana Karma (Purgative property) e.g. Danti

(3) Rakshoghna Karma (Antimicrobial activity) e.g. Guggulu, Jatamansi.

(4) Manasa Karma (Psychotropic activity) e.g. Kushta, Rakta Chitraka.

All the examples of non-specific activity may be considered as Prabhavajanya karma.

4. Vichitra Pratyayarabdhatwam

On the basis of the Panchabhuta composition, Dravyas are divided into two groups viz.[1]

(i) Samana Pratyayarabdha dravyas- drugs which exhibit structure related pharmacological activities and therapeutic effects.

(ii) Vichitra Pratyayarabdha dravyas- drugs which do not have structural similarity among the constituents.

Charaka explained about two types of dravyas in the context of relation between Rasas and doshas.

They are:

(a) Prakriti Sama Samaveta

(b) Vikriti Vishama Samaveta

Basically there is no difference between Samana Pratyayarabdha dravyas and Prakriti Sama samaveta dravyas. But Vikriti Vishama samaveta differs from Vichitra pratyayarabdhatwa. Vikriti vishama samaveta dravyas will have similarity among the constituents but exhibit a special therapeutic effect independent of constituents. Thus Prabhava may be tentatively divided into two categories:

(1) Vikriti Vishama Samaveta- structurally similar but functionally similar.

(2) Vichitra Pratyayarabdhatwa- Structurally dissimilar but functionally similar.

* **Note:–** Charaka did not use the term Vichitra pratyayarabdha.

---

१. इति सामान्यतः कर्म द्रव्यादीनां पुनश्च तत् । विचित्रप्रत्ययारब्धद्रव्यभेदेन भिद्यते ॥
स्वादुर्गुरूश्च गोधूमो वातजिद्वातकृद्यवः । उष्णा मस्त्याः, पयः शीतः, कटुः सिंहो न शूकरः ॥
(अ.हृ.सू. ९)

Arunadatta described that the dravyas which are formed by similar bhutamses (bhoutika sanghatana) along with their constituents like Rasa, Virya etc., are Samanapratyayarabdhatwa dravyas. The vice versa are denoted as Vichitra pratyayarabdha dravyas. Some scholars questioned this concept by objecting that- "Dravya and Dravya constituents are formed only at once. Therefore there should not be any dissimilarity between their Bhoutika Sanghatana"[1]. The author clarify that Vichitra pratyayarabdha concept of Arunadatta is scientific from ancient and modern perspective also.

In second chapter Vyavasthitatwa, Swajatyavasthanatwa, Kramapekshitawa have denoted that Vipaka, Rasa, Virya etc, are unstable in the dravya. Similarly in Rasa chapter reasons for Rasa transformation are explained. Even seasonal formation of different Rasas was also described. These references indicate that though the original dravaya remains as it is its constituents will vary depending upon various factors. e. g. Ārdra Pippali is Seeta Veerya and Sushka Pippali is Ushna Virya; Bāla Āmra is sour and Pakwa Āmra is sweet; Nava guggulu is Medo kara and Purana guggulu is Medo hara.

The following examples are quoted by Laghu Vagbhata for Vichitra pratyaya rabdhatwa:

1.	Godhuma (wheat)	Madhura rasa	Guru guna	Vata hara	Samana
	Yava (Barley?)	Madhura rasa	Guru guna	Vata kara	Vichitra
2.	Ksheera Matsya (fish)	Madhura rasa	Guru guna	Ushna Virya	Vichitra
3.	Sukara (pork)	Madhura rasa	Guru guna	Madhura Vipaka	mamsa Samana

१. तदेवं द्रव्याणां द्वैविध्यं यत: क़ानिचित् द्रव्याणि यैरेव महाभूतैर्यथाविधै: रसादय: आरब्धास्तैरेव तथाभूतैर्महाभूतै: तदाश्रयाणि द्रव्याण्यारब्धानि तानि रसादिसमानप्रत्ययारब्धान्युच्यन्ते तानि च यथायथं तत् कर्म रसाद्यनुगुणं सामान्यत् कुर्वते यथा क्षीरेषु शर्करादीनि । कानिचित् पुनस्तदाश्रितरसादिसमारम्भकमहाभूतान्यन्यानि, तदाश्रयद्रव्यारम्भकाण्यन्यानि च महाभूतानि तैरारब्धानि तानि विचित्रप्रत्ययारब्धानि द्रव्याणि, तानि ये यथायथं रसाद्यनुगुणं कर्म न कुर्वन्ति, भिन्नत्वाद्धेतुभावस्य-यथा मकुष्ठ-यव-मत्स्य-सिंहादीनि । (अरुणदत्त:)

Simha mamsa (lion meat)	Madhura rasa	Guru guna	Katu Vipaka	Vichitra

Hemadri stated that the Vata hara and Vata Kara properties of Godhuma and Yava respectively are due to Prabhava or Vichitra pratyayarabdhatwa only.

Charaka mentioned certain Rasa viruddha Viryas (incompatible potencies). They are the examples of Vikriti Vishama Samaveta only[1].

(i) Maha Pancha mula	- Madhura, Kashaya, Tikta Rasas	- Ushna Virya
(ii) Anupa mamsa	- Madhura, Kashaya, Tikta Rasas	- Ushna Virya
(iii) Saindhava lavana	- Lavana Rasa	- Seeta Virya
(iv) Āmalaki	- Amla Rasa	- Seeta Virya
(v) Arka, Aguru, Guduchi	- Tikta Rasa	- Ushna Virya

While commenting upon Prakriti sama samaveta and Vikriti vishma sameveta Chakrapani quoted certain examples[2]:

(a) Madhura Rasa dravyas should act as Sneha and Vrishya. But Tanduliya is not exhibities these properties in spite of being Madhura.

(b) Tila should act as either Kapha-pitta hara or Tridosha hara, for possessing Kashaya, Katu, Tikta & Madhura rasas. But it is acting as pitta and Kapha vardhaka.

(c) Vārtāka (Brinjal) acts as Vāta hara even though it is having Katu, Tikta Rasas.

---

१. मधुरं किञ्चिदुष्णं स्यात् क़षायं तिक्तमेव च । यथा महत्पञ्चमूलं यथाऽब्जानूपमामिषम् ॥
लवणं सैन्धवंनोष्णमम्लमामलकं तथा । अर्कागुरूगुडूचीनां तिक्तानामुष्णमुच्यते ॥
तस्माद्रसोपदेशेन न सर्वं द्रव्यमादिशेत । दृष्टं तुल्यरसेऽप्येवं द्रव्ये द्रव्ये गुणान्तरम् ॥

२. तत्र रसस्य विकृतसमवायो यथा- मधुरे तण्डुलीयके मधुरो हि प्रकृत्या स्नेहवृष्यत्वादिकरः, तण्डुलीयके तु विकृतिविषमसमवेतत्वेनतन्नकरोति विषमसमवेतास्तु तिले कषायकटुतिक्तमधुराः, यदि हिमे रसाः समया मात्रया समवेताः स्युस्ततस्तिलोऽपि पित्तश्लेष्महरस्त्रिदोषहरो वा स्यात् पित्तकफकरत्वयं तेनात्ररसानां क्वचित् कर्त्तुत्वमकर्त्तुत्वं च क्वचिदिति वैषम्यमुन्नीयते । नानान्मकानामित्यादि हेतुत्रयं तु विकृतिसमवायविषमसमवायोरेवोपलभ्यकं । यत्र वार्तकि कटुतिक्तत्वेन वातरक्तत्वं प्राप्तमपि च विकृतिविषमसमवायात्तन्न भवति, तत्राचार्येण "वार्ताकं वातघ्नं इत्युक्तमेव ।"(चक्रपाणि- च.वि.१.अ)

Gangadhara mention that Dravya, Guna and Karma will have similarity in genesis usually. This is because similar will produce similar. However it need not be compulsory always. When ever there is equality or similarity then Sajātiya Karma will occur (Samana pratyayarabdhatwa). Other wise Vijatiya Karma will occur (vichitra pratyapratyaya rabdhatwa)[1]. In this context Acharya P.V. Sharmaji questions that "Gangadhara considers Prabhava as Karma. But Karma can not produce another Karma. Then how Prabhava can be considered as Karma?". Hence it is concluded that Prabhava is Shakti and it is Sadhana (means) for a particular Karma (effect).

5. Superiority of Prabhava

Vagbhata concluded that the drug action is ultimately controlled by Prabhava and it is superior among the durg constituents[2].

Badhanta Nagarjuna proposed the following factors to high-light the superiority of Achintya Virya (Prabhava)[3].

1. **Achintyata** ***(unpredictable):*** It effects are quite unpredictble and therefore it is considered as superior.

2. **Daiva Pratighata** ***(super natural power):*** It exhibits super natural power. Hence it is important.

3. **Visha Pratighata** ***(anti-dotal effects):*** It helps in anti-dotal activity irrespective of drug constituents. Hence it is superior.

4. **Darsana** ***(practically visible):*** Its extra-ordinary effect are practically seen.

---

१. स्वस्वारम्भकद्रव्यसंयोगे समवेतानां तेषां द्रव्यगुणकर्मणां द्रव्यगुणयो: सजातीयारम्भकत्वात् तत्र द्रव्यात् सजातीयद्रव्यान्तरं जायते, गुणात् सजातीयगुणान्तरं जायते, कर्मणां तु सजातीयकर्मारम्भकत्व-नियमाभावात् कर्मसाध्यकर्माभावाच्च यत्र विजातीयं कर्म तदारम्भकद्रव्याणां कर्मण्यारभते, तद् विजातीयं कर्म खल्वचिन्त्यं, स प्रभाव उच्यते । कार्यभूतं कर्मेदं, कर्मपदार्थ: प्रभाव: । कार्यद्रव्यं दन्त्यादिकं तत्कर्मविशेषेण स्वीयेन प्रभावेण विरेचादि कर्म करोति इति । (गङ्गाधर:)

२. अप्रधाना: पृथक् तस्माद् रसाद्या: संश्रितास्तु ते ।
प्रभावाश्च यतो द्रव्ये, द्रव्यं श्रेष्ठमतो मतम् ॥ (अ.सं.सू. १७)

३. अचिन्त्यात्, दैवप्रतीघातात्, विषप्रतीघातात्, दर्शनात्, श्रवणात्, तुल्यरसगुणेषु
विशेषात्, दर्शनाच्चाद्भुतादीनां कर्मणां, आगमाच्च ॥ (र.वै.१.सू. १३२-१४०)

5. **Sravana** *(praise):* Many scholars praise its efficacey and superiority.
6. **Tulya Rasa guna Visesha** ***(non-specificity):*** It will exhibit very special action independent of other drug constituents or their qualities.
7. **Adbhuta Karma** ***(magic effects):*** Using precious stones, hypnotism, hymns chanting etc., will yield some magic effects. Hence Prabhava is superior.
8. **Āgama** ***(classical treatises):*** All the classical texts high-lighted Prabhava as the main quality of a Dravya. Therefore Prabhava is considered as superior.

✵

[Part - B]

Chapter-IX

Relation between Rasādi Gunas

Mutual Relation between Rasadi Gunas

Usually the drug action of any dravya will depend upon either Rasa or Virya or Vipaka or Prabhava according to Charaka[1].

Sushrita described his view that the variation in increase or decrease in Panchabhutas results in the variation of Rasa, Virya and Vipaka[2].

Generally the dravyas with Madhura Rasa will have Madhura Vipaka and Seeta Virya. Similarly, Amla Katu Rasa dravyas will have corresponding Vipaka and Ushna Virya. Their qualities can be assessed on the basis of Rasas. These are known as Samana Pratyayarabdhas[3].

By accepting a leaf each from charaka and Sushrita's views Vagbhata said that Rasa, Virya etc., may be similar (Eka rupa) or dissimilar (Virupa) in a dravya. For example, (Eka rupa) or dissimilar (Virupa) in a dravya. Rasa, Virya Vipakas while Ānupa mamsa (meat of water animals & birds) will be presented with dissimilar qualities[4].

Normally, in a drug Vipaka will supersed Rasa; Rasa and Vipika will be superseded by Virya and finally Prabhava will supersede all the three. That means when ever there is equality in strength of different qualities, the naturally potent or powerful quality is mainly active e.g., though Madhu (honey) is Madhura Rasa its Vipaka is

---

१. किञ्चिद् रसेन कुरुते कर्म बीर्येण चापरम् ।
द्रव्यं गुणेन पाकेन प्रभावेण च किञ्चन ॥ (च.सू. २६) और (अ.सं.सू. १७)

२. तद्द्रव्यमात्मना किञ्चित् किञ्चिद्वीर्येण सेवितम् ।
किञ्चिद्रसविपाकाभ्यां दोषं हन्ति करोति वा ॥ (सु.सू. ४०)

३. शीतं वीर्येण यद्द्रव्यं मधुरं रसपाकयो: । तयोरम्लंयदुष्णं च यद्द्रव्यं कटुकं तयो: ॥
तेषां रसोपदेशेन निर्देश्यो गुणसंग्रहः । वीर्यतोऽविपरीतानां पाकतश्चोपदेक्ष्यते ॥ (च.सू. २६)

४. रसवीर्य प्रभृतयो भूतोत्कर्षापकर्षतः एकरूपा विरूपा वा द्रव्यं समधिशेरते । माधुर्य-शैत्य-पैच्छिल्य-स्नेह-गौरव-मन्दताः सहवृत्त्या स्थिताः क्षीरेवानूपौदिकामिषे ॥ (अ.सं.सू. १७)

Katu and therefore it acts as Kapha hara instead of Kapha vardhaka; Sura (beverage) is Amla Rasa and Amla Vipaka but acts as Stanya janana because of its Prabhava[1].

Therefore it is concluded that when ever there is association of dissimilar qualities, the more potent quality will supersede the quality of lower potency and exhibits its own effects or qualities e.g., Ksheera (milk) which is Seeta virya in nature does not aggravate Vata but subsides it by means of other qualities like Madhura Rasa, Snigdha-Guru Gunas etc[2].

Though these qualities i.e., Rasa, Guna, Virya, Vipaka etc., are opposite to one another, they do not interfere with the therapeutic effects of drugs. Just like Tridoshas which are possessing different qualities are maintaining the homoeostasis of human body. The dissimilar constituents of body will also have mutual balance and produce good effect[3].

In the previous chapters, the individual constituents of dravyas were discussed in detail. Here the mutual relation between Rasa, Guna, Virya, Vipaka and Prabhava are explained. These qualities generally exhibit a balanced interplay to produce the therapeutic effect. There fore all the constituents of Dravya are of equal importance.

✸

---

१. रसं विपाकस्तौ वीर्यं प्रभावस्तान्व्यपोहति । बलसाम्ये रसादीनामिति नैसर्गिकं बलम् ॥ (च.सू. २६)

२. यद्द्रव्ये रसादीनां बलवत्वेनवर्तते ।
अभिभूयेतरांस्तत्तत् कारणत्वं प्रपद्यते ॥
विरूद्धगुणसंयोगे भूयसाऽल्यं हि जीयते । (अ.सं.सू. १७)

३. विरुद्धा अपि चान्योन्यं रसाद्या: कार्यसाधने ।
नावश्यं स्युर्विघाताय गुणदोष मिथोयथा ॥ (अ.सं.सू. १७)

*इन्दुकर:- गुणा: सत्त्वरजस्तमांसि परस्परं भिधान कार्यसाधने, विरुद्धयापि यथा विघाताय न भवन्ति दोषाश्च, वात-पित्त-कफ:, देह-रोगादि साधने यथा मिथो विघाताय न भवन्ति तद्वद्रसादयोऽपि ।

Chapter - X
Concept of Karma

1. Etymology of Karma: (कर्म निरूक्ति)

The element which is responsible for the action of a drug is known as 'Karma'[1].

2. Definition of Karma: (कर्म लक्षणम्)

The factor which is responsible for the association (Samyoga) and dissociation (Vibhaga), and which resides in the drug (dravya) with inherent relation is known as 'Karma'[2].

Badhanta Nagarjuna considered action as the main property of Karma[3].

Pharmacological action of a drug is defined as the action which is aimed to obtain a specific therapeutic effect. e.g., an analgesic drug is administered to obtain analgesia through its analgesic action.

3. Characteristics of Karma: (कर्म स्वरूपम्)

Activity or action is the characteristic feature of Karma. In other words, 'Karma' is the *cause* and 'Karya' is the *effect*[4].

Charak considered Vamana (emesis), Virechana (purgation) etc, actions as Karmas. Chakrapani in this context opined that Brimhana (nourishment) etc., shall also be considered as Karmas[5]. Prayatna, Chetana etc., were also treated as actions by Charaka[6]. Suśruta

---

१. क्रियते इति कर्म । (द्र.गु.वि.)

२. संयोगे च विभागे च कारणं द्रव्यमाश्रितम् ।
कर्तव्यस्य क्रिया कर्म कर्मनान्यदपेक्षते ॥ (च.सू.१अ.)
*चक्रपाणि:- संयोगे च विभागे च युगपत्कारणं ।

३. क्रियालक्षणं कर्म । (र.वै.१.अ.१७१सू.)

४. यत् कुर्वन्ति तत् कर्म । (च.सू.२६अ.)

५. कर्म पञ्चविधमुक्तं वमनादि । (च.सू.)
*चक्रपाणि:- एतच्च प्राधान्यादुच्यते तेन बृंहणाद्यपि बोद्धव्यम् ।

६. प्रयत्नादि कर्म चेष्टितमुच्यते । (च.सू.१अ.)

considered the following as drug actions viz., Urdhwabhaga-sodhana, Adhobhaga Sodhana, Ubhayabhaga Sodhana, Somsamana, Sangrahika, Agni deepana, Peedana, Lekhana, Brimhana, Rasayana, Vajikarana, Swayathukara, Vilayana, Dahana, Dārana, Mādana, Pranaghna, Visha prasamana etc. These Karmas are based upon the Veerya[1].

According to Vaiseshika darsana Utkshepana (lifting of hands), Apakshepana (folding the shoulders), Akunchana (flexion), Prasarana (extension), Gamana (walking) etc., are all considered as Karmas[2].

4. Types of Karma

Generally it is stated that drug action may be the result of either of the following viz.,

(i) Dravya Prabhava (natural property of a drug)

(ii) Guna Prabhava (property of ingredients of a drug)

(iii) Dravya Guna Prabhava (a combination of both factors)

Though there is no specific typing among the Karmas in the ancient texts. However the following five catogories may be made for practical purpose. They are:

(I) Sodhana (curative effect)
Samana (palliative effect)

(II) Samanya (generalized effect)
Visishta (specialized effect)

(III) Antah parimarjana (internal action)
Bahih parimarjana (external effect)

(IV) Sthanika (local action)
Sarva dehika (systemic effect)

(V) Mukhya (major effects) & Gouṇa (minor effects)

---

१. इहौषधकर्माणि ऊर्ध्वाधोभागोभयभागसंशोधन-संशमन-सांग्राहिक-अग्निदीपन-पीडन-लेखन-बृंहण-रसायन-वाजीकरण-श्वयथुकर-विलयन-दहन-दारण-मादन-प्राणघ्न-विषप्रप्रशमनादीनि वीर्यप्राधान्यात् भवन्ति ॥ (सु.सू. ४०)

२. उत्क्षेपणं ततोऽपक्षेपण माकुञ्चनं तथा । प्रसारणं च गमनं कर्माण्येतानि पञ्चच । भ्रमणं रेचनं स्यन्दनोर्ध्वज्वलनमेव च । तिर्यग्गमनमप्यत्र गमनादेव लभ्यते ॥ (कारिकावली)

Drug actions may be assessed on the basis of their effects/ actions on Doshas. Dhatus, Malas, Srotas etc.

On the doshas the drug action may be either Kopana (Vardhava) or Kshapana (Samaka). On the dhatus and malas also the drugs may act either as Vriddhikara or Kshaya kara. While the action of a drug on the Srotas is more important since it provides a comprehensive effect e.g. Sukrala drug on Sukravaha Srotas, Sonita Sthapana drug on Rakta vaha Srotas, Hridya drugs on Prana Vāha Srotas.

The classification of drug actions on the basis of their end effect will be discussed under the coming sub-heads. In this context the brood categorization of Karma according to the mechanism of action are duscussed. Acharya P.V. Sharmaji opine that direct and reflex actions are Mukhya and Gouna Karmas respectively.

5. Discussion on the Modality of Karma from Ancient and Modern Perspective

Many times the terms 'action' and 'effects' of a drug are being used as synonyms. However, it is useful to term the initial consequences of drug-cell interaction as "action of the drug" and the remaining events that follow are called as "drug effects".

Charaka explained different modalities of drug action in the following way:

(i) which perform a particular activity is called as 'Karma'

(ii) which is the means of performing the karma is called as 'Virya'

(iii) the site of action is known as 'Adhikarana'.

(iv) the time taken for drug action is known as 'Kāla'.

(v) the particular type of activity through a specific path way is known as 'Upāya'.

(vi) the result obtained through the effect of drug over the body is called as 'Phala''[1].

---

१. यत् कुर्वन्ति तत् कर्म । (action of the drug)
येन कुर्वन्ति तत् वीर्यं । (potency of the drug)
यत्र कुर्वन्ति तदधिकरणम् । (site of action)
यदा कुर्वन्ति स कालः । (time for bioavailability)
यथा कुर्वन्ति स उपायः । (mode of action)
यत् साधयन्ति तत् फलम् । (specific therapeutic effect) (च.सू.२६)

With this view only, Charka explained that a drug may act either by means of "natural property" (Dravya Prabhava) or by means of "individual characteristics" (Guna Prabhava). Some time both may help together in drug action[1].

Chakrapani in this context elaborated that Parthiva dravyas are usually explained on the basis of their properties like Guru, Khara etc. But it is not sufficient to claim all its actions are due to Guna Prabhava. It is to remember that the purgative property of Danti etc., are the examples for *Dravya Prabhava*. Utility of Tikta Rasa in Jwara etc., are examples for *Guna Prabhava*. Krishnajina is the suitable example for *Dravyaguna Prabhava*[2].

Chakrapani further explained the modalities of Karma by taking 'Nasya' (nasal administration of drugs) as an example:

1. Dravya - Sirovirechana dravya.
2. Karma - Sirovirechna karma.
3. Virya - Ushna, Seeta etc., Potent Gunas/dravyas.
4. Adhikarana - Sirah (head)
5. Kāla - different seasons or the time when heaviness of head is experienced (i.e., useful time)
6. Upāya - Various measures like positioning the patient supine on the bed, extending the neck etc. while performing Nasya.
7. Phala - Obtaining relief from heaviness of head, head ache[3] etc.

---

१. न तु केवलं गुणप्रभावादेव द्रव्याणि कार्मुकाणि भवन्ति; द्रव्याणि हि द्रव्यप्रभावात् गुणप्रभावात् द्रव्यगुणप्रभावाच्च तस्मिंस्तस्मिन् काले तत्तदधिकरणमासाद्य तां तां च युक्तिमर्थं च तं तमभिप्रेत्य यत् कुर्वन्ति तत् कर्म ....। (च.सू. २६)

२. पार्थिवादिद्रव्याणां गुरूखरादिगुणयोगाद्भेषजत्वमुक्तं, तेन गुणप्रभावादेव भेषजं स्यादिति शङ्कां निरस्यन्नाह- न तु केवलमित्यादि । द्रव्यप्रभावद्यथा- दन्त्या विरेचकत्वं, तथा मणीनां विषादिहन्तृत्वमित्यादि । गुणप्रभावाद्यथा- ज्वरे तिक्तको रसः, शीतेऽग्निरित्यादि । द्रव्यगुणप्रभावाद्यथा- कृष्णाजिनस्योपरीति, अत्रापि कृष्णत्वं गुणोऽजिनं च द्रव्यमभिप्रेतं । (चक्रपाणि- च.सू. २६/१३)

३. यत् कुर्वन्तीत्यादावुदाहरणं यथा- शिरोविरेचनद्रव्याणि यच्छिरोविरेचनं कुर्वन्ति, तच्छिरोविरेचनं कर्म; येनोष्णत्वादिकारणेन शिरोविरेचनं कुर्वन्ति, तद्वीर्यं, वीर्यं शक्तिः, सा च द्रव्यस्य गुणस्य वा; यत्र

क्रमशः पृष्ठ १८९ में.............

The final traget achieved by administering a drug is considered as 'Uddesya' or 'Sādhya'. The means of achieving a particular Phala is known as 'Karma'.

As already explained every drug (dravya) will possess constitunets viz., Rasa, Guna, Virya, Vipaka and Prabhava. All these five will perform their individual actions.

Mode of drug action according to Ayurveda

In the modern pharmacology the mode of drug action is explained through 'pharmacodynamics' and 'pharmacokinetics'. The former will elucidate the mode of action of a drug in relation to its chemical structure and the later will denote the absorption, fate and excretion of drugs in relation to its pharmacological response. The resulting effects are used in the therapeutics (Chikitsa) i.e., pharmacotherapeutics[1].

Ayurveda explained the sturctural and functional aspects of human body on the basis of Panchabhutas. Similarly the drugs are considered as the composite units of Panchabhutas.

(a) Pharmacodynamics in Ayuraveda

The drug action is many times explained on the basis of Panchabhoutik conbination or configuration i.e., structure related activity. This may be treated as pharmacodynamics of Ayurveda. All the five ingredients of Dravya shall be proved with individual pharmacodynamic activities.

पृष्ठ १८८ से क्रमशः...........

शिरोविरेचनं कुर्वन्ति तदधिकरणं शिरः, नान्यत्राधिकरणे शिरोविरेचनद्रव्यं प्रभवतीत्यर्थः, यदेति वसन्तादौ शिरोगौरवादियुक्ते च काले, एतेनाकाले शीते शिरोविरेचनं स्तब्धत्वात्र कार्मुकं, किन्तु स्वकाल एव; यथा येन प्रकारेण प्रधमनावपीडनादिना तथा "प्रसारिताङ्गमुत्तानं शयने संस्तरास्तृते ईषत्प्रलम्बशिरसं संवेश्य चावृतेक्षणम्"- इत्यादिना विधिना कुर्वन्ति, स उपायः; यत् साधयन्ति शिरोगौरवशूलाद्युपरमं, तत् फलं; फलम् उद्देश्यम् । कर्म कार्यं साधनम् उद्देश्यं फलं साध्यं; यथा- यागनिष्पाद्यो धर्मः कार्यतया कर्म, तज्जन्यस्तु स्वर्गादिरूद्देश्यः फलम्; एवं वमनादिष्वपि कर्माधिकरणाद्युन्नेयम् ॥

(चक्रपाणि- च.सू. २६/१३)

१. (i) द्रव्ये रसो गुणो वीर्यं विपाकः शक्तिरेव च । पदार्थाः पञ्च तिष्ठन्ति स्वं स्वं कुर्वन्ति कर्म च ॥ (भा.प्र.)

(ii) किञ्चिद्रसेन कुरुते कर्म वीर्येण चापरम् ।
द्रव्यं गुणेन पाकेन प्रभावेण च किञ्चन ॥ (अ.सं.सू. १७)

(1) Dravya

Akasa + Vayu + Agni ⟶ Vamana (emesis)

Apya + Prithivi ⟶ Virechana (purgation)

(2) Rasa

Amla (e.g. CH_3 COOH) is claimed to be Hridya since vit. C helps in preventing atherosclorosis and therefore helps to heart and CVS.

Madhura (e.g. $C_6H_{12}O_6$) is claimed to be Preenana since glucose nourishes all the tissues.

(3) Guna

$MgSO_4$ acts as osmotic purgative.

(4) Virya

Seeta virya — Prithvi + Ap → Pitta Samaka

Laghu virya — Agni + Vayu + Ākasa → Kapha samaka

(5) Vipaka

Madhura Vipaka < Madhura rasa (Ap+Pr), Lavana rasa (Ag+Ap) > Srishta Vit & Mutra, Vrishya

Katu Vipaka < Katu rasa (Ag+Va), Tikta rasa (Ak+Va), Kashya rasa (Pr+Va) > Baddha Vit & Mutra, Avrishya

(6) Prabhava

(i) Vikriti vishama Samaveta:

Tanduliya - Madhura rasa but Avrishya

(ii) Vichitra pratyayarabdhatva:

Godhuma	-	Madhura rasa (Ap+Pr)	Guru guna (Ap+Pr) Vata hara
Yava	-	Madhura rasa (Ap+Pr)	Guru guna (Ap+Pr) Vata kara

[**Note:** Among the above aspects, Prabhava does not fall under structure ralated activity group since it is non-specific activity]

(b) Pharmacokinetics in Ayurveda

The absorption and fate of the drug (which is orally administered) is well explained by Charaka. While its journey inside the body each one of the pharmacologically active ingredients of the dravya will supercede the other in the following order:

Rasa ⟶ Vipaka ⟶ Virya ⟶ Prabhava

when it is found that virya is superior than Rasa and Vipaka, "VIRYANTU KARMANISHTAYA" may not be a questionable concept. It is to be finally concluded that vipaka is a process but not a pharmacologically active ingredient.

Fate of the five ingredients of a drugs is well known to the ancient acharyas:

(i) Raso Nipate Dravyanam	-	effect or rasa is percieved on contact with the tongue which is mainly local action.
(ii) Viryam Yāvadadhivasta Nipatat Cha Upalabhyate	-	effect of virya assessed either when it is applied externally on the body or when it exhibits its activity on the receptor internally[1].
(iii) Vipakah Karma Nisht-Aya	-	vipaka is assessed after observing the final action of the metabolized ingredient of a drug.
(iv) Visishta Karmanam Chaiva Prabhava	-	the non-specific effects of a drug are stated to be due to Prabhava.

[* **Note:** As Guna is physical property its fate was not mentioned in the classics]

---

१. अधीवास: सहावस्थानं, यावदधीवासादिति यावच्छरीरनिवासात्; एतच्च विपाकात् पूर्वं निपाताच्चोर्ध्वं ज्ञेयम् । निपाताच्चेति शरीरसंयोगमात्रात्; तेन किञ्चिद्वीर्यमधीवासादुपलभ्यते।

(चक्रपाणि-च.सू. २६/६६)

Drug absorption

According to Ayurveda, Amashaya is the place for Kapha. Thus Snigdha (lipid soluble), Seeta (non-ionized) and Guru (heavy in molecular weight) are supposed to be absorbed there.

Grahani is the place for Pitta and substances having properties like Snigdha (lipid soluble), Ushna (ionized) and Laghu (smaller in molecular weight) are absorbed there through the Pitta-dhara kala.

Pakwashaya is the site for Vata and thus, Ruksha (water soluble), Seeta (non-ionized) and Laghu (smaller in molecular size) are absorbed here.

For easier under-standing the following correlation of the anatomical correlation is made:

Amashaya	-	oral cavity to 1st part of duodenum
Grahani	-	2nd part of duodenum to caecum
Pakwashaya	-	Ceacum to rectum

In modern pharmacology it is explained that crystalloids are easily obserbed than colloids. Gases are absorbed through respiratory system and solids & liquids are absorbed through G.I.T. These concepts are already existing in Ayurvedic system of medicines. It is well known fact that bhasmas (mineral ashes) are in the colloidal state. Where ever the sustained release effect or delayed effect is required either the mineral or herbomineral drugs were used. Dhupa (fumes) and Dhumapana (medicated smoking) etc., were used to introduce the drug for respiratory problems and infectuous conditions. Otherwise most of the drugs were administered orally for their action on G.I.T.

Receptor Theory in Ayurveda

The drug will act either by guna or Prabhava or by both by taking required time and by acting on respective site of action by respective means of action. It is also posturated that the site of action is nothing but the receptor (Adhikarana).

It is generally accepted that the Dosha-dushya sammurchana (etiopathogenesis) occurs in the srotas in a disease process.

Therefore, a drug may act in either of the following ways:

(i) If the effect of the drug is on cell membrance, that may be compared to the action of the drug on Srotas.

(ii) If the drug acts outside the cell (extracelluar), it can be considered as effect on *Poshaka dhatu.*

(iii) If it is inside the cell (intracellular), the effect is on *Poshya dhatu.*

(iv) If the effect of the drug is on the cell metabolism, then it shall be considered as the effect on *Dhatwagni.*

Basing upon the site of action or receptors, different actions have been confirmed in the ancient texts e.g.: Twachya, Varnya, Chakshushya, Medhya, Pleehagna, etc.

The mode of action of a drug in relation with the state of Samprapti

Late Prof. S.C. Dhyaniji explained the mode of drug action on the basis of relation between drug constituents, site of action and the state of pathogenesis.

S.N.	Rasa Panchaka	Site of Action	State of Pathogenesis
1.	Rasa & Vipaka	Koshta	Chaya & Prakopa
2.	Guna	Rasa samvahana	Prasara
3.	Virya & Prabhava	Dushyas & Srotas	Sthanasamsraya & Vyakti

The above concept may be substantiated with the help of the prarmacotherapy of Atisara (diarrhoea). In Atisara, Vata is the main dosha and Purisha is the dushya. Purisha Vata srotas is the srotas involved. Atipravritti is the type of Srotodushti. In this condition, Sunthi acts on vata, Bhanga acts on purisha and Ahiphena acts on purishavaha srotas. Therefore either of these three drugs or combination of them are to be administered in Atisara to prevent the samprapti at different levels and to cure Atisara.

To explain the Ayurvedic perspective vis-a-vis modern pharmacology, opium will be a fine example. Opium contains two important ingredients viz., morphine and papavarine. The former is narcotic and the later is non-narcotic due to Prabhava. Morphine/opium is bitter in taste (Rasa). Due to Vyavayi guna is first stimulates and then depresses the CNS. Its Ushna virya causes erythema, urticaria and itching dermatitis on Nipata (on contact with the skin) while on oral administration exhibits two states of narcosis (stage of excitement & stage of stupor) at Adhivasa. The third stage i.e., stage of coma is due to Vipaka wherein morphine is conjugated with glucuronic acid. Thence morphine causes constipation (i.e., Baddha vit & Mutra = Katu vipaka).

Before we further discuss about the mode of drug action according to Ayurveda, it is essential to realize that all the drugs under go Agni paka i.e., digestion as well as metabolism. Being the drugs of herbal origin they will undergo both the phases. The Jataragni paka represents digestion while Bhutagni & Dhatwagni paksa represent the metabolism of drug. Vipaka therefore is the process of conversion of different drug constituents. Chakrapani while elaborating his concept-Virya pradhana and Rasa pradhana dravyas concluded that the food material (Āhara dravya) is mainly concerned with Dhatwagni vyapara. While drug (Oushadha dravya) is mainly concerned with Bhutagni vyapara e.g., Vyavayi acts before Jataragni paka.

It is the Gunas (Rasa, Virya etc.), which will surface different pharmacological actions. Being the Utkrishta chintya Guna 'Virya' will perform the drug action mainly. Achintya virya on the otherhand is Prabhava and part of Virya again.

Usually the treatment aims at rectifying the imbalance between the dosha-dhatu-malas i.e., Samprapti Vighatana. The Samprapti can be dismantled by instituting either dosha pratyanika chikitsa (antagonistic measures to dosha) or Vyadhi pratyanika chikitsa (antagonistic measures to disease). Therefore drugs are classified into certain groups basing upon their actions on Dosha, Dhatus, Malas and Vyadhis. More and more pharmacological actions have been enumerated by the Acharyas of later period. But the definitions and implications of these actions are lacking in the Brihat-trayee. Sarngdhara attempted to fill those lacunae and defined many actions with suitable examples.

Drug Action in Modern Pharmacology

(I) Local Action

When the drug is applied locally or direct to a tissue or organ it combines to form an albuninate with the cell's albumins.

(1) Astringent action	-	When a drug can not act because the albuminate does not dissolve.
(2) Corrosive action	-	When the drug is strong enough to destroy cells.
(3) Irritating action	-	When too much of the drug combines with cells to impair them.

(I) General or Systemic Action

When the drug enters the blood stream by absorption or direct injection affecting tissues and organs not near the site of entry. This action may be:

(1) Specific	-	When specific in the cure of a certain disease.
(2) Substitutive	-	When it supplies substances deficient in the body.
(3) Physical	-	When some of the constituents of a cell are dis solved by the action of the drug in the blood stream.
(4) Chemical	-	When the drug or some of its principles com bine with the constituents of cells or organs to form a new chemical combination.
(5) Salt	-	Osmosis caused by dilution of salt (also acids, sugars & alkalies) in the stomach or intestines by fluid with drawn from the blood and tissues, or cells from the lymph.
(6) Selective	-	Action produced by drugs which only affect certain tissues or organs.

(7) Synergistic - The stimulating of the action of one drug by another drug.

(8) Antagonistic - Counteraction of one drug by another one.

(9) Physiological - The effect of a drug on normal animal body.

(10) Therapeutic - The effect upon diseased organs or tissues.

(11) Side Action - Creating an effect not desired.

(12) Emperic - An effect produced but not proved by laboratory experiment.

(13) Toxicological- A poisonous effect generally from result of an overdose.

Cumulative Effect

The effect of drugs too slowly exerted or absorbed so that an accumulation of the drug in the body produces a poisonous effect. Such drugs should not be administered continuously.

Incompatible Drug Action

Ill effects produced by two or more drugs antagonistic to each other.

Mechanism of Drug Action

The terms 'action' and 'effect' are often used as synonyms. How ever it will be appropriate to define the initial consequences of drug-cell interaction as 'action' of the drug and the remaining events are called as the 'effects;' of the drug. A drug may act in either of the following ways:

1. Extracellularly - e.g. osmotic diuretics, and plasma expanders
2. Intracellularly - e.g. antimalignency compounds, and steroid hormones.
3. On the cell surface - e.g. digitalis, penicillin, and insulin.

Drugs may produce their effects through:

(1) Stimulation: Increase in the activity of specialized cells. But, excessive stimulation produces depression e.g. morphine stimulates the vagus and occulomotor nuclei, and the CTZ but depresses the vomiting

	and cough centres. Example for pure stimulation is leptazol produced respiratory stimulation.
(2) Depression:	Decrease in the activity of specialized cells is called depression e.g. myocardial depression by quinidine; CNS depression by barbiturates.
(3) Irritation:	It indicates that a drug produces effects on the growth, nutrition and morphology of living tissues. It is not restricted to specialized cells but can occur in all the body tissues. Irritation may produces changes in cell structure, inflammation, corrosion and necrosis of cells.
(4) Replacement:	Endogenous deficiencies may be managed by replacement e.g. insulin in diabetes mellitus, thyroxine in hypothyroidism etc.
(5) Anti-infective:	Specific action against the causative organisms may be required to prevent, arrest or eradicate the infections. e.g. usage of antibiotics.
(6) Modification: of immune Status	Vaccine, sera and certain other agents (tetramisole & corticosteroids) act by altering (enhancing or depressing) the immune status.

Site of Drug Action

The site of drug action and the mechanism of drug action are two most fundamental aspects of pharmakodynamics. The usual sites for drug action are:

(a) at the point of application e.g. corticosteroid ointment etc.

(b) using transport in the body e.g. osmotic diuretics like mannitol and urea.

(c) by reflex effects through nerves e.g. skin irritants like turpentine oil.

(d) by reaching a definite concentration in a particular tissue, e.g. volatile general anaesthetics like either, and

(e) by reaching a definite concentration in a particular cell, e.g. digitalis.

Drug Receptors

Langley (1905) introduced the idea of a specific 'receptor substance' to explain the action of nicotine and curare. The site (either on the cell membrane or inside the cell) at which a drug molecule attaches itself to produce action is called a 'receptor'. Recent studies indicate that receptors are proteins or enzymes, and a number of receptors have now been identified by ligand binding techniques using radioactive labelled agents and tissue homogenates. Although receptors are dynamic in nature they can be regarded as definite structural entities interacting with the active principle. The selective binding of drugs to receptors is specific and complimentary with their physico-chemical structures.

A drug combines with a receptor to form a drug receptor complex and that brings about the final action. The drugs which produce effect combine with the receptors and this combination is rapidly broken to facilitate further combination to take place. When a drug occupies a receptor and remains there, further action through that receptor is blocked.

Therapeutic Index

It is an approximate assessement of the safety of the drug. It is expressed as the ratio of the median laethal dose to the median effective dose:

$$TI = \frac{LD_{50}}{ED_{50}}$$

LD_{50} (Median Lethal Dose)– is the dose (mg/kg) which would be expected to kill one-half of an unlimited population of the same species and strain.

ED_{50}(Median Effective Dose)– is the dose (mg/kg) which produces a desired response in 50% of the test population.

Adverse Reactions for Drugs

"Any response to a drug that is noxious and unintended and that occurs at doses used in man for prophyloxis, diagnosis or theraphy" is known as adverse reaction- (W.H.O.).

(i) Side effects - pharmacological effects produced with therapeutic doses of the drugs e.g. dryness of mouth with atropine.

(ii) Untoward effects - they develop with therapeutic dose of a drug which are undesirable e.g. vomiting and diarrhoea with para-amino salicylic acid.

(iii) Toxic effects - are seen when a drug is administered repeatedly and or in large doses e.g. paralysis of res piration with morphine or deafness following dihydrostreptomycin.

6. Classification of Karma

Drugs may exert their actions on Doshas, Dhatus, Malas, Srotas, Ashaya, Vyadhi, Agni etc. Usually every drug will exhibit some selective affinity towards a specific organ or organ system. For example, Pramathi dravya removes Sroto Sanga; Āmalaki etc., mainly acts on Rasa and Rasa vaha Srotas; Manjishta acts on Rakta vaha Srotas; Palamkasha acts on Mamsa and Mamsavaha Srotas; Shilajit acts on Medas and Medovaha Srotas; Asthisamharaka acts on Asthi and Asthivaha Srotas; Sobhanjana acts on Majja and Majjavaha Srotas; Musali acts on Sukra and Sukra vaha Srotas etc.

(I) Effect on Doshas

1. Vāta Prakopaka - Mudga, Jambu, Syamaka, Sushka Saka etc.
2. Vāta Sāmaka - Bala, Kushta, Rasna, Erandamula etc.
3. Pitta Prakopaka - Tila taila, Aguru, Sarshapa, Kulutha etc.
4. Pitta Sāmaka - Chandana, Useera, Sariva, Manjishta etc.
5. Kapha Prakopaka - Masha, Godhuma, Dadhi, Ksheera, Kaseruka etc.
6. Kapha Sāmaka - Satapushpa, Kāravellaka, Shilajatu, Bhallataka etc.

[**Note:** Prakopaka = aggravating and samaka = subsiding.]

(II) Effect on Dhatus

1. Rasa Vriddhikara - Ksheera, Seeta guna Rasayanas like Satavari, Snigdha and Āpya dravyas etc.

2. Rasa Kshaya kara - Yava, Ushna guna Rasayanas like Shilajit, Ruksha and Vayaviya dravyas etc.
3. Rakta Vriddhikara - Punarnava, Agnimantha, Yakrit, Kumari Loha, Mandura etc.
4. Rakta Kshaya kara - Sarshapa (vidahi), Amla dravyas, Lavana, Madya, Mrittika, Kshara, Gandhaka etc.
5. Mamsa Vriddhikara- Mamsa rohini, Pacham pacha, Kharjura, Āmra etc.
6. Mamsa Kshayakara- Vacha, Ativisha, Mustha, Palam Kasha, etc.
7. Medo Vriddhikara - Navina guggulu, Vasa, Medas, Ghrita etc.
8. Medo Kshayakara - Purana guggulu, Shilajit, Madhu, Ushna Jala, Yava etc.
9. Asthi Vriddhikara - Asthi samharaka, Rāsna, Pravala, Mukta etc.
10. Asthi Kshayakara - Vata vardhaka dravyas etc.
11. Majja Vriddhikara- Shigru, Majja, Tikta- Madhura Rasas etc.
12. Majja Kshayakara - Ruksha padarthas etc.
13. Sukra Vriddhikara- Kapikachchu, Kokilaksha, Musali, Aswagandha, Ksheera, ghrita, Sarkara etc.
14. Sukra Kshayakara - Haritaki, Chanaka, Kshara, Lavana, etc.

[**Note:** Vriddhikara = enhancing & kshayakara = reducing]

Certain actions like Jeevaniya, Balya, Brimhana, Medohara, Rakta prasadana, Sonita Sthapana, Sukrala etc. are mentioned in the ancient texts which denotes the effect on dhatus.

(III) Effect on Malas

1. Purisha vriddhikara - Masha, Isabgol, Yava etc.
2. Purisha kshayakara - Mudga, Sunthi, Pippali etc.
3. Mutra vriddhikara - Palandu, Gokshura, Useera, Udichya etc.
4. Mutra kshayakara - Aswatha, Asana, Jambu, Dhava etc.
5. Sweda vriddhikara - Sigru, Punarnava, Vatsanabha, Maricha, Madya, Hingula etc.
6. Sweda kshayakara - Parasika Yavani, Useera, Yasada etc.

Classical references about the effect of drugs on Malas are as following:

Purisha— Purisha Sangrahaniya, Purisha virajaniya, Bhedaniya, Sramsana, Anulomana.

Mutra— Mutra virechaniya, Mutra Sangrahaniya, Mutra virajaniya, Ashmarighna, Prameha hara etc.

Sweda— Sweda janana, Sweda Samgrahaka, Swedopaga etc.

(IV) Effect on Upadhatus

(1) Sthanya janana (galactogogues)- Jeevanti, Shatavari etc.

(2) Sthanya Sodhana- Katuki, Tiktalabu etc.

(3) Artava janana (emmenogogues)- Kumari, Ashoka etc.

(4) Artava nasana (anti-ovulatory)- Haritala etc.

(V) Effect on Srotas

1. Pranavaha Srotas	-	Vibhitki, Yashti madhu, pushkaramula, Bharngi, Tulasi, Kantakari, etc.
2. Udakavaha srotas	-	Dhanyaka, Useera, Chandana, Musta etc.
3. Annavaha Srotas	-	Sunthi, Pippali, chitraka, Jeeraka, etc
4. Rasa vaha Srotas	-	Āmalaki, Arjuna, Guduchi, Jeevanti, Nirgundi etc.
5. Raktavaha Srotas	-	Vāsa, Manjishta, Chakramarda, Nimba, Laksha, Karanja, Haridra etc.
6. Mamsavaha Srotas	-	Mamsa rohini, Palam kasha, Lasuna, Bhallataka, Chavya, Madhuka, Agaru etc.
7. Medovaha Srotas	-	Karpoora, Guggulu, Kanchanara, Shilajit, Apamarga, Vacha, Musta etc.
8. Asthivaha Srotas	-	Bakula, Asthisamharaka, Snuhi, Chanaka etc.
9. Majjavaha Srotas	-	Chopchini, Habusha, Shalmali etc.
10. Sukravaha Srotas	-	Dasamula, Kasturi, Kapikachchu, Patalagarudi, Mundi etc.
11. Artavavaha Srotas	-	Lodhra, Ashoka, Kumari, Lakshmana, Sariva, Lajjalu, Dugdhika etc.

12. Purishavaha Srotas - Haritaki, Jatiphala, Bilwa, Mocha rasa, Kutaja, Āragwadha etc.

13. Mutravaha Srotas - Pashanabheda, varuna, Gokshura, Kulutha etc.

14. Swedavaha Srotas - Vatsna nasha, Shigru, Nagakesara, Priyangu, Punarnava etc.

The classical pharmacological properties on the individual Srotas are as following:

(i) Pranavaha - Hridya, Ahridya etc.

(ii) Udakavaha - Trishna nigrahana, Trishna janana etc.

(iii) Annavaha - Deepana, Pachana, Vidahi, Vishtambhi, Vamana, Vamanopaga, Chardi nigrahara, Rochana, Grahi, Sthambhana, Sula prasamana etc.

(VI) Effect on Āshaya or Srotomula

1. Chakshushya
2. Plihari
3. Netrarogari
4. Kantya
5. Hridya
6. Vrishya

(VII) Effect on Vyadhi or Lakshana

1. Arsoghna - Kutaja, Chavya etc.
2. Kushtaghna - Bakuchi, Āragwadha etc.
3. Jwaraghna - Sariva, Patha etc.
4. Vishaghna - Sirisha, Maricha etc.
5. Krimighna - Vidanga, Sigru, Palasa etc.
6. Kandughna - Chandana, Sarshapa etc.
7. Udarda prasamana - Haridra.
8. Angamarda prasamana - Katphala.

9. Vedana sthapana - Ashoka, Saptaparna, Mahanimba etc.
10. Seeta prasamana - Agaru,
11. Daha prasamana - Chandana, Useera etc.
12. Sotha hara - Dosamula, Punarnava etc.
13. Kasa hara - Bhumyamalaki, Vasa, Tulasi etc.
14. Swasa hara - Bhumyamalaki, Sathi, Pushkaramula, Kantakari etc.

(VIII) Effect of Agni

1. Deepana
2. Pachana
3. Deepana-Pachana
4. Rochana

7. Different tests of Drug Action

According to the philosophy of Ayurveda the mode of drug action may be assessed by three means viz., Pratyaksha, Anumana and Aptopadesa.

(i) Pratyaksha (direct observation)- assessement of Rasa, Virya etc., by means of orgonoleptic methods and practical observation.

(ii) Anumana (inference)- Virya and Vipaka are usually assessed through inference by observing the actions.

(iii) Āptopadesa (classical references)- e.g. wearing the root of Datura metel (Krishna Dhattura) as waist band while participating in coitus will prevent conception. Similar references are available as the famous sayings of the elders.

Usually the drugs will be utilized for human administration and basing upon their therapeutic effect the pharmacological properties are inferred. For example, a drug resulting in loss of weight may indicate the Lekhana property; increased urination will indicate the diuretic effect etc. Sushrita quoted that the authority of Acharyas or Sastra are unquestionable and are to by followed without any doubt. Reasons for non-specific action of a drug need not be searched.

Now a days there is a trend to assess the action of a drug by means of animal experimentations. Though there are many references about the study of drugs on animals in Ayurveda, they were not intended for pharmaco-therapeutics. e.g.

1. Aswa mara (Thevesia peruviana) - which kills horses
2. Kakaghna (Pongamia sps.) - which kills crows
3. Krimighna (Embelia ribes) - which kills intestinal worm etc
4. Kapikachchu (Mucuna prurieta) - which causes itching to monkeys.
5. Sarpagandha (Rauwalfia serpentina) - which causes agony to snakes

There are references that several animals and birds are used to test the poisonous foods etc., of royal families and kings. Monkey, Peacock are important among them. In Bhava Prakasha it is mentioned that the milk of a cow which is fed with the leaves of Black gram will be the best Rasayana & Vrishya. Similarly the meat of animals which will eat the flesh of other animals will be best in providing strength. These are some of the references about utilizing animals in assessing pharmacological properties of Ayurvedic drugs etc.

Today we have different animal models for the assessement of biological activities and toxicological studies. The modern experimental pharmacology developed various animal models.

The table shows Tests done by CDRI for the study of different biological activities

	Activity		Test done
(A)	Antiviral	1.	Ranikhet disease virus, chorioallantoic membrane (CAM), chick embryo fibroblast monolayers (CEF), in vitro
		2.	Vaccina virus - CAM & CEF
		3.	Semliki forest virus (mouse, in vivo)
		4.	Interferon inducers (mouse)

(B)	Antibacterial (In vitro unless mentioned otherwise)	1.	Streptococcus faecalis
		2.	Klebsiella pneumoniae
		3.	Mycobacterium laprae (in vivo, mouse)
		4.	Mycobacterium tuberculosis (in vivo also)
		5.	Staphylococcus aureus
		6.	Salmonella typhi
		7.	Escherichia coli
		8.	Pscudomonas aeruginosa
		9.	Baeillus subtilis
(C)	Antifungal (In vitro unless mentioned otherwise)	1.	Candida albicans (in vivo also)
		2.	Tricophyton metagrophytes (in vivo also)
		3.	Aspergillus fumigatus
		4.	Cryptococcus neoformans
		5.	Sporotrichum schenckii
		6.	Fusarium solani (in vivo)
		7.	Curvularia lunata (in vivo)
		8.	Acrophialophora fusispora (in vivo)
(D)	Antiprotozoal		
	(a) Antiamoebic	1.	Axenic culture in vitro
		2.	Intestinal infection in rat
		3.	Hepatic infection in rat
		4.	Meningeoencephalitis in mouse
	(b) Antimalarial	1.	Blood schizonticide (i) in vitro-P. falciparum (ii) in vivo- mouse, rat, monkey, mastomys
		2.	Causal prophylactic - mastomys, mouse, monkey
		3.	Antirelapse - monkey in vitro and in vivo (hamster)

(E)	Anthelminitc		
	(a) Filaria	1.	Litmosoides carinii (cotton, rat, mastomys)
		2.	Brugia malayi (cat, mastomys)
		3.	Dipetalonema viteae (mastomys)
	(b) Hook worm		Ancylostoma ceylanicum (rat, hamster)
	(c) Tape worm		Hymenolepis nana (mouse, rat)
(F)	Anti-cancer		In vitro cell line
(G)	Endocrinal		
	(a) Antifertility	1.	In vivo
	In female		anti-implantation (rat, hamster)
			abortifacient (rat)
			Tubal occluding (monkey)
			Blastotoxic (rat)
			Oxytocic (cat)
		2.	In vitro
			Abortifacient (rate uterus)
	In male	1.	Antispermatogenic (rat)
		2.	Spermicidal in vitro
		3.	Semen coagulant in vitro
	(b) Hypoglycaemic		Rabbit, rat
(H)	CNS activity	1.	Gross effects on behaviour
	(mouse & rat)	2.	Body temperature
		3.	Analgesia
		4.	Supramaximal electroshock seizure pattern
		5.	Barbiturate potentiation and antagonism
		6.	Amphetamine hyperactivity and toxicity
		7.	Strychnine/metrazol seizures
		8.	Antireserpine

		9.	Phenylquinone writhing
		10.	Rota rod
		11.	Learning and memory
(I)	CVS and autonomic effects (cat, dog)	1.	Blood pressure
		2.	Respiration
		3.	E.K.G.
		4.	Antiarvhythmic in vitro-guinea pig auricle in vivo-rat, aconitine arrhythmia
(J)	Hypolipidaemic (a) Lipid lowering in vivo triton (rat, rabbit, monkey)		Serum cholesterol, triglycerides and lipoproteins in normal and high fat fed/treated animals.
	(b) Cholesteral biosynthesis		Rat liver slices
	(c) Inhibition of platelet aggregation		in vitro and in vivo
(K)	Anti-inflammatory		Carrageenin paw edema (mouse, rat) Granuloma pouch (rat) Adjuvant arthritis (rat) Ulcerogenic index (rat)
(L)	Miscellaneous		
	(a) Acute toxicity (LD_{50})		Mouse, rat (i.p., oral)
	(b) Diuretic		Rat
	(c) Spasmolytic		Isolated guinea pig ileum
	(d) Neuromuscular conduction		Cat
	(e) Hepatoprotective		Liver damage by ccl_4 Lanthanum and galoctosamine in rats
	(f) Antiallergic		PCA (mouse, rat) Haemagglutination cell mediated immunity (rat).

8. Detailed study of Pharmacological actions deleniated in Ayurvedic texts

(1) Deepana: ***(Appetizers)***

Deepana drugs will stimulate or enhance the Agni[1]. This agni may be either Jataragni or Bhutagni or Dhatwagni. Sarngdhara defined it as the drug which enhances the Agni without performing Āma pāchana e.g., Misi (Satapushpa)[2].

Charaka mentioned Pippali, Pippali mula, Chavya, Chitraka, Nagara, Amlavetasa, Maricha, Ajamoda, Bhallataka & Hingu as Deepaniya Dasaimani[3].

Sushrita considered Agni predominant dravya as Deepaniya while others quote Prithi & Vayu predominant drug as Deepaniya[4].

Arunadatta stated that Deepaniya drug may also perform Āma pachana sometimes. This may be the reason for not mentioning Pachaniya Dasaimani in Charaka Samhita[5].

Arunadatta mentioned Ghrita as the example for Deepana[6].

(2) Pachana: (Digestives)

The drug which under take digestion of Ama alone without causing Agni deepana is known as 'Pachana' e.g. Nagakesara[7].

Arunadatta considered Pachana as the part of activity of Agni and the drug which improves digestion is known as Pachana. He also

---

१. दीपनीयं वह्नेरूद्दीपनाय हितम् । (गङ्गाधर: च.सू.४अ.)

२. पचेन्नामं वह्निकृच्च दीपनं तद्यथा मिशि: । (शा.सं.पू.खं.४)

३. पिप्पली-पिप्पलीमूल-चव्य-चित्रक-शृङ्गवेर-अम्लवेतस-मरिच-अजमोद-भल्लातकास्थि-हिङ्गुनिर्यास इति दशैमानिदीपनीयानि भवन्ति । (च.सू.४अ.)

४. (i) दीपनमग्निगुणभूयिष्ठं तत्समानत्वात् । (सु.सू.४१)
(ii) पृथिव्यनिलबाहुल्याद्दीपनं परिचक्ष्महे ।। (र.वै.४ भाष्यं)

५. क्षारपाणिनाऽप्युक्तम् - पाचनं पाचयेद्दोषान् सामान् शमनमेव तु ।
दीपनं ह्याग्निकृत्वामं कदाचित्पाचयेन्न वा । (अरुणदत्त-अ.हृ.सू. १४/६-७)

६. यदग्निकृत् पचेन्नामं दीपनं तद्यथा घृतम् । दीपनं ह्यग्निकृत्वामं कदाचित् पाचयेन्न वा ।। (अरुणदत्त-अ.हृ.सू.७)

७. पचत्यामं न वह्निं च कुयाद्यत्तद्धि पाचनम् ।
नागकेसखत् विद्यात् .... ।। (शां.सं.प्र.ख.४/)

mentioned it as a type of Samana action[1].

Sarangdhara made specific definition for Pachana, which is digestive property in modern pharmacology. Another related action Sula prasamana may be equal carminative, rather than spasmolytics.

Sushrita explained Pippalyadi and Dasamula ganas act as Ama pachaka; Vachadi and Haridradi ganas act as Dosha pachaka; Mustadi gana act as Pachaka.

At later times Jarana & Jaraniya terms were used to denote Pachana e.g. Souveeraka, Tushodaka[2]. Chakrapani opined Pachana dravya as predominant of Vayu & Agni bhutas while Arunadatta considered it as predominant of Agni bhuta.

Probably the utility of Deepana and Pachana is elaborated in detail during the period of Laghutrayee where in the description of Agnimandya and Ajeerna are found seperately. The former condition is treated with Deepaniya drugs while the later is treated with Pachaniya drugs.

Concept of Deepana- Pachana

After mentioning Deepana and Pachana properties, Sarngdhara mentioned Chitraka as Deepana as well as Pachana (i.e. appetizer as well as digestive)[3]. In this context it will be essential to find out the difference between these actions. Charaka mentioned Deepaniya dasaimani alone.

However Charaka mentioned deepana, Pachana properties seperately as well as combinedly for different drugs:

(i) In Upakalpaniya chapter Deepana and Pachana properties are mentioned seperately[4].

(ii) Pippalimula is Deepana-Pachana-Ānahahara[5].

---

१. पचतोऽग्नेः पक्तुं शक्तिमधिकां यदुत्पादयति तद् द्रव्यं क्रिया वा पाचनमुच्यते । (अरुणदत्त)
पाचनं पाचयेद्दोषान् सामान् शमनमेव तु । (अरुणदत्त-अ.हृ.सू.१४)
२. जरणीयं पाचनम् । (योगेन्द्रनाथः)
३. चित्रो दीपनपाचनः । (शा.सं.म.ख.४)
४. ....संग्रहणीय-दीपनीय-पाचनीय-उपशमनीय-वातहारि-समाख्यातानि चौषधानि । (च.सू.१५/७)
५. पिप्पलीमूलं दीपनीयपाचनीयानाहप्रशमनानां । (च.सू. २५)

(iii) Chitramula is deepana-pachana-guda sotha-Arsohara-Sulahara[1].

(iv) Mustha is sangrahi-deepana-pachana[2].

(v) Udichya is nirvapana-deepana-pachana-chardighna-Atisarghna[3].

(vi) Katwanga is Sangrahi-pachana-deepana[4].

(vii) Amrita is sangrahi-vatahara-deepaniya-kapharakta hara[5].

(viii) Bilwa is sangrahi-deepaniya-vatakapha hara[6].

(ix) Haritaki is deepana-pachana[7].

Above references indicate that the Deepaniya dasaimani of Charaka includes deepana-pachama drugs like: Pippali mula & Chitraka. But it is essential to realize that only Pachana activity is rarely seen. Therefore emphasis was only made on Deepana while classifying the drug groups.

The practical utility of Deepana-Pachana will be seen in the management of Amavata where the line of treatment denotes 'Tikta deepana' and 'Katu deepana'. Tikta rasa dravyas may be pitta Samakas while being Agnivardhakas. Vice-versa may be the mode of action of Katu rasa dravyas[8].

Modern Perspective

(a) Appetizers: They are the agents employed commonly to stimulate appetite. Usually the bitters will augment the flow of gastric juice and increase the appetite. Symptomatically, appetite can be improved by varying diet and by the use of such simple preparations

---

१. चित्रमूलं दीपनीयपाचनीयगुदशोथार्श:शूलहराणां । (च.सू. २५)

२. मुस्तं सांग्राहिकदीपनीयपाचनीयानाम् । (च.सू. २५)

३. उदीच्यं निर्वापणदीपनीयपाचनीयच्छर्द्यतीसारहराणां । (च.सू. २५)

४. कट्वङ्गं सांग्राहिकपाचनीयदीपनीयानाम् । (च.सू. २५)

५. अमृता सांग्राहिकवातहरदीपनीयश्लेष्मशोणितविबन्धप्रशमनानाम् । (च.सू. २५)

६. बिल्वं सांग्राहिकदीपनीयवातकफप्रशमनानां । (च.सू. २५)

७. हरीतकीं पञ्चरसामुष्णामलवणां शिवम् ।
दोषानुलोमनीं विद्याद्दीपनपाचनीम् ॥ (च.चि. १/१/२९)

८. .....ततो दीपनपाचनं दीपनमग्निदीपनं पाचनं आमादिशमनं । (आढमल्लः-शा.सं.प्र.खं.१/७)

** According to Charaka 'Langhana-Pachana' is a specific procedure advised under Langhana for Madhyama Bala.

as lemon, pickles & soup. Small quantities of Alcohol, Insulin are also used as appetizers.

(b) Digestants: They are the drugs that are claimed to aid digestion in the GIT e.g. HCl, Bile, Pancreatin etc.

(c) Carminatives: They are the drugs used to expel gas from the stomach or the intestines in the treatment of flatulance and of colics. They act by mild irritation, thereby increasing the GI motility and causing relaxation of sphincters. They produce the feeling of warmth in the stomach. It is important to note that they do not affect the gastric acid secretion significantly.

(3) Samsodhana

The drug which seperates the Malasanchaya (doshas as well as malas) from their respective sites and expel upwards (through mouth) or downwards (through anus) is known as "Deha-Samsodhana". e.g. Devadali (Jeemutaka).

Though Charaka considered Sodhana is of four types (viz., Vamana, Vireshana, Sirovirechama & Niruha Vasthi)[1,2], Deha Samsodhana includes only Vamana (emesis) and Virechana (purgation)[3] according to Dalhana.

Sushrita mentioned four dosha Samsodhana vargas viz.;

(i) Kapha Samsodhana or Vamana or Urdhwabhagahara dravyas.

(ii) Pitta Samsodhana or Virechana or Adhobhagahara dravyas.

---

१. स्थानाद्बहिर्नयेदूर्ध्वमधश्च मलसञ्चयम् ॥
देहसंशोधनं तत् स्याद्देवदालीफलं यथा । (शा.सं.प्र.खं. ४/८-९)
* आढमल्लः- यद्द्रव्यं प्रकुपितस्थानात् मलसञ्चयं दोषादीनां स्वस्थानादूर्ध्वमधो वा बहिर्नयेत् बहिः करेति तद्देहे शरीरे शोधनं कथितम् ।.....ऊर्ध्वं मुखनासिकाभ्यां, अधः पायुमेढ्रमार्गेण, देहग्रहणेन शोणितावसेचनमपि गृह्यते शोधनत्वात् । यतः शोधनं 'द्विविधमाचक्षते बहिराश्रयमभ्यन्तराश्रयं च । तत्र बहिराश्रयं शस्त्रक्षाराग्निप्रलेपादयः । अभ्यन्त्रराश्रयं तु चतुःप्रकारं वमनविरेचनास्थापनशोणितमोक्षणं च । डाके शिरोविरेचनं मन्यन्ते । तच्चात्र वमनान्तर्भूतं बोद्धव्यम्, ऊर्ध्वशोधनत्वात् ।

२. चतुष्प्रकाराः संशुद्धिः । (च.सू.)

३. तत्र द्विविधं संशोधनं-वमनं, विरेचनं च । (डल्हण-सू.सू. ३९/३)

(iii) Kapha-pitta Samsodhana or Vamana - Virechana or Ubhayabhagahara dravyas.

(iv) Nasya or Sirovirechana dravyas.

[**Note:** Sushrita did not mention Vasti dravyas under Samsodhana varga descreptions]

Among the treatment procedures, Sodhana and Shamana were mentioned as the varieties of Langhana[1]. Laghu Vagbhata considered 'Pancha Karmas' as Sodhana procedures[2].

(4) Samsamana

The drug which expel the doshas neither upwards nor downwards and which does not aggravate the doshas but brings the doshas to normal state is known as 'Samsamana'. e.g. Guduchi[3].

Sushrita consdered these drugs as predominent of Akasha bhuta while Badhanta Nagarjuna considered them as Vayu, Jala & Prithvi predominent[4].

He mentioned three dosha Samsamana group of drugs viz.,

(i) Vata Samsamana varga

(ii) Pitta Samsamana varga

(iii) Sleshma Samsamana varga.

Vagbhata indicated Brimhana as Vata Samaka as well as Vata-pitta Samaka[5].

These drugs are usually administered for the palliative management of various diseased conditions. While Sodhana drugs perform

---

१. शोधनं शमनं चेति द्विधा तत्रापि लङ्घनम् ॥ (अ.हृ.सू. १४/७)

२. यदीरयेद्बहिर्दोषान् पञ्चधा शोधनं च तत् ।
निरूहो वमनं कायशिरोऽस्रविस्रुतिः ॥ (अ.हृ.सू. १४/५)

३. (i) न शोधयति न द्वेष्टि समान् दोषांस्तथोद्धतान् ॥
समीकरोति विषमान् शमनं तद्यथाऽमृता । (शा.सं.प्र.खं. ४/)

(ii) न शोधयति यद्दोषान् समान्नोदीरयत्यपि ।
समीकरोति विषमान् शमनं तच्च सप्तधा ॥
पाचनं दीपनं क्षुत्तृड्व्यायामातपमारूताः । (अ.हृ.सू. १४/६-७)

४. आकाशगुणभूयिष्ठं संशमनम् । (सु.सू. ४१

५. बृंहणं शमनं त्वेव वायोः पित्तानिलस्य च । (अ.हृ.सू. १४/७

the action of expulsion of the vitiated/aggravated doshas, these drugs will exert the action of suppressing the aggravated doshas.

(5) Anulomana

The drug which will do Mala pāka and removes the bandha (sphincter relaxation) to expel them downwards is known as 'Anulomana' e.g. Haritaki[1]. Some scholars consider Mala paka as subsiding the aggravated/vitiated doshas and malas.

Sushrita quoted Anulomana as the specific property of 'Sara guna'. In this context Dalhana mentioned Anulomana as Vata (flatus?) and Mala (feces?) Anulomana[2].

Acharya Yadavji Trikamji called Anulomana as Saraka (Sara) which is a Adhobhagahara variety. Similarly 'Sramsana' is also considered as a type of Adhabhagahara property.

Acharya P.V. Sharmaji considered Anulomana dravyas as carminatives. They are expected to remove the flatulance (vayu) formed in the Amashaya. Usually these drugs should be Ushna veerya & Snigdha guna e.g. Hirgu & Yavani. Other examples are: Katu dravya, Karpoora, Madya, Nadi hingu, Teja patra, Misreya, Putiha etc.

The author is of the openion that carminative drugs are described under the Sulahara dasaimani is Charaka Samhita. Hingu, Yavani etc, are there in that group. Anulomana group of drugs will possess digestive as well as laxative property.

Prof. S.G. Dhyaniji attributed four actions to sara guna viz.,

(i) Anulomana, (ii) Vāta pravartaka, (iii) Mala pravartaka & (iv) Pitta vardhana.

---

१. कृत्वा पाकं मलानां यद्भित्वा बन्धमधो नयेत् ॥
तच्चानुलोमनं ज्ञेयं यथा प्रोक्ता हरीतकी । (शा.सं.प्र.खं. ४/३-४)
* आढमल्लः- यद्द्रव्यं मलानां दोषाणां पाकं कोपशान्तिं कृत्वा बन्धं निबन्धं च भित्त्वा भिनत्ति नीत्वा अधो नयेत् अधः करोति वातादिकमिति शेषः प्रतिलोमादनुलोमं करोतीत्यर्थः ।........कोष्ठ इति पाचकस्थाने ।

२. (i) सरोऽनुलोमनः प्रोक्तः ॥ (सु.सू. ४६)
*डल्हणः- अनुलोमनोवातमल प्रवर्तनः ।
(ii) अनुलोमनं वातादीनामधः प्रवर्तनं सरगुणत्वात् । (आढमल्लः-शा.सं.प्र.खं. ४/८)

Prof. Viswanath Dwivedi considered that the action of Anulomana drugs will be there on the intestinal walls and clearly quoted it as the GIT action. However some scholars are of the openion that Anulomana may be systemic action also.

The utility of Anulomana action is observed in various conditions e.g.

1. Atisara	:	Samgrahi drug shall not be given in Āmātisāra. Initially Anulomana to be administered for mala pachana and Āma nirharana.
2. Agnimandya	:	Virechana is indicated as Pitta pratikara.
3. Ajeerna	:	Mala vata Apravritti is the main picture in Ajeerna. Therefore Anulomana will be more useful. Hence its management possess Pathyadi churna, Amrita Haritaki etc.
4. Udavarta	:	The line of treatment contains Vata Anulomana and therefore Haritakyadi churna is indicated in Udavarta.
5. Ānaha	:	In Ānaha also Udavarta chikitsas i.e., Anulomana is useful.
6. Gulma	:	Vātanulomana is specifically indicated in the line of treatment of Gulma (Yo.Ra.)

Sramsana

The malas which remain attached to the Koshta will be expelled without paka (digestion) by the action of Sramsana drugs. e.g. Āragwadha[1]. But according to Yogendranath Sen Sramsana means Virechana[2].

The main difference between Anulomana and Sramsana is that "the former will perform Malapaka while the later does not".

Charaka quoted that expulsion of Pitta or Pitta-Kapha from Pittasaya is known as 'Sramsana'[3].

---

१. पक्तव्यं यदपक्वैव शिलष्टं कोष्ठे मलाधिकम् ।
नयत्यधः स्रंसनं तद्यथा स्यात् कृतमालकः ॥ (शा.सं.प्र.खं. ४/)

२. स्रंसनं विरेचनम् । (योगेन्द्रनाथ-च.चि.)

३. पित्तं वा कफपित्तं वा पित्ताशयगतं हरेत् - स्रंसनं । (च.चि.३अ.)

Sri Vamana Ganesh Desai made the following comparisions between various purgative drugs:

(a) Sramsana = simple purgative e.g. Eranda Taila, Eluva
(b) Bhedana = drastic purgative e.g. Trivrit, Revand chini
(c) Virechana = hydrogogue purgative e.g. Jamalghota
(d) Anulomana = laxative e.g. Haritaki
(e) Pitta Saraka = chologogue purgative e.g. Katuka rohini

Prof. S.C. Dhyaniji explained the mode of action of different purgative properties according to Ayurveda in the following manner:

	Mode of action	Anulomana	Sramsana	Bhedana	Rechana
1.	Effect on Mala or dosha	digests	without digesting	-	-
2.	Effect on incre-ased Mala	breaks	-	breaks	-
3.	Effect on Mala	-	-	liquifies	liquifies
4.	Effect on sticked Mala	-	removes at-tachement	-	-
5.	Effect on expu-lsion of Mala	+	+	+	+

(6) Bhedana

The action by which solid or liquid Purisha and malas i.e., Baddha malas or Abaddha malas etc., will be expelled downwards (through guda marga) is called as 'Bhedana' e.g. Katuki[1].

These drugs are simile to Choleretics or Chologogues. Chologogues effect constriction of gall bladder and expulsion of

---

१. मलादिकमबद्धं च बद्धं वा पिण्डतं मलैः ।
भित्त्वाधः पातयति तद्भेदनं कटुकी यथा ॥ (शा.सं.प्र.खं. ४/५-६)
*आढमल्लः-यन्मालादिकमबद्धं मलबद्धं वा अत एव मलैर्दोषैश्च कृत्वा पिण्डितपरिपाकात् पिण्डीभूतम् । ईदृशं मलादिकं भित्वा स्थानात् सञ्चाल्याधः पातयति तद्भेदनं ज्ञातव्यमिति शेषः । बद्धं, विबद्धं, शुष्कं, ग्रथितं च । तत्र शुष्कं पुरीषविषयं ग्रथितं दोषादीनाम् । अबद्धमपि द्विविधं । तथा एकं द्रवरूपं पुरीषविषयं स्वतन्त्रमेकं मलादिकमिति, मलोऽत्र दोषः । आदिग्रहणात् रूक्षदूषितादीनामपि ग्रहणम् । भित्वेति तत्पुरीषं भित्त्वा विदार्याधः पातयति द्रव्यमिति शेषः ॥

excessive bile into GIT which causes increased perstalytic movements leading to purgation.

Charaka mentioned 10 drugs under the Bhedaniya group of drugs. As already mentioned, Chitraka among this group must be Dravanti i.e., Jatropa gossypifolium. Sushrita described Shyamadi gana as 'Vid bhedi'. While Vriddha Vagbhata accepted both the views.

(7) Rechana

The drug which will exerete the Pakwa or Apakwa malas/doshas downwards in the liquid form is known as "Rechana" e.g., Trivrit[1]. The Virechana dravyas are usually Prithvi and Jala bhuta predominant[2].

Charaka considered that expulsion of doshas in the downward direction as 'Virechana'. He also mentioned that both Vamana and Virechana together are called as 'Rechana'[3]. This is because both have the similarity of expelling the vitiated doshas. According to him there are three grades of Virechana dravyas:

(i) Sukha virechana - Trivrit

(ii) Mridu virechana - Āragwadha

(iii) Tikshna virechana - Snuhi ksheera

The mode of action of Virechana dravya is explained in the following manner: 'the drugs which have Ushna, Teekshna, Sukshma, Vyavayi, Vikasi gunas will reach the heart through vessels by means their Virya initially. Due to Sukshma and Vyavayi properties they reach macro and micro channels (Sthula and Sukshma Srotas). After spreading all over the body, they break and liquify the complexes of doshas by means of Agni and Tikshna gunas. Thence the drava rupa (liquid) mala will reach the koshta i.e. Amasaya and expelled in the

१. विपक्वं यदपक्वं वा मलादि द्रवतां नयेत् ॥
रेचयत्यपि तज्ज्ञेयं रेचनं त्रिवृता यथा । (शा.सं.प्र.खं. ४/६-७)
* आढमल्लः- यद्द्रव्यं विपक्वमपक्वं वा मलादि दोषादिकं द्रवतां नयेत्
द्रवभावं करोतीत्यर्थः । न केवलं द्रवतां नयेत् रेचयत्यपि च तद्रेचनं ज्ञेयं.......।

२. विरेचनद्रव्याणि पृथिव्यम्बुगुणभूयिष्ठानि । (सु.सू.)

३. तत्र दोषहरणं उर्ध्वभागं वमनसंज्ञकं; अधोभागं विरेचन संज्ञकम् । उभयं वा
शरीरमलरेचनात् विरेचनमिति संज्ञां लभते ॥ (च.क.१.अ.)

downward direction (through anus) because of Prithvi- Jala bhuta dominance[1].

Pharmacological Actions on Peristaltic Movements

(1) Laxative: *(Anulomana)*

Laxative effect suggests the elimination of soft, formed stool without griping and without much loss of water.

(2) Bulk Laxative: *(Sramsana)*

The natural or semisynthetic polysachcharides and cellulose derivatives, which when given orally are not absorbed and increase the indigestible residue are known as bulk-laxatives.

(3) Emollient Laxative: *(Bhedana)*

They are not significantly absorbed and exerts a softening as well as lubricating effect on faeces.

(4) Cathartics: *(Rechana)*

Drugs which are used to promote defication are called 'cathartics'. *Osmotic cathartics* are not much absorbed and retained in GIT. They exert an asmotic effect and, therefore, hold considerable amounts of water, thus increaing the intestinal bulk. Thus mechanical stimulus causing evacuation.

(5) Choleretics: *(Bhedana)*

Any agent that increase excretion of bile by the liver. The excessive bile may lead to purgation.

Note: Yogendranath considered that the drug which expels the Pindita mala in the Drava rupa (liquid form) as the Bhedana drug, which is not coinsiding with the definitions of Bhedana or Rechana[2].

(8) Lekhana

The drug which will reduces or scrapes away the unwanted tissues (dhatus) and metabolic wastes (malas) is known as 'Lekhana'

---

१. तत्रोण-तीक्ष्ण-सूक्ष्म-व्यवायि-विकासीन्यौषधानि स्ववीर्येण हृदयमुपेत्य, धमनीरनुसृत्य स्थूलाणु स्रोतेभ्यः केवलं शरीरगतं दोषसङ्घातमाग्नेयत्वाद्विष्यन्दयन्ति, तैक्ष्याद्विच्छिन्दन्ति

२. भेदनं पिण्डितमलानां द्रवीकृत्य बहिःसारंण, तस्मैहितम् । (योगेन्द्रनाथः)

e.g., Vacha, Yava, honey, hot-water[1].

A lekhana drug is usually Vayu and Agni bhuta predominant[2]. Dalhana defined lekhana drug as the one which removes the Kapha and Medas[3]. While Gangadhara explained it as the drug which causes cracks in the skin by rubbing the skin with it[4]. In surgery (Salya Tantra) Lekhana means scraping with instruments or alkalies[5].

Charaka mentioned Lekhaniya group of ten drugs e.g. Musta, Chitraka, Haridra, Vacha, Kushta etc. Sushrita indicated Sālasāradi gana as kapha-medo visoshana.

There is another property which is similar to lekhana i.e.; Chedana.

Chedana

The drug which forcefully detaches the malas and doshas that are stick to (or deeply attached to) the body is known as "Chedana" e.g. Maricha, Silajatu[6]. Kasiram specially mentioned that Chedana drug will destroy the sticky nature of vitiated malas and doshas. Gangadhara mentioned that Amla, Lavana & Katu Rasa dravyas will cut through the Sareera kleda etc[7]. Charaka described Chedana as one of the actions of Hingu. He did not mention any group of drugs possessing this property.

---

१. धातून् मलान् वा देहस्य विशोष्योल्लेखयेच्च यत् ॥
लेखनं तद्यथा क्षौद्रं नीरमुष्णं वचा यवाः । (शा.सं.प्र.खं. ४/१०-११)
*आढमल्लः- यद्द्रव्यं धातून् रसादीन् मलान् वा । अत्र मलान् वा यद्ग्रहणं कृतं तन्मनोदोषव्यवच्छेदार्थम् । यतो मनोदोषप्रतीकारमन्यदप्यस्तीति ।

२. लेखनमनिलानलगुणभूयिष्टम् । (सु.सू. ४१)

३. लेखनं कफमेदसोः । (डल्हण-सु.सू. ४१)

४. लेखनम् ईषच्चर्मविदरणं घर्षणेन, तस्मै हितं लेखनीयम् । (गङ्गाधरः)

५. शल्यतन्त्रे कठिनोत्सन्न मांसानां व्रणानां शस्त्रेण क्षौमादिभिर्वा घर्षणं लेखनमित्युच्यते ॥(सु.चि. १ अ.)

६. शिलष्टान् कफादिकान् दोषानुन्मूलयति यद्बलात् ॥
छेदनं तद्यथा क्षाराः मरिचानि शिलाजतु । (शा.सं.प्र.खं. ४/९-१०)
*काशीरामः- यद्द्रव्यं शिलष्टान् मलादिकान् दोषान् बलादुन्मूलयति स्वभावान्नाशयति तच्छेदनं ज्ञेयम् ।
** आढमूल्लः- यद्द्रव्यं शिलष्टान् संचितान् - परस्परग्रथितानित्येके, अत्यर्थं कुपितानित्यपरे, कफादिकान् दोषान्, आदिग्रहणेन वातपित्तशोणितकृमिग्रहणंनतु दूष्यदूष्यतादिकं, यतः दोषानिति पुनर्ग्रहणं कृयिशोणितयोरपि दोषसंज्ञा ।......कृमिस्तु गग्गुलुकल्पे यथा पञ्चादिदोषान् शमयेदित्यादिप्रश्ने कृमिदोषनिबर्हणादित्यादिना तन्मने कृमेस्तु दोषसंज्ञा ।

७. द्रव्याणि हि अम्ल-लवण-कटूनि शरीरक्लेदादीनि छिन्दन्ति । (गङ्गाधरः)

From the above description a conclusion may be drawn that Chedana is more powerful action compared to Lekhana. For example, Chedana drugs may be used in conditions like obesity when excessive/unwanted adipose tissue is to be removed from the body. Similarly Lekhana will be more useful in reducing the serum cholesterol levels in hyperlipaemia where in circulating fats are usually removed. The concept of Poshya & Poshaka dhatus or Sthula & Sukshma dhatus will support this view.

At the broad sense, Chedana drug will cut-through the tissues. while Lechana drug scrapes away the surface of interior or exterior of body or organ systems.

(9) Grahi

The drug which acts both as appetizer and digestive (Deepana & Pachana) while absorbing the fluids is known as Grahi e.g. Sunthi, Jeeraka, Gaja Pippali[1].

The Grahi or Sangrahi dravya is predominent in Prithvi and Vayu bhutas usually[2]. Sushrita pointed out Vayu bhuta as the responsible factor for Drava soshana while sarngdhara considers Ushna virya as responsible.

Adhamalla is of the view that Grahi is two types viz., Pakwa (Seeta) and Āma (Ushna) Sangrahis. The former will digest the Āma in the Grahani and absorbs the fluids. Therefore it is known as *Ushna Sangrahi* or *Āma Sangrahi*. While the later will stop the Pakwa malas in Atisara etc., and stops their excretion. Therefore it is known as *Seeta Sangrahi* or *Pakwa Sangrahi*[3]. In otherwords "Grahi" may be

---

१. दीपनं पाचनं यत् स्यादुष्णत्वात् द्रवशोषक़म् ।
ग्राहि तच्च यथा शुण्ठी जीरकं गजपिप्पली ॥ (शा.सं.प्र.खं.४/११-१२)
सांग्राहिकं विजानीयात् पृथिव्यनिलसम्भवम् । (र.वै.)

२. यद्द्रव्यं दीपनमग्निकरं पाचनमामादीनां, द्रवशोषकमिति द्रवसवरूपाणां दोषधातुमलादीनां शोषकमित्यर्थः, उष्णत्वात् उष्णवीर्यत्वात् ।.....ननु संग्राहकमनिलगुणभूयिष्ठं यतोऽनिलस्य शोषणात्मकत्वात्। तत् कथमुष्णत्वादिति। उच्यते-पक्वामग्राहकत्वेन द्विविधं हि संग्राहकत्वं तत् यद् ग्रहण्यामामं सम्पाच्य वह्निं कृत्वा तत्रस्थं द्रवं च शोषयित्वा स्तम्भनं करोति तदुष्णग्राहकं ज्ञेयम् । यद्द्रव्यमतीसारादौ पक्वमलादिकं स्तम्भनं संग्रहं करोति तच्छीतग्राहकं ज्ञेयमेतदनिलगुणभूयिष्ठमित्यदोषः ॥ (आढमल्लः-शा.सं.प्र.खं.४/४-१२)

३. स्तम्भनं स्तम्भयति यद् गतिमन्तं चलं ध्रुवम् । (च.सू.२२)

considered as Ushna Sangrahi and "Sthambhana" may be considered as Seeta Sangrahi.

By and Large the drug which prevents or stops further excretion of malas is called as Purisha Sangrahaniya, Vidgraha, Sangrahika or Grahi dravya.

We come across Purisha and Mutra-Sangrahaniya vargas in Charaka but not the Sthambhana Varga.

(10) Sthambhana

The drug which prevents the expulsion of fluids or malas which have either upward or downward movement is known as 'Sthambhana'. Seeta Guna is said to be Sthambhana by Hemadri[1].

Sarngdhara described it as the drug which causes Vata Vriddhi through Ruksha, Seeta gunas; Kashaya rasa and Laghu paka. By this mechanism it will act as Sthambhana e.g. Kutaja, Shyonaka[2].

Therefore a clear demarcation is made between Grahi and Sthambhana. The former will be ushna in nature and is involved with Drava Soshana. While the later is Seeta in nature and produced Sthambhana through Vāta Prakopa.

Basing upon the above descriptions a comparision may be made between Ayurvedic perspective of anti-diarrhoeals and that in modern medicine:

(i) Grahi - GI protectives and adsorbents.

(ii) Sthambhana - Drugs affecting intestinal motility.

(iii) Purisha Sangrahana - Miscellaneous agents.

Antidiarrhoeals

1. some of them act locally, by producing a protective coating on the gut.
2. by decreasing the propulsion of the intestinal contents e.g., morphine.

---

१. स्तम्भनो हिम: । (हेमाद्रि)

२. रौक्ष्याच्छैत्यात्कषायत्वाल्लघुपाकाच्च यद्भवेत् ॥
वातकृत्स्तम्भनं तत्स्याद्यथा वत्सकटुण्टुकौ । (शा.सं.प्र.खं.४/१२-१३)
*आढमल्ल:- अनिलस्य शोषणात्मकत्वेनानिलगुणभूयिष्ठं द्रव्यं स्तम्भनं भवति इत्यभिप्राय: ।

3. by acting on intestinal microcirculation and lowering the hydrostatic pressure in favour of water absorption.
4. by acting directly on mucosal transport process thus reducing fluid accumulation in the intestinal lumen (anti-secretary action)

[**Note:** The first two groups may be similar to Sthambhana action; while the last two groups represent the Grahi action.]

(11) Madakari

The drug which affect the clear sensorium owing to its Tamo guna and produces Mada (depression) is known as Madakari e.g. Madya, Sura etc[1].

In Yogaratnakaram we find Dhattura, Ahiphena & Bhanga as Madakari drugs along with other properties. Therefore it may be defined that the drugs which affect the sensorium are Madakari durgs.

Alcohol depresses the CNS in a descending order. In small doses it causes euphoria, freedom from anxiety and worry and may improve social communication. This action may be beneficial therapeutically by relieving pathological nervours tension and by improving appetite in anorexia. The initial effect of alcohol is due to a depression of the reticular activating system. The cortex is thus released from the integrating control or inhibitions required for purposeful activity.

Adhamalla clarified that the first stage of Madyapana is only promoting sensorium the other three states are destroying the sensorium.

Madya will badly affect the Ojus with its properties like Ushna, Tikshna, Ruksha, Vyavyayi, Asukari etc. It may even reach the Hridaya along with Jataragni and spreads in the upward direction through the

---

१. बुद्धिं लुम्पति यद्द्रव्यं मदकारि तदुच्यते ॥
तमोगुणप्रधानं च यथा मद्यं सुरादिकम् । (शा.सं.प्र.खं.४/२१-२२)
*आढमल्लः- यद्द्रव्यं बुद्धिं ज्ञानविषयं लुम्पति आचज्छादयति तन्मदकारि कथ्यते ....। बुद्धिस्तु मेधाधृतिस्मृतिमतिप्रतिपत्तिषुवर्तते ।.....तद्यथा मेधा ग्रन्थाकर्षणसामर्थ्यं, धृति सन्तुष्टिः, अन्ये नियमात्मिकां बुद्धिमाहुः । स्मृतिः पूर्वानुभूतस्य स्मरणम् । अर्थधारणशक्तिरित्यन्ये । मतिरनागतविषयोपदेशः, त्रिकालविषया बुद्धिरित्यन्ये; पतिपत्तिरर्थावबोधप्रागल्भ्यमिति.....।

Dhamanis. Therefore it effects the Indriyas (organs) & Manas (mind)[1].

(12) Pramathi

The drug which will expel the malas (digestive or metabolic waste product) from various channels or systems because of its potency (virya) is known as Pramathi e.g. Maricha, Vacha etc[2].

It is very important to note that this property of Maricha is different from Chedana. In other words Chedana may be general effect of Maricha while Pramathi is specific effect which is directly linked up with its Virya alone. Similarly, Lekhana is the general effect of Vacha while Pramathi is specific effect.

These drugs will act upon the Sanchaya of doshas i.e., during early state of pathogenesis.

Adhamalla considers mainly Bahirmuka Srotas viz; karna, mukha, nasa etc; while Kasiram accepts all Abhyantara Srotas viz; Rasa vaha etc.

(13) Vyavayi: ***(CNS stimulation followed by depression)***

The drug which spreads all over the body first and then undergo paka (metabolism) at a later time is known as Vyavayi e.g. Bhanga, Ahiphena etc[3].

---

१. मदस्य चत्वार: पानावस्था: कथिता: तत्र प्रथमं मदपानं बुध्यादिकं करोति, शेषास्तुबुध्यादिकं लुम्पन्तीत्यदोष: । (आढमल्ल: शा.सं.प्र.खं.४)

२. (i) निजवीर्येण यद्द्रव्यं स्रोतेभ्यो दोषसंचयम् ॥
निरस्यति प्रमाथि स्यात्तद्यथा मरिचं वचा । (शा.सं.प्र.खं.४/२३-२४)

(ii) यद्द्रव्यं निजवीर्येण स्वप्रभावेन स्रोतोभ्यो रसवाहिशिरामार्गेभ्य: दोषसंचयं निरस्य दूरीकरोति तत्प्रमाथि स्यात् । (काशीराम्- शा.सं.प्र.खं.४/२३-२४)

(iii) यद्द्रव्यं निजवीर्येण स्वप्रभावेण कृत्वा स्रोतेभ्य: कर्णमुखनासादीनां अन्यविवरेभ्यश्च वा दोषबाहुल्यं निरस्यति तत् प्रमाथि संज्ञं कथितम् । यथा मरिचं वचा । दोषशब्दोत्र व्याधिष्वपि वर्तते कारणे कार्योपचारात्, तेन व्याधिसञ्चयमपीत्यर्थ: ।

३. (i) व्यवायी चाखिलं देहं व्याप्य पाकाय कल्पते । (सु.सू.४६) और (अ.सं.)

(ii) पूर्वं व्याप्याखिलं कायं तत: पाकं च गच्छति ।
व्यवायी तद्यथा भङ्गा फेनंचाहि समुद्भवम् ॥ (शा.सं.प्र.खं.४)

(iii) अपक्व एवाखिलं देहं व्याप्नोति पश्चन्मद्य विषवत् पाकं याति । (डल्हण-सु.सू.४६)

(iv) यत्तु त्वचि पित्तं तस्मिन् भ्राजकोऽग्निरिति संज्ञा, सोऽभ्यङ्गपरिषेकावगाहालेपादीनां क्रियाद्रव्याणां पक्ता, छायानां च प्रकाशक: ॥ (सु.सू.२०/११)

* ल्हण:- त्वचीति अवभासिनीनामधेयायां बाह्यत्वचीत्यर्थ: ।
अभ्यङ्गादीनां क्रियाद्रव्याणां क्रियानिमित्तानां कर्मनिमित्तानामित्यर्थ: ।

क्रमश: पृष्ठ २२३ में.......

These are the drugs which will act by initial stimulation of CNS followed by depression e.g. morphine, Cannabis etc. It is already discussed that the unmetabolized morphine produces first two states of narcosis and conjugated morphine produces the last two states of narcosis.

Some scholars opine that all the drugs should under go Agni paka at one level or the other since Agni is present all over the body. Arunadatta and Hemadri quoted that Upadhatus and Malas will also have Agnis.

In this context, the Vyavayi drug may not undergo the routine Jataragni paka as is the case with other drugs. Owing to its quick absorption it exhibits some of the pharamcological properties immediately and then under goes Agni paka (Bhutagni or Jataragni)

Bhrajaka pitta is meant for the metabolism of drugs used in Abhyanga, Parisheka, Avagaha, Alepa etc. This is an indication that Agni paka is possible apart from Jataragni paka.

(14) Vikasi

The drug which seperatus ojus from the dhatus and results in the laxity of tissue unions (Sandhi bandha), is known as Vikasi e.g., Kramuka, Kodrava etc[1].

In this context Sandhi or Sandhi bandha means the joints or union between different tissues especially connective tissues.

पृष्ठ २२२ से क्रमशः........

(v) ......त्वक्स्थं भ्राजकं भ्राजनात्त्वचः ॥ (अ.हृ.सू.१२/१४)

* अरुणदत्तः- त्वचो भ्राजनात्- दीपनात्, भ्राजकं नाम पित्तम् ।
एतच्च पित्तमभ्यङ्गलेपपरिषेकादीन् पाचयति ।

१. (i) विकासी विकसन्नेवं धातुबन्धान् विमोक्षयेत् । (सु.सू.४६)

(ii) विकासी विकसन्नेवं सन्धिबन्धान् विमोक्षयेत् । (अ.सं.सू.१)

(iii) सन्धिबन्धास्तु शिथिलान् यत् करोति विकाशि तत् ।
विश्लिष्योजश्च धातुभ्यो यथा क्रमुक कोद्रवाः ॥ (शा.सं.प्र.खं.४)

विकसन् प्रसर्पन्, एवमिति अपक्व एव सकल देहं व्याप्य धातुबन्धान्,
विमोक्षयेत् धातुशैथिल्यं करोतीत्यर्थः । (डल्हण-सु.सू. ४६)

अन्ये तु सरविशेषो व्यवायी तीक्ष्णविशेषो विकाशीति ब्रुवते, तत्र सर्वमतम् ।
(आढमल्लः- शा.सं.प्र.खं.४)

......व्यवायित्वात् स्थिरत्वं, श्लक्ष्णतामपि विकसिभावात् । (च.चि.२४)

These drugs may stimulate the CNS directly without further depression e.g. laptazol.

According to Dalhana the vikasi drug spreads all over the body without Agni paka and causes the dhatu saithilya (laxity of tissues).

Adhamalla quoted that Vyavayi and Vikasi are nothing but Sara guna visesha and Teekshna guna visesha as per some Acharyas view.

Charaka in the context of Madya (alcoholism) explained that the Vyavayi and Vikasi properties will effect the Sthira and Slakshna properties of ojus respectively.

Above descriptions indicates that Vikasi affects the Ojus directly while Vyavayi is not. Ojus (immunity) is the essence of all tissues and related to Kapha mainly. Therefore vikasi dravya may affect connective tissues since Skeshaka Sleshma is present in the Sandhis.

Some of the important Karmas missing in the CCIM syllabus:

(1) Abhishyandi

The drug which causes obstruction in the Rasa vaha siras (channels of propagation of plasma/ECF) due to its Pichchila, Guru gunas producing heaviness (Gurutwa) in the body is known as "Abhyis—hyandi" e.g. Dadhi (curd)[1].

Chakrapani considered it as the drug which will break the complexes formed by doshas[2] while Dalhani opined it as the one which produces Kledatwa (moisture) in Doshas, Dhatus, Malas & Srotas[3].

(2) Āsukari

The drug which spreads all over the body within no time simile to oil drop on water e.g. Visha (poison), Madya (alcohol) etc[4].

This action will be the answer to many who consider that Ayurvedic drugs act very slowly. The properties like Vyavayi, Vikasi,

१. पैच्छिल्याद् गौरवात् द्रव्यं रूद्धा रसवहा: सिरा: ।
धत्ते यद् गौरवं तत् स्यादभिष्यन्दि यथा दधि ॥ (शा.सं.प्र.खं.४)
२. दोषसङ्घातविच्छेदकारकम् । (च.सू. १३ चक्रपाणि)
३. अभिष्यन्दि- दोषधातुमलस्रोतसां क्लेदप्राप्तिजननम् । (डल्हण-सु.सू.४६)
४. आशुकारी तथाऽऽशुत्वाद्धावत्यम्भसि तैलवत् । (सु.सू.४६)

Asukari, Sukshma etc., will indicate the immediate actions of a given drug/material.

(3) Yogavāhi

The drug which will enhance the properties of other drugs used along with it is known as "Yoga vāhi" e.g. Madhu (honey)[1].

They can be either analogues or prodrugs the former increases the potency (i.e., they act directly on original drug) and the later increases the pharmacological activity (i.e., they act on the body directly).

(4) Sukshma

The drug which can enter even into the minutest of channels is known as "Sukshma" e.g., Saindhava lavana, Honey, Nimba tailam, Eranda tailam[2].

(5) Prana hara

The drug which possess Vyavayi, Vikasi, Sukshma, Chedi, Mada & Yagovahi gunas and which kills a person owing to the Agni bhuta dominance is known as "Pranahara" e.g., visha (poison)[3].

(6) Vidahi

The drug which will be digested very lately because of its Guru guna or due to its original nature while generating burning sensation is called as Vidahi e.g. Sarshapa[4].

(7) Jeevaniya

Indukara defined it as essential for maintanance of life. Dalhana considered it as basis of survival of life[5].

---

१. निजवीर्येण यद्द्रव्यं स्रोतोभ्यो दोषसञ्चयम् ।
निरस्यति प्रमाथि: स्यात् तद्यथा मरिचं वचा ॥ (शा.सं.प्र.खं.४)

२. देहस्य सूक्ष्म छिद्रेषु विशेद्यत् सूक्ष्ममुच्यते ॥
तद्यथा सैन्धवं क्षौद्रं निम्बतैलं उरूबूद्भवम् । (शा.सं.प्र.खं.४)

३. व्यवायि च विकाशि स्यात् सूक्ष्मं छेदि मदावहम् ॥
आग्नेयं जीवितहरं योगवाहि स्मृतं विषम् ॥ (शा.सं.प्र.खं.४)

४. द्रव्यस्वभावादथ गौरवाद्वा चिरेणपाकं जाठराग्नियोगात् ।
पित्तप्रकोपं विदहत् करोति तदन्नपानं कथितं विदाहि ॥ (सु.सू.४५)

५. (i) जीवनीयानां प्राणानां सन्धारकम् । (इन्दुकर:-अ.सं.सू.३४)
(ii) जीवन: प्राणाधार: । (डल्हण-सु.सू.३८)

The word Jeevaniyam has been interpreted by Chakrapani as that is good (hita) for Ayu (life). The milk is best among Jivaneeya dravyas. Dr. Vaman Ganesh Desai has given the term restoratives for Jeevaniya drugs. Jivanam is the main function of Rakta dhatu and therefore they may act particularly on Rakta dhatu. e.g., Ashta varga, Kākolyadi varga, Jeevaniya dasaimani etc.

(8) Brimhana: *(nourishing)*

The drug which provides strenght (Pushti) and addition (Brihatwa) to the body tissues in known as "Brimhana"[1].

The word 'Brimhana' implies that action which can give good muscular tone and imparts strong built. The drugs possessing guru, Seeta, Pichchila, Sthira gunas can cause Brimhana. It is formed by Prithvi Jala bhutas. Brimhana karma implies the action on mamsa dhatus which brings out good muscle tone. Therefore mamsa is best among brimhana dravyas.

(9) Balya: *(tonic)*

The drug which provides strength to the body is known as "Balya" e.g. Kukkuta mamsa (chicken)[2].

It also connotes the action which increases the bala of the dhatus. Deha bala depends on Sleshma which is otherwise known as 'ojus'. Therefore the action of Balya drugs could be interpreted on five dhatus which are related to kapha i.e., Rasa, Mamsa, Medas, Majja and Sukra.

(10) Sandhaniyam

The drug which promotes the process of fracture healing (of bones) is usually known as Sardhaniyam[3]. It can otherwise be defined as the drug which is effective against the subluxation of connective tissues.

---

१. बृहत्वं यच्छरीरस्य जनयेत्तच्च बृंहणम्, गुरु शीतं मृदुस्निग्धं बहुलं स्थूलपिच्छिलम्,
प्रायो मन्दं स्थिरं श्लक्ष्णं द्रव्यं बृंहणमुच्यते । (च.सू. २२)

२. बलाय हितं बल्यम् । (गङ्गाधरः)

३. सन्धानीय भग्नसंयोजनाय हितम् सन्धानीयम् । (गङ्गाधरः)

Note:- Analeptic action i.e., analepsis is "gaining strength after an illness. It provides restoration to health. This action may be similar to Balya.

(11) Vayah Sthapana

The drug which prevents ageing process is known as Vayasthapana. Others may call it as one which provides more than 100 years of healthy life[1].

The question of restoration of youth comes only in old age. Senility or Jara is the result of dhatukshaya (degeneration of tissues) and vayasthapana prevent the same.

Charaka considered Āmalaki (P-embelica) as the best vayasthapana drug. Sushrita mentioned Seeta daka (cold water), Kshira (milk), Kshoudra (honey) & Sarpi (ghee) as vayasthapana dravyas.

(12) Rasayana

The word Rasayana has been defined by Sarngdhara as that which ameliorates, Jara (senility) and Vyadhi (disease). charaka explicitly stated that rasayana imparts youth (Tarunam vayah), Deha bala (body strength), Indira bala (strength to organs), Ayu (life), Medha (intelligence), Smriti (memory), Prabha (complexion) etc[2].

Dalhana while commenting on rasayana chapter of Sushrita chikitsa interpreted the actions of rasayana as "Ayu Bala" etc., which clearly indicates that rasayana incorporates the actions like Ayushya, Balya, Vayasthapana etc.

In Rasayana "Medhya rasayanas" (e.g., Sankhapushpi, Mandukaparni etc.) are different from "Doshaghna rasayanas (e.g. Bhallataki, Hareetaki etc.) and "Dhatu rasayanas" (e.g. Aswagandha, Āmalaki etc.).

---

१. वयःस्थापनं वर्षशतमायुः स्थापनम्, आयुष्करं शताधिकमपि करोति, अन्ये तु
वयःस्थापनं जरापहरणं तारूण्यं बहुकालं स्थापयतीत्यर्थः । (डल्हण-सु.सू.१)

२. (i) रसायनं च तज्ज्ञेयं यज्जराव्याधिनाशनम् ।
यथाऽमृता रूदन्ती च गुग्गुलुश्च हरीतकी ॥ (शा.सं.प्र.खं.४)

* आढमल्लः- जरावार्धक्य व्याधयो ज्वरादयो रोगा ग्राह्याः ।

(ii) दीर्घमायुः स्मृतिं मेधामारोग्यं तरुणं वयः ।
प्रभावर्णस्वरौदार्यं देहेन्द्रियबलं परम् ॥
वाक्सिद्धिं प्रणतिं कान्तिं लभते ना रसायनात् ।
लाभोपायोहि शस्तानां रसादीनां रसायनम् ॥ (च.चि.१/१)

(13) Vajikarana

The drug which produces orgasm and libido in males as well as females is known as Vajikarana according to Ādhamalla. e.g., Nagabala, Kapikachchu etc[1].

It is usually believed that Vajikarana or Vrishya is meant for aphrodisiac activity and exclusively for males. It is a wrong notion. Commenting on the management of Rajo doshas (eight types) in Sushrita Sareera Sthana, Dalhana mentioned Rasayana and Vajikarana dravyas for their treatment. In the chapter on Yoni vyapats (gynaeic disorders), Charaka described eight types of Sukra doshas (seminal disorders) where in several drugs used in Yonivyapats are indicated. In Sushrita Uttara sthana Yoni vyapat chikitsa consists of many Vajikarana dravyas and their utility. This concludes without controversy that Vajikarana is meant for both males and females if we strongly believe the concept "Sukra is commonly present in both the sex".

Keeping the above concepts in view probably Sarngdhara did try to differentiate between Vajikarana and Sukrala drugs etc. We find the following actions on Sukradhatu in the Ayurvedic texts.

1. Sukrala	-	which acts on spermatogenesis e.g. Aswagandha, Musali, Sarkara, Satavari etc[2].
2. Sukra rechaka	-	which helps in emission and ejacula tory disorders e.g. Brihati phala etc.
3. Sukra sthambhaka	-	which helps in premature ejaculation e.g. Jati phala.
4. Sukra soshana	-	which prevents spermatogenesis e.g. Haritaki
5. Sukra janaka-pravartaka	-	Ksheera, Masha, Bhallataka etc.

---

१. यस्माद्द्रव्यात् भवेत् स्त्रीषु हर्षो वाजीकरं च तत् ॥
यथा नागबलाद्याः स्युर्बीजं च कपिकच्छुजम् । (शा.सं.प्र.खं.४)

२. यस्माच्छुक्रस्य वृद्धिस्याच्छुक्रलं तु तदुच्यते ॥
यथाऽश्वगन्धा मुसली शर्करा च शतावरी । (शा.सं.प्र.खं.४)

6. Sukra pravartaka - which stimulates ejaculation prychologically e.g. woman[1].

(14) Prajāsthapana

The drug which rectifies the defects of Garbha Samagri (Rutu, Kshetra, Ambu, Beeja) etc., and helps in fertilization/nidation is known as 'Praja Sthapana', e.g. Brahmi, Durva[2].

Usually these drug are used in female infertility treatment while Vajeekarana drugs are used in male infertility.

(15) Vedanasthapana: *(anodynes)*

The drug which is used to remove the pain (vedana) of a particular part of the body and which restores nomal state is known as 'Vedana Sthapana'[3]. Indukara also considered it as anodyne e.g. Guggulu, Kat phala etc.

However, Gangadhara in this context opined that Vedana Sthapana drugs will re-establish the lost sensation or Vedana in the body. If it is so, the anasthetic areas/patches etc., may be treated by this group of drugs.

(16) Sonita Sthapana

The drug which will rectify the vitiated blood and provides normalcy is known as Sonita sthapana. These are two releted activities viz., Sonitā Sthapana and Rudhira Samsthapana[4].

Sonitāsthapana - act as anti-haemorrhagic.

Rudira Samsthapana - acts as nourishing and haemetenic.

(17) Sanjna Sthapanam

The drug which will restore the lost conciousness is known as "SanjnaSthapana" e.g. Vacha, Hiugu etc. These drugs may be used in

१. प्रवर्तनी स्त्री शुक्रस्य, रेचनं बृहतीफलं ॥
जातीफलं स्तम्भकं च, शोषणी च हरीतकी । (शा.सं.प्र.खं.४)
२. प्रजोपघातकं दोषं हृत्वा प्रजां स्थापयतीति प्रजास्थापनम् । (चक्रपाणि-च.सू. ४)
३. (i) वेदनायां संभूतायां तां निहत्य शरीरं प्रकृतौ स्थापयतीति वेदनास्थापनम् । (चक्रपाणि-च.सू. ४)
(ii) वेदनायाश्चिच्छक्तेः संतर्पकं वेदनास्थापनम् । (इन्दुकर- अ.सं.सू. १५)
(iii) वेदनानां यत्र निवृत्तौ व्यापत् स्यात् तत्र वेदनां स्थापयतीति । (गङ्गाधर- च.सू. ४ अ.)
४. (i) शोणितस्य दुष्टस्य दुष्टिमपहृत्य तत् प्रकृतौ स्थापयतीति शोणितस्थापनम् । (चक्रपाणि-च.सू. ४)
(ii) शोणितास्थापनम् शोणितातिप्रवृत्ति स्तम्भनम् । (डल्हण- सु.चि. १)
(iii) रूधिरसंस्थापनं पुरुषस्य रूधिरवृद्धि-स्थैर्यकरम् । (इन्दुकरः- अ.सं.)

condtions like Mada, Murcha, Sanyasa, Apasmara etc[1].

(18) Hridya

It is generally stated that Hridya is the drug which is excellent for the heart. Some commentators quote it as good for mind. e.g. Amlavetasa, Badara, Amra[2] etc.

The Hridya dasaimani of Charaka contains Āmla dravyas (sour materials) and he claimed Amla rasa as the best among Hridya. It is well known fact that sour substances occuring in nature are full of vit-C is useful in preventing atherosclerosis and angina pectoris.

(19) Kaṇtya

The drug which is good for throat problems is known as 'Kantya'[3]. These are the group of drugs which are useful in the treatment of laryngitis or pharyngitis (Swarabhanga), URTI (Vataja kasa) etc. The drugs like Simhi and Vyaghri are the drugs which are named after their effect on larynx. But, unripen Kapitha is mentioned as 'Akantya'.

(20) Vamana

The process by which the doshas (i.e., Kapha mainly) are expelled out in the upward direction i.e., through mouth is called as 'emesis'. The drug which performs Vamana Karma is known as "Vamana dravya' (emetics).

Sarngdhara defined it as "the dravya which will forcefully expel the indigested Pitta and Slesha through the mouth" e.g. Madana phala etc[4].

The term 'Vamana' is used physiologically and 'Chardi' is the term used under pathological conditions in Ayurveda which will in-

---

१. संज्ञां ज्ञानं स्थापयतीति संज्ञास्थापनम् । (चक्रपाणि- च.सू. ४)

२. (i) हृदयाय हितम् हृद्यम् । (चक्रपाणि- च.सू. ४)
(ii) हृदयाय मनसोहितम् । (गङ्गाधरः, योगेन्द्रनाथः- च.सू. ४)
(iii) अम्लम् हृद्यानाम् । (च.सू. २५)

३. (i) कण्ठाय हितम् कण्ठ्यम् । (योगेन्द्रनाथः- च.सू. ४)
(ii) कण्ठस्थितस्वराय हितं कण्ठ्यम् । (गङ्गाधरः- च.सू. ४)

४. (i) तत्र दोषहरंण ऊर्ध्व भागं वमनसंज्ञकं । (च.क.१ अ.)
(ii) अपक्वपित्तश्लेष्माणौ बलादूर्ध्वं नयेत्तु यत् ॥
वमनं तद्धि विज्ञेयं मदनस्य फलं यथा । (शा.सं.प्र.खं. ४)

dicate vomiting. Chardi Nigrahana group of drugs are the anti-emetics described by Charaka.

In modern pharmacology emetics acts by three means:

(i) Central emetics	- acting on CTZ
(ii) Peripheral emetics	- acting reflexly through vagus
(iii) Central as well as peripharal	- both mechanisms involved.

(21) Purisha Sangrahaniya: *(Anti-diarrhoeal)*

The drug which prevents the repeated excretion of stools is known as Purisha Sangrahaniya[1]. The anti-diarrhoeal cencept according to Ayurveda is explained in detail in the context of Grahi and Sthambhana.

(22) Purisha Virajaniya

The drug which rectifies the discouloration of feces is known as Purisha virajaniya[2]. For example in Ruddha pada kamala the stools are Tila pishta nibha in Sannipata Atisara it is Mechakagara dhunabha etc. under these conditions the drugs will act on feces i.e., on stircobilin.

(23) Āsthapana

The drug which when administered in the form of enemata will expel the vitiated doshas and restores the normal health to the body[3].

Though Prajasthapana, Vayasthapana are mentioned seperately, Āsthapana term exclusively and seperately used in Vasthi karma only.

(24) Anuvasana

The drug which when administered in the form of enemata will strengthen the body[4].

---

१. पुरीषस्य अतिसरतः संग्रहणं संग्रहः तत्र हितं पुरीषसंग्रहणीयम् । (योगेन्द्रनाथः- च.सू. ४)

२. पुरीषस्य विरजनं विगतं रजनं (रागः) रागसंबन्धनिरासः तस्मै हितं पुरीषविरजनीयम् । (योगेन्द्रनाथः- च.सू. ४)

३. शरीरं दोषसंशोधनेन स्थिरं कर्वन्ति इति आस्थापनानि । (चक्रपाणि- च.सू. ४)

४. अनुवासयन्ति अनुबध्नाति शरीरं बलदानेन इति अनुवासनादि । (चक्रपाणि- च.सू. ४)

Some of the Important Pharmacological Properties deleniated in Ayurvedic Texts

(1) Anulomana

1. Vatanulomana
2. Kaphanulomana
3. Doshanulomana
4. Varchonulomana
5. Garbhanulomana

(2) Avasādana

1. Vatavasadana
2. Pittavasadana
3. Sleshmavasadana
4. Kledavasadana
5. Mamsavasadana
6. Vranavasadana
7. Koshtavasadana
8. Agni sadana
9. Bala-varna-Agni sada krit

(3) Āpaha

1. Vāta gulmapaha
2. Vātajwarapaha
3. Yakshmapaha
4. Udara vishapaha
5. Kamalapaha
6. Viplutapaha
7. Kasāpaha
8. Hikkapaha
9. Sukramayapaha
10. Timirapaha
11. Dourbalyapaha
12. Trishnapaha
13. Mutrakrichchrapaha
14. Swasapaha

(4) Āpādana

1. Sirahsulamāpādana
2. Arditamāpādana
3. Pumstwopaghatamāpādana

(5) Eraṇa

1. Vāta Sameeraṇa
2. Dosha Sameeraṇa

(6) Uttejaka

1. Āmasayottejaka
2. Netrottejaka
3. Hridyottejaka
4. Yakriduttejaka

(7) Upaga

1. Snehopaga
2. Swedopaga

3. Vamanopaga	6. Anuvāsanopaga
4. Virechanopaga	7. Sirovirechanopaga
5. Āsthapanopaga	

(8) Upachaya krit

1. Raktopachaya krit	2. Mamsopachaya krit

(9) Kara/Krit

1. Anila kara	21 Cheshta kara
2. Kapha kara	22. Smriti kara
3. Pitta kara	23. Buddhi kara
4. Ādhmana kara	24. Mangala kara
5. Stanya vriddhi kara	25. Murcha kara
6. Ojaskara	26. Purisha krit
7. Sroto mardava kara	27. Dosha krit
8. Chardi kara	28. Dosha mardava krit
9. Dhatu sosha kara	29. Mamsasthairya krit
10. Mada kara	30. Asthi sthairya krit
11. Indriyopatapa kara	31. Sukra krita
12. Medo vriddhi kara	32. Jwara krit
13. Vishtambha kara	33. Supti krit
14. Kandu kara	34. Ayu krit
15. Krimi kara	35. Oorja krit
16. Ruja kara	36. Swapna krit
17. Peeda kara	37. Kārsya krit
18. Daha kara	38. Jadatā krit
19. Sula kara	39. Ghrana Srava krit
20. Swayathu kara	40. Rakta krit

(10) Karshana *(Apakarshana)*

1. Pitta karshana	3. Sthoulyapa karshana
2. Sleshma karshana	4. Puti malapakarshana

(11) Kopana

1. Vāta prakopana
2. Pitta prakopana
3. Kapha prakopana

(12) Kledana ***(Prakledana)***

1. Vrana kledana
2. Mamsa kledana
3. Kaphotkledana

(13) Ghati

1. Vyāḍhi ghati
2. Prāṇa ghati
3. Pāka ghati
4. Dosha ghati

(14) Ghna

1. Kandugha
2. Doshaghna
3. Vishaghna
4. Kushtaghna
5. Arshoghna
6. Jwaraghna
7. Krimighna (Jantughna)
8. Sulaghna
9. Trishnaghna
10. Kanthaghna
11. Swayathughna
12. Atisāraghna
13. Dahaghna
14. Soshaghna
15. Akshisulaghna
16. Kasaghna
17. Swasaghna
18. Vātaghna
19. Pittaghna
20. Sleshmaghna

(15) Janana

1. Nidra janana
2. Tandra janana
3. Sthanya janana
4. Swapna janana
5. Purisha janana
6. Udavarta janana
7. Mutra janana

(16) Jit

1. Kaphajit
2. Vātajit
3. Urahsūla jit
4. Vranasula jit
5. Parswa sula jit
6. Angavasada jit
7. Mutra vibandha jit
8. Visarpa jit
9. Vishamajwara jit
10. Twagroga jit

(17) Tarpaṇa

1. Akshi tarpana
2. Karna tarpana
3. Sirastarpana

(18) Dushana (Pradushana)

1. Dhatu pradushana
2. Dosha pradushana
3. Pittasrik dushana
4. Sonita pradushana
5. Basti dushana
6. Drishti pradushana

(19) Nāsana

1. Sukra nasana
2. Dosha nasana
3. Kesa vinasana
4. Sidhma nasana
5. Gulma nasana
6. Bhagandara nasana
7. Mukharoga nasana
8. Udarvarta nasana
9. Pandu nasana
10. Ardita nasana

(20) Nigrahana

1. Vata Nigrahana
2. Varcho nigrahana
3. Chardi Nigrahana
4. Hikka Nigrahana
5. Trishna Nigrahana
6. Nidra Nigrahana

(21) Nirvahaṇa

1. Kushta Nirvahana
2. Sarva vyadhi Nirvahana

(22) Nivarana

1. Galamaya Nivarana
2. Dosha Nivarana

(23) Nuth

1. Apasmara nut
2. Mutra vibandha nut
3. Mala vibandha nut
4. Supti nut
5. Jwara-Daharti nut

(24) Pachana

1. Dosha Pachana
2. Pitta Pachana
3. Ama Pachana
4. Vrana Pachana

(25) Prabodhana *(Bodhana)*

1 Indriya Bodhana
2. Buddhi Prabodhana
3. Swara Prabodhana
4. Sanjna Prabodhana

(26) Pravartana

1. Rajah Pravartaka
2. Sukra Pravartaka
3. Varchah Pravartaka
4. Visha roga Pravartana

(27) Prahladana

1. Jihwa Prahladana
2. Oshta Prahladana

(28) Baddha

1. Baddha mutra/prabaddha mutra
2. Baddha purisha

(29) Bala Prada

1. Mamsa bala prada
2. Sukra balaprada
3. Hanyobala prada

(30) Bhedana

1. Ashmari bhedana
2. Ānaha bhedana
3. Sarkara bhedana
4. Rakta Vibhedana
5. Vid bhedana
6. Sandhi bhedana

(31) Mardava krit

1. Dosha Mardava krit
2. Dhatu Mardava krit
3. Kesa Mardava krit

(32) Vardhana

1. Vata Vardhana
2. Pitta Vardhana
3. Sleshma Vardhana
4. Stanya Vardhana
5. Ojo Vardhana
6. Dhatu Vardhana
7. Sukra Vardhana
8. Agni Vardhana
9. Bala Vardhana
10. Rakta Vardhana

(33) Vidahi

1. Koshta vidahi
2. Udara vidahi

(34) Vicchedana

1. Kapha vicchedana
2. Mamsa vicchedana

(35) Virajaniya

1. Mutra virajaniya
2. Purisha virajaniya

(36) Ranjana

1. Kesa ranjana

(37) Lekhana *(vilekhana)*

1. Jihwa vilekhana
2. Mamsa vilekhana

(38) Soshanam

1. Puya soshana
2. Medo soshana
3. Sukra soshana
4. Mutra soshana

(39) Sodhana *(Visodhana or Samsodhana)*

1. Vamana
2. Virechana
3. Ubhayabhagahara
4. Vasthi
5. Sirovirechana
6. Ārtava sodhana
7. Sukra sodhana
8. Stanya sodhana
9. Sroto sodhana
10. Hrid visodhana
11. Yoni visodhana
12. Garbhasaya sodhana
13. Vasthi visodhana
14. Vrana sodhana
15. Udgara sodhana
16. Deha visodhana
17. Pakwasaya visodhana

(40) Samsamana *(Samana or Doshaprasamana)*

1. Vata Samasamana
2. Pitta Samasamana
3. Sleshma Samsamana
4. Udarda Prasamana
5. Angamarda Prasamana
6. Jwara Prasamana
7. Daha Prasamana
8. Seeta Prasamana
9. Sula Prasamana
10. Visha Prasamana

(41) Syandana

1. Mukha Syandana
2. Akshi Syandana

(42) Sangrahi *(Grahi)*

1. Purisha Sangrahana
2. Mutra Sangrahana
3. Sleshna Sangrahana
4. Pitta Sangrahi

(43) Sthambhana

1. Sukra Sthambhana
2. Purisha Sthambhana
3. Mutra Sthamshana
4. Rakta Sthambhana

(44) Sthāpana

1. Sonita Sthapana	4. Garbha Sthapana
2. Vayah Sthapana	5. Sanjna Sthapana
3. Praja Sthapana	

(45) Hara

1. Srama hara	8. Sotha hara
2. Switra hara	9. Kāsa hara
3. Mutra dosha hara	10. Swāsa hara
4. Dāha hara	11. Krimi hara
5. Jawara hara	12. Ashmari hara
6. Abhishyandi hara	13. Unmada hara
7. Tridosha hara	14. Agnimandya hara

Drugs used in various conditions in Ayurveda on the basis of pharmacological action

(1) Jwara: ***(fevers)***

1. Jwaraghna or Jwara hara - antipyretic
2. Dāha prasamana - cooling agents
3. Seeta prasamana (in hypothermia) - drugs increasing temp.
4. Trishna nigrahana (in hyperpyrexia)
5. Deepana & Pachana (appetizers & digestives)
6. Virechana (laxatives)

(2) Atisara & Grahani: ***(diarrhoeal disorders)***

1.	Anulomana	- in Āmatisara
2.	Sthambhana	- in Pakwati sara, Pravahika
3.	Grahi	- in Grahani
4.	Sonita Sthapana	- in Raktatisara
5.	Trishna nigrahana	- in Dehydration
6.	Dāha Prasamana	- in Pittatisara, Pittaja Grahanı
7.	Deepana & Pachana	- in Grahani & Āmātisara
8.	Purisha Sangrahaniya	- in Sannipatatisara, Grahani
9.	Purisha Virajaniya	- in Sannipatatisara, Grahani

(3) Aruchi, Agnimandya & Ajeerna: ***(digestive disorders)***

1. Rochaka - improves the feeling of hunger
2. Deepana - appetizers
3. Pachana - digestives
4. Sula prasamana - carminatives and those relieve abdominal colic.

(4) Pandu: ***(Anaemias)***

1. Sonitaasthapana } Haemetinics
2. Rudira Samsthapana } Haemetinics
3. Sotha hara - oedema induced by reduced Hb%
4. Medo Vardhaka - in aplastic anaemias?
5. Deepana & Pachana.

(5) Arsas: ***(haemorrhoids)***

1. Arshoghna
2. Mridu rechaka
3. Rakta pitta hara
4. Deepana
5. Sonitaasthapana

(6) Raktapitta

1. Sonitaasthapana
2. Rakta sthambhaka
3. Pitta samsamana (Daha prasamana)

(7) Kāmala, Yakritodara & Pleehodara

1. Pitta Samsamana
2. Bhedana - Ruddha pada kāmala
3. Pleehaghna
4. Virechana dravyas

(8) Unmada, Apasmara, Murcha & Sanyasa

1. Medhya Rasayana
2. Sanjna sthapana
3. Nidrajanana

(9) Mutra krichchra, Mutraghata, Ashmari & Prameha

1. Mutra virechaniya - in Mutra krichchra
2. Mutra virajaniya - in Avilatwa caused by Prameha

3. Mutra sangrahaniya - in Bahu mutra caused by Prameha
4. Ashmarighna - in Ashmari & Ashmarija mutra krichchra
5. Vata Vardhaka - in sthula Madhumahi

(10) Amavata, Varta rakta, Urusthambha & Vata vyadhi

1. Sotha hara
2. Deepana-pachana
3. Medo hara
4. Vata hara
5. Vedana sthapana
6. Angamarda prasamana
7. Sodhana dravyas

(11) Sotha & Udara

1. Mutra virechaniya
2. Deepana
3. Sotha hara
4. Virechana

(12) Kushta: *(skin discases)*

1. Kushtaghna
2. Kandughna
3. Udarda prasamana
4. Varnya
5. Twachya
6. Krimighna
7. Virechana
8. Rakta sodhaka

(13) Chardi

1. Chardi nigrahana
2. Trishna nigrahana

(14) Swasa, Kasa & Hikka

1. Swasa hara
2. Kasa hara
3. Hikka nigrahana
4. Vamana
5. Rakta sthambhaka - in Urah kshata or kshata ksheena

Modern Approach to Pharmacological Activities of Ayurvedic Drugs Proved through Experimental Studies

1. Action on Reproductive System

(1) Spermatogenic/aphrodisiac property

1. Asterecantha longifolia
2. Mucuna prurieta
3. Pureria tuberosa
4. Withania somnifera
5. Trivanga bhasma

(2) Antifertility action *(male)*

1. Plumbago zeylanica - anti androgenic (Bhargav et al., 1984)
2. Sapindus trifoliatus - reduces spermatogenesis (Dixit & Gupta, 1982)
3. Azadirachta indica - spermicidal (Sinha et al., 1984)

(3) Antifertility activity *(female)*

1. Abrus precatorium
2. Aloe indica
3. Areca catechu
4. Butea frondosa/B. monosperma
5. Caesalpina bonducella
6. Carica papaya
7. Curcuma longa
8. Daucus carota
9. Embalia ribes - anti-implantation, anti-estrogenic (Prakash, 1981)
10. Hibiscus rosa-sinensis - anti-implantation, abortifacient (Singh et al., 1982)
11. Plumbago zeylanica - antiovulatory (Chaudhuri et al., 1982)
12. Thespesia populnea - anti-implantation (Murthy et al., 1981)
13. Adhatoda vasica - vasicine is abortificient and has oxitocin like activity (Gautam & Sharma, 1982; Lal & Sharma 1981)

(4) Uterine activity

1. Abroma augusta - oxytocic activity
2. Abrus precatorius
3. Annona squamosa
4. Areca catechu
5. Aristolochia bracteata
6. Asparagus racemosus
7. Bombax malabarica
8. Carica papaya
9. Costus speciosus
10. Cyperus rotundus
11. Gloriosa superba

(5) Emmanogogues

1. Aloe vera
2. Saraca asoca
3. Ferula asefoetida

2. NSAID activity

(1) Anit-inflammatory & Anti-arthritic activity

1. Allium sativum - allin
2. Acacia catechu (Chakravarthy et al. 1983)
3. Azadirachta indica (Pillai & Santhakumari, 1981)
4. Berberis aristata - berberine
5. Boerhavia diffusa
6. Cassia fistula
7. Calophyllum inophyllum (Saxena et al., 1982)
8. Clerodendrum phlomidis
9. Commiphora mukul
10. Costus speciosus - saponin mixture
11. Crataeva nurvala - sterols
12. Curcuma longa - Curcumin
13. Cyperus rotundus/C.scariosus
14. Dalbergia lanceolaria-phytogenic crystalline principle
15. Desmodium gangeticum (Ghosh & Ananda kumar, 1983)
16. Glycyrrhiza glabra
17. Mesua ferra (Gopalakrishnan et al., 1980c)
18. Randia dumetorum (Ghosh et al., 1983)
19. Symplocos spicata (Frotan et al., 1983)
20. Tylophora indica (Gopalakrishnan et al., 1980b)
21. Tinospora cordifolia (Pendse et al., 1981)
22. Nyctanthes arbor-tristis (Saxena et al., 1984)
23. Hedychium spicatum (Srimal et al., 1984)

(2) Analgesic activity

1. Abutilon indicum (Bagi et al., 1984)
2. Cannabis indica (Ghosh & Bhattacharya, 1980a)
3. Cissus quadrangularis (Singh et al., 1984c)
4. Desmodium gangeticum (Ghosh & Ananda kumar, 1983)
5. Embelia ribes (Atal et al., 1984)

6. Hedychium spicatum (Srimal et al., 1984)
7. Randia dumetorum (Ghosh et al., 1983)
8. Sisymbrium irio (Vohora et al., 1980b)
9. Taxus buccata (Vohora et al., 1980a)
10. Trianthema portulacastrum (Vohora et al., 1984b)

(3) Antipyretic activity

1. Cyperus rotundus (Gupta et al., 1980b)
2. Sisymbrium irio (Vohora et al., 1980b)
3. Taxus buccata (Vohora et al., 1980a)
4. Trianthema portulacastrum (Vohora et al., 1984b)

(4) Analgesic anti-inflammatory

1. D. ganeticum
2. R. Dumetorum
3. H. spichatum

(5) Analgesic- antipyretic

1. Taxus buccata
2. Sisymbrium irio
3. T. portulacastrum

(6) Antipyretic- anti-inflammatory

1. C. rotundus
2. Corchorus depressus

3. Action of GIT

(1) Anti-peptic ulcer activity

1. Asparagus racemosus
2. Emblica officinalis

(2) Purgative property

1. Capparis decidua
2. Cassia fistula

(3) Hepatoprotective property

1. Eclipta alba (Mogre et al., 1981)
2. Acacia catectu (Rege et al., 1984c)
3. Phyllanthus amarus
4. Piper longum (Rege et al., 1984c)
5. Picrorhiza kurroa (Mogre et al., 1981)
6. Tinospora cordifolia (Rege et al., 1984a & Singh et al., 1984a)

4. Action on CVS

(1) Cardiac stimulents

1. Asclepias curassavica
2. Asterecantha longifolia
3. Bacopa monniera
4. Berginia ligulata
5. Lagerstroemia speciosa
6. Melia azaderach (Srivastava et al., 1981)

(2) Cardiac depressents; antihypertensives & diuretics

1. Acorus calamus
2. Azadirachta indica (nimbidin)
3. Boerhavia diffusa

(3) Antianginal & hypocholesterolaemic

1. Allium sativun
2. Carum copiticum
3. Commiphora mukul
4. Inula racemosa
5. Saussurea lappa
6. Terminalia chebula

(4) Antihypertensive & antiatherogenic

1. Curcuma longa
2. Ipomea batatas

(5) Hypolipideamic & hypoglyceamic

1. Mucuna prurieuce
2. Piper nigrum
3. Zingiber officinale

(6) Hypolipideamic, hypoglycaemic & antihypertensive

1. P. marsupium

(7) Antihypertensive; hypoglycaemic & diuretic

1. Achyranthus aspera
2. Barleria cristata

(8) Digitalis like

1. Thevetia peruviana

(9) Antihypertensive & hypoglycaemic

1. Hedychium spicatum
2. Luffa echinata
3. Musa paradisiaca
4. Ocimum sanctum

(10) Antihypertensives (hypotensive)

1. Ailanthus excelsa
2. Allium cepa
3. Cynodon dactylon
4. Eclipta alba
5. Mesua ferrea
6. Moring pterigosperma

7. Withania somnifera
8. Costus speciosus
9. Hedychium spicatum
10. Holerrhina antidysenterica
11. Achyranthes aspera
12. Alangium lamarkii
13. Aristolochia bracteata
14. Bacopa monniera
15. Carissa carandas
16. Butea superba
17. Carum copticum
18. Cassia absus (chaksine)
19. Catharanthus roseus (alkoloid fraction V-22)
20. Cocculus hirsutus
21. Convolvulus pluricaulis
22. Curcuma longa (curcumin)
23. Emblica officinalis
24. Costus speciosus (Benerji et al., 1981)
25. Withania coagulan (Budhiraja et al., 1983)

(11) Hylolipaemic & anti-atherosclerotic

1. Commiphora mukul (Srivastava et al., 1984)
2. Curcuma amada
3. Curcuma longa
4. Emblica officinalis (Thakur & Mandal, 1984)

(12) Other cardioactive drugs

1. Acacia farnesiana
2. Aconitum sps. (Aconite) producing arrhythmia.
3. Aegle marmelos
4. Artemisia vulgaris
5. Calophyllum inophyllum (calophyllolide, coumarin)
6. Calotropis procera

7. Carica papaya
8. Carissa carandas
9. Catharanthus roseus
10. Cissampelos pariera (hayatin)
11. Cissus quadrangularis
12. Crotalaria juncea
13. Dacus carota
14. Digitalis lanata
15. Evo-lvulus alsinoides

5. Drugs Acting on Blood

(1) Antiatherogenic

1. C. mukul
2. Curcuma amada
3. Ipomea batatas

(2) Anti-coagulant

1. Litsea umbrosa
2. Ocimum americanum
3. Plumbago zeylanica
4. Calotropis procera
5. Carica papaya

(3) Haemostatic

1. Jatropha curcus
2. Rubia cordifolia

(4) Haematenics

1. Cleistanthus collinus (Cleistanthin-glycoside)

6. Action on CNS

Acacia arabica, Aconitum ferox, Acorus calamus (asarone), Anogeissus latifolia, Apium graveolens, Areca catechu, Atropa sps, Bacopa monniera (hersaponin), Barleria cristata, Boeswellia serrata, Cannabis indica (cannabinol), Carum roxburghianum, Cassia fistula, Celastrus paniculatun, Centella asiatica (brahmosides), Cissampelos pariera, Convolvulus pluricaulis, Curcuma amada, Curcuma aromatica, Cyperus rotundus, Dillenia indica, Emblica officinalis (phyllemblin), Euphorbia tirucalli, Ficus religiosa, Glycyrrhiza glabra (glycyrrhitic acid), Grewia hirsuta.

(1) Depressants

1. Hedychium spicatum
2. Indigofera tinctoria
3. Jatropha curcus
4. Leucas aspera
5. Luffa echinata
6. Melia azaderach

7. Mesua ferrea
8. Momordica charantia
9. Morus indica (Pal et al., 1983)
10. Mucuna pruriens
11. Nerium indicum
12. Ocimum sanctum
13. Pisum sativunm
14. Psoralia corylifolia

(2) Stimulants

1. Justacia simplex
2. Kalanchoe integra
3. Mangifera indica
4. Piper longum

(3) Autonomic effects

1. Hedychium spicatum
2. Leptadaenia reticulata
3. Melia azaderach
4. Nigella sativa
5. Nyctanthes arbor-tristis
6. Plantago ovata.

(4) Muscle relaxants

1. Jatropha curcas
2. Lepidium satvum
3. Nordostachys jatamamsi
4. Inula royleana (curariform activity)
5. Mucuna pruriens (like M-dopa)
6. Merremia gangetica (muscuranic activity)

(5) Spasmolytics *(anti-spasmodics)*

1. hedychium spicatum
2. Luffa echinata
3. Melia azarderach (Srivastava et al., 1981)
4. Mumusops elengi
5. Pterocarpus santalinus
6. Symplocos spicata (Rao et al., 1983)

(6) Spasmogeneics

1. Helictera isora
2. Mimosa pudica
3. Moringa oleifera
4. Nerium indicum
5. Piper longum
6. Psoralea corylifolia

(7) Anaesthetics

1. Tephrosia purpusea
2. Anacyclus pyrethrum
3. Sansviera roxburghiana
4. Gynandropsis gynandra

(8) Hypoglycaemic Activity: ***(Anti-diabetic activity)***

1. Achyranthus aspera
2. Aegle mormelos leaves (G. satyavati; 1983)
3. Alangium salvifolium
4. Allium cepa (Herbs Polonica, 1990)
5. Atropa belladona
6. Barleria cristata/B. prenoites
7. Berberis aristate - berberine
8. Cassia auriculata
9. Cassia fistula
10. Coccinia indica
11. Erythrina suberosa
12. Eugenia jambolana
13. Euphorbia hirta
14. Ficus bengalensis
15. Ficus glomerata - bark
16. Ficus religiosa
17. Gmelina arborea
18. Gymnema sylvestve (Shanmuga Sundaram et al., 1983)
19. Acacia catechu (Chakravarty et al., 1983)
20. Pterocarpus marsupium (Chakravarty et al., 1980, 1981a, 1981b)
21. Momordia charantia (Khanna et al., 1981b)
22. Allium sativum
23. Aloe barbedences/A. vera (Jrl. of Ethnopharma, 1990, 28 (2)
24. Annona squamosa - leaves
25. Asparagus racemosus - (UNI Do, April 1985)
26. Astercantha longifolia
27. Azaderachta indica - leaves (I.J. of Pharmacy, 1970)
28. Cinnamomum tamala - leaves
29. Clerodendrum phlomidis - root

30. Curcuma longa
31. Emblica officinalis - fruit
32. Enicostemma littorate - whole plant
33. Grewia asiatica - fruit
34. Inula racemosa - root
35. Saussurea lappa - root
36. Morus alba - root
37. Momordica charantia - fruit

(9) Anti-cancer Activity

1. Abrus precatorius (Subba Reddy V.V. & Sirsi M., 1968 & 1969)
2. Albezzia lebbeck (Dhar et al., (1968)
3. Alstonia scholaris (Dhar et al., 1968)
4. Amura rohitaka (Prad G.C. & Deshpande P.J., 1968)
5. Annona squemosa (Bhakuni et al., 1969)
6. Asparagus racemosus (Dhar et al., 1968)
7. Bacopa monniera (Bhakuni et al., 1969)
8. Boswellia serrata (Dhar et al., 1968)
9. Calotropis procera (Dhar et al., 1968)
10. Cedrus deodara (Dhar et al., 1968)
11. Erythrina suberosa (Dhar et al., 1968)
12. Euphorbia hirta (Dhar et al., 1968)
13. Datura metel (Dhar et al., 1968)
14. Plumbago zelanica
15. Semicarpus anacardium (chintil et al., 1980 & Indap et al., 1983)
16. Taxus buccata (Melado et al., 1984)
17. Vinca rosea (Cancer Res., 1960,20,1016) & (Rastogi et al., 1993)
18. Withania somnifera (G.ilter et al., 1967).
19. Allium sativum (Chem. Abst. 1961, 55, 9643b)

20. Aloe vera (Hoffman 1998)
21. Baliospermum montanum (Ogura M., 1978)
22. Bahunia racemosa
23. Berberis aristata - (Bhakuni D.S. et al., 1968)
24. Centella asciatica (Babu et al., 1995a & 1995b)
25. Curcuma longa (Leela Sinivas, 1993)

(10) Carcinogenic Activity

1. Argemone mexicana

(11) Anti-microbial Activity

(1) Anti-bacterial

1. Amura rohitaka
2. Areca catechu
3. Argemone mexicana
4. Asteracantha longifolia
5. Azadirachta indica
6. Bryophyllum calycinum
7. Capparis deciduda
8. Carissa carandas
9. Cassia fistula
10. Cassia occidentalis
11. Cocos nucifera
12. Crotolaria juncea
13. Curcuma longa
14. Cyperus rotundus
15. Desmodium gangeticum
16. Emblica officinalis
17. Euphoriba prostata
18. Hedychium spicatum
19. Hemedismus indicus
20. Leucas aspera
21. Madhuca longifolia
22. Mallotus philippensis
23. Mangifera indica
24. Pterocarpus marsupium
25. Punica granatus
26. Plumbago zeylanica

(2) Anti-viral

1. Amura rohitaka
2. Azadirachta indica
3. Caesalpinia bonducella
4. Capparis sepiaria / c. decidua
5. Cassia auriculata
6. Cassia tora
7. Celastrus paniculatum
8. Cynodon dactylon
9. Eclipta alba
10. Emblica officinalis
11. Gmelina arborea
12. Grewia hirsuta
13. Grewia latifolia
14. Hemedismus indicus

15. Ocimum sanctum
16. Phyllanthus niruri var. amarus
17. Madhuca longifolia
18. Nyctanthes arbor-tristis

(3) Anti-fungal

1. Asteracantha longifolia
2. Cassia fistula
3. Cocos nucifera
4. Desmodium gangeticum
5. Euphorbia thymifolia
6. Hedychium spicatum
7. Hibiscus rosa-sinensis
8. Holarrhina antidysenterica
9. Indigofera tinctoria
10. Inula racemosa
11. Lawsonia inermis
12. Leptadin reticulata

(4) Anti-tubercular

1. Acorus calamus
2. Alpinia galanga
3. Cucurbita maxima
4. Eucalyptus citroidora (citriodorol)
5. Grewia populifolia
6. Lawsonia inermis (Lawsone)
7. Ocimum americanum
8. Piper longum (Isobutylamide)

(5) Anti-lepromatous

1. Achyranthus aspera
2. Ocimum sanctum

(6) Anti-cholera

1. Berberis aristata
2. Myristica fragrans

(7) Amoebicidal & anti-protozoal

1. Acacia arabica
2. Alangium salvifolium
3. Asparagus racemosus
4. Atropa belladonna
5. Berberis aristata
6. Centella asiatica
7. Clerodendron inferturatum
8. Coceinia indica
9. Curcuma longa
10. Euphorbia hirta
11. Euphorbia tirucalli
12. Ficus racemosa
13. Ficus religiosa
14. Holerrhina antidysenterica
15. Murraya koenigii
16. Nardostachys jatamansi
17. Nigella sativa
18. Oroxylum indicum

(8) Anthelmintic

1. Aegle marmelos - marmelosin
2. Amura rohitaka
3. Artemisia martima - santonin
4. Butea frondosa
5. Capparis decidua
6. Carica papaya - benzylthiourea
7. Dalbergia latifolia
8. Datura metal
9. Embelia ribes
10. Ficus religiosa
11. Hedychium spicatum
12. Inula racemosa
13. Melia azaderach
14. Pterocarpus-marsupium

(9) Antimalarial

1. Alstonia scholaris
2. Andrographis paniculata
3. Caesalpinia bonduc
4. Pichrorrhiza kurroa
5. Swertia chirata
6. Somyda febrifuga

(10) Insecticidal

1. Acorus calamus
2. Annona squamosa
3. Euphorbia nerifolia

*** Note:** Insecticidal property is not used for clinical purposes.

(11) Action on Urinary System

(1) Anti-diuretic activity

1. Glycyrrhiza glabra (glycyrrhizin)

(2) Diuretic activity

1. Achyranthes aspera (saponins)
2. Azadirachta indica (sodium nimbidinate)
3. Barleria prionites
4. Boerhavia diffusa
5. Cassia occidentalis
6. Dolichos biflorus
7. Grewia hirsuta
8. Toddalia asiatica (Rastogi & Dhawan, 1982)
9. Hemedismus indicus
10. Oroxylum indicum
11. Picrorrhiza kurroa

(3) Anti-urolithiatic activity

1. Crataeva nurvala
2. Berginia ligulata
3. Coleus amboinicus

(4) Potassium sparing diuretics

1. Musa paradisiaca

(12) Action on Respiratory System

(1) Bronchodilator

1. Alpinia galanga
2. Inula racemosa
3. Saussurea lappa
4. Solanum xanthocarpum
5. Allium cepa (Handa et al., 1983)
6. Hedychium spicatun
7. Glycirrhiza glabra
8. Allium sativum

(2) Antitussive

1. Adathoda vasica
2. Solanum indium
3. Piper longum
4. Ocimum sanctum
5. Phyllanthus amarus
6. Terminalia chebula

(3) Anti-asthmatic & Anti-histaminic

1. Allium sativum
2. Citrullus colosynthis (coloside-A-glycoside)
3. Clerodendron serratum (saponin)
4. Curcuma longa
5. Tylophora indica (Geetha et al., 1981)
6. Albezzia lebbeck (Tripathi et al., 1983) antihistaminic
7. Piper longum (Dahanukar & Karandikar, 1984

Modern Perspective of Different Drug Actions

(1) Drugs acting on the CNS

(I) Central Transmitter Substances

(1) **Fast point-to-point signalling:** Ach and nicotinic effects. Except for a few cholinergic synapses with nicotinic receptors. the transmitters used in fast, point-to-point neural circuits are *amino acids* e.g. glutamate, aspartate, GABA, glycine.

(2) **Slow regulating signalling:** Ach and muscarinic effects.

(i) Neuropeptides– substance P. met-enkephalin, leu-enkephalin, angiotensin, somatostatin, LHRH, Calcitonin gene-related peptide (CGRP) etc.

(ii) Monoamines– dopamine, noradrenaline, adrenaline, serotonin (5HT).

(II) Autonomic nervous system

Preganglionic autonomic nerves release Ach for its effects on parasympathetic system and they also release *noradrenaline* for its effects on sympathetic system. Noradrenaline and adrenaline produce their actions on effector organs by acting on a, b or b_2- adrenoceptors. The nerve endings of postganglionic parasympathetic fibres release Ach which produces its action on the effector organs by activating muscarinic receptors. Ach released at synapses is increased by the enzyme, acetylcholinesterase.

Some of the important features related to autonomic nervous systmes are:

(i) Adrenaline mimics most sympathetic effects i.e., sympathomimetic agents. (Noradrenaline is more effective than adrenaline).

(ii) Effects of sympathetic stimulation are: pupillary dilation, bronchiolar dilatation, increase in rate & force of heart. raise in B.P., vasoconstriction in skin & viscera and vasodilatation in skeletal muscles, contraction of spleen, glycogenlysis in stimulated and blood glucose increases etc.

(iii) Adrenoceptors are mainly of two types

[a] **α-receptors–** mediate exitatory effects of sympathomimetic amines. Their inhibitary effects are mediated by β-receptors generally. They are again two types viz., post and presynaptic (α_1 &α_2).

[b] **β-receptors–** are not homogeneous e.g. noradrenaline is an effective stimulant of cardiac β-receptors, but has little or no action on the β-receptors mediating vasodilatation. They are also two types viz., β_1(heart, intestinal smooth muscle) β_2(bronchial, vascular and uterine smooth muscle)

(iv) Ach action–

[a] **Muscarinic effects**–are mainly parasympathetic and generally opposite to those caused by sympathetic stimulation. The effects are constriction of pupil, accommodation for near vision, profuse watery salivation, bronchiolar constriction, bronchosecretion, hypotension, increased GI motility and secreting contraction of urinary bladder and sweating.

[b] **Nicotinic effects**– include stimulation of all autonomic ganglia. But the action of Ach on ganglia is relatively weak compared with its effect on muscarinic receptors and so parasympathetic effects predominate.

(v) Acetylcholine receptors are divided into muscarinic and nicotinic receptors

Choline esterases– They are the quaternary compounds, that do not penctrate the blood-brain barrier e.g., methacholine, carbachol, bethanechol.

Anticholinesterases– They act directly on cholinomimetics e.g., physostigmine. Their effects are generally similar to those produce by the directly acting muscarinic agonists.

(1) Autonomic drugs acting at cholinergic synapses (cholinomimetics)

(i) Muscarinic agonists: They have relatively few uses, but pilocarpine is used to reduce introcular pressure in glaucoma e.g. methacholine, carbachol, bethanechol, pilocarpine.

(ii) Anti-cholinesterases: They have relatively little effect at ganglia and are used mainly for their nicotinic effects on the nueromuscular junction. They are used in myasthenia gravis etc. e.g., edrophonium, neostigmines physostigmine.

(iii) Nicotinic agonists: They stimulate nicotine receptors on both parasympathetic and sympathetic ganglionic neurones. e.g., nicotine, carbacol, antic-holinesterases.

(iv) Ganglion blockers: Such as hexamethonium are apparently not competitive antagonists of Ach, but are cation-channel blockers. Their effects include hypotension, mydriasis, dry mouth, anhydrosis, constipation, urinary retention & impotence.

(v) Muscarinic antagonists: They block the effects of Ach released from post-ganglionic parasympathetic nerve terminals. e.g., atropine, scopalamine, ipratropium tropicanide, benzhexol etc.

(2) Drugs acting on the sympathetic system

(i) Sympathomimetics

a. Indirectly acting: ephedrine, amphetamine, cocaine

b. Directly acting:

α-Agonist– α_1/α_2e.g.; noradrenaline, adrenaline.

α_2e.g.; clonidine, α-methyl-nor.

α_1e.g.; phenylephrine, methoxamine.

β-Agonists– β_1/β_2e.g.; adrenaline, isoprenaline.

β_2- solbutamol, terbutaline.

β_1- noradrenaline, dobutamine.

(ii) Adrenergic neurone blockers

reserpine, guanathidine, bethanidine

(iii) Adrenoceptor Antagonists

a. α-blockers: α_1/α_2- e.g.; phenoxybenzamine, phentolamine

α_1 e.g..prazosin.

b. β-blockers: β_1/β_2e.g.; propranolol, nadolol, timolol, oxprenolol, pindolol, alprenolol.

β_1 (cardioactive) e.g.; metaprolol, atenolol, acebutolol.

(iii) Drugs acting at the neuromuscular junction

Action potentials are conduted along the motor nerves to their terminals where they are controlled by Ach and cations like Ca^{2+} Na^+ & K^+. NM transmission can be increased by anticholinesterase drugs like Neostigmine and pyridostigmine which are used in Myasthenia gravis.

NM blocking drugs are used as anaesthetics to relax skeletal muscles during surgical operations and to prevent muscle contractions during electroconvulsant therapy (ECT).

(1) **Agents that reduce Ach release-** hemicholinium; botulinum toxin; Mg_2^+, Co_2^+ ions.

(2) **Agents that potentiate Ach transmission** ***(anticholinesterases):*** pyridostigmine, neostigmine, edrophonium, distigmine, ambenonium, phytostigmine, (eserine).

(3) **NM blocking drugs**

(i) Competitive- tubocurarine, gallamine, pancuronium, alcuronium, atracurium, vecuronium.

(ii) Depolarizing: suxamethonium.

(iv) Local anaesthetics

The drugs used to prevent pain by causing reversible block of conduction along nerve fibres. Most local anaesthetics are weak bases that exist at body pH mainly in a protonated form. Though all nerve fibres are sensetive to local anaesthetics, small-diameter fibres are more sensitive than large.

They are mainly divided into two categories viz., Amides and Esters.

(1) **Amides-** lignocaine, prilocaine, mepivacaine, bupivacaine.

(2) **Esters-** cocaine, benzocaine, amethocaine, procaine.

[**Note:** The local anaesthetic effect of Sarapunkha (Tephrosia purpurea) was studied and reported by Dr. P.V. Raj of Andhra Pradesh in 1975-76]

(v) General Anaesthetics

(1) **Premedication:** muscarinic antagonists, anxiolytics/sedatives narcotic analgesics, antiemetics

(2) **Inhalation anaesthetics:** nitrous oxide, halothane, iaoflurane, enflurane, ether, methoxy flurone, cyclopropane, trichlorethylene.

(3) **Intravenous induction agents**

(i) **Barbiturates:** thiopentone, methohexitone

(ii) **Non-barbiturates:** propanidid, althesin, ketamine, etomidate

(vi) Hypnotics and anxiolytics

(1) BDZS marketed as hypnotics

(i) **Short acting:** triazolan, temazepam, lormetagepam.

(ii) **Longer acting:** flunitrazepam, nitrazepam, flurazepam.

(2) Other drugs used as hypnotics

barbiturates, chloral hydrate, chlomethiazole.

(3) BDZS marketed as anxiolytics

diazepam, chlordiazepoxide, oxazepam, lorazepam etc

(4) Other drugs used as anxiolytics

barbiturates, benzoctamine, meprobamate, β-adrenergic blockers.

(vii) Anticonvulsants

(1) **Drugs used in status epilepticus:**

nitrazepam, diazepam, clonazepam

(2) **Drugs used in Grand mal epilepsy:**

phenobarbitone, phenytoin, carbamazepine, valproate.

(3) **Drugs used in Petitmal epilepsy:**

ethusuximide, valproate.

(viii) Drugs used in Parkinsonism

(1) **Muscarinic antagonists:**

benztropine, benzhexol, orphenadrine

(2) **Dopaminergic drugs:**

(i) Dopamine agonists - bromcriptine

(ii) Release dopamine - amantidine

(iii) Dopamine precursor - levodopa

(3) **MAO_B Inhibitors:**

Selagiline & (deprenyl)

(ix) Drugs used in psychosis- neuroleptics

(1) **Phenothiazines:**

(i) Propylamine side-chain - chlorpromazine

(ii) Piperidine side-chain - thioridazine

(iii) Piperazine side-chain - fluphenazine, prochlorperazine and trifluroperazine.

(2) **Butyrophenones:** e.g. haloperidol.

(3) **Thioxanthides:** e.g. fluphenthixol.

(4) **Diphenyl butylpiperidines:** e.g. fluspirilene & pimozide.

(x) Drugs used in affective disorders

(1) Noradrenaline and /or 5HT uptake blockers

(i) **Tricyclics**– amtriptyline, dothiepin, clomipramine, imipramine, desipramine.

(ii) **Non-tricyclics**– maprotiline, nomifensine, viloxazine.

(2) MAOIs: phenelzine, isocarboxazid, tranylcypromine.

(3) Atypical antidepressants: They do not block the amine up take. e.g.; mianserin, iprindole, trozodone.

(2) Drugs acting on the CVS

(I) Antihypertensive (hypotensive) drugs

(1) Centrally acting– lonidine methyldopa, reserpine.

(2) Ganglion blockers– rimetaphan, haxamethonium, pempidine

(3) β-blockers–	β_1/β_2 e.g. propranolol, nadolol, timolol, oxiprenolol, pindolol, sotalol.
	β_1 selective e.g. metaprolol, atenolol, acebutalol
(4) Adrenergic neurone blockers–	gaunethidine, bethanidine, debrisoquine, reserpine.
(5) Thiazide diuretics:	chlorthiazide, bendropfluazide etc.
(6) Converting enzyme inhibitors:	captopril, enalopril.
(7) Vasodilators:	
(i) α_1-blockers:	prazosin, indoramin
(ii) α/β blocker:	labetalol
(iii) Calcium antagonists:	nefidipine, diltiazem
(iv) Unknwon mechanism:	hydralazine, minoxidil, diazoxide, nitroprusside.

(II) Drugs used in angina

(1) β-blockers:	Propranolol, atenolol etc.
(2) Calcium antagonists:	nifedipine diltiazem verapamil
(3) Nitrates:	glyceryl trinitrate, isosorbide dinitrate, isosorbide -5-mononitrate

(III) Antiarrhythmic drugs

(1) Class IA:	ventricular and Supra ventricular e.g., disopyramide, procainamide, quinidine, flecainide, lorcainide, encainide.
(2) Class IB:	Ventricular e.g., lignocain, (phenytoin) mexiletine, tocainide
(3) Class II:	β– blockers (for specific problems)
(4) Class III:	Amiodarone (for specific probems)
(5) Class IV:	Supraventricular e.g.; verapamil, (digoxin).

(IV) Drugs used in heart failure

(1) Inotropic agents: digoxin, digitoxin, amrinone, milrinone, aminophylline, glucagon, dobutamine, dopamine.

(2) Vasodilators

(i) To decrease preload - nitrates

(ii) to decrease afterload or both preload & afterload e.g., hydralazine, nifedipine, prazosin, captopril.

(3) Drugs acting on Blood and Blood forming organs

(I) Drugs affecting blood coagulation

(1) Anticoagulants: They are used to prevent venous thrombosis e.g. heparin & vit. K antagonists like: warfarin, dicoumarol.

(2) Antiplatelet drugs: They are used to try and prevent arterial thrombosis e.g., aspirin, dipyridamole, sulphinpyrazone, prostacyclin (PGI2 epoprostenol).

(3) Fibrinolytic drugs: Streptokinase, urokinase.

(4) Antifibrinolytic drugs: Aminocaproic acid, tranexamic acid.

(II) Agents used in anaemias

(1) Vit. β_{12}: hydroxocobalamin, cynocobalamin

(2) Iron preparations: (i) oral- ferrus sulphate, ferrus gluconate, ferrus fumerate, ferrus glycine sulphate

(ii) Parenteral- iron dextran, iron sorbitol.

(4) Drugs used in Respiratory disorders

(I) Pharmacotherapy of cough

(1) Pharungeal demulcents: lozenges, troches, cough drops or linctuses made by using menthol etc.

(2) Expectorants: They are the drugs which increase the production of demulcent respiratory tract fluid that covers and protects the irritated mucosa.

(i) Direct stimulants: eucalyptus oil, lemon oil, alcohol, cederwood oil used orally or by inhalation other drugs are: creosotes, guaiacol (glyceryl guaiacolate).

(ii) Reflex expectorants: act by stimulating gastric reflexes which help to increase respiratory secretions.

(i) **Saline Expectorants**

a. Ammonium salts - NH_4Cl etc.

b. Potassium salts - KI

(ii) **Ipecacuanha:** contains emetine

(iii) **Vasaka alkaloids:** vasicine, vasicinone

(3) Central cough suppressants

(1) Opium derivates and related drugs: codeine, noscapine & dextramethorphin.

(2) Antihistaminic antitussives: diphenhydramine, chlor-cyclizine & dimethoxante.

(3) Local anaesthetic antitussives: benzonatate

(4) Miscellaneous antitussives: piperidone, ethyl dibunate and pimetine.

(4) Mucolytic agents:

They are used to make the sputum thin and less viscid, so that it can be easily expectorated. e.g., acetylcysteine, bromhexene, pancreatic dornase.

(5) Bronchodilators

Discussed later

(II) Pharmacotherapy of Asthma, hey fever & Anaphylaxis

The allergic manifestations are involved with two aspects mainly- "Allergins" and "Mediators".

Allergins	Mediators
Pollen	Histamine
Animal hair	Serotonin
Stings	Prostaglandins

Drugs e.g.	leukotrienes
antibiotics	bradykinin
iron injections	platelet aggregating factor (PAF)
aspirin	others

(1) Used in Asthma

(i) Bronchodilators

a. β_2- stimulants - solbutamol, terbutaline, rimiterol

b. xanthines - theophylline, aminophylline

c. Muscarinic antagonist - ipatropium (acrosol)

(ii) Steroids

a. inhaled - beclomethasone, dipropionate

b. oral - prednisolone

(2) Antitistaminics: astemizole, terfenadine promethazine, chlorpheniramine, mepyramine

(3) Anaphylaxis: bronchospasm, CV collapse, skin rashes, oedema in nose & throat, vomiting etc., are the common symptoms. The treatment includes drugs like: adrenaline, antihistamines, steroids.

(5) Drugs acting on the GIT

(I) Ulcer healing drugs

(1) Acid secretion reducers: cimitidine, rantidine, pirenzepine, omeprazole

(2) Mucosal strengtheners: sueralfate, bismuth chelate, carbenoxolone

(II) Antacids: $NaHCo_3$, $CaCo_3$, Mg $(OH)_3$, $Al(OH)_3$

(III) Laxatives

(1) Bulk: methyl cellulose, lactulose, $MgSo_4$ $(+H_2o)$

(2) Stimulant: bisacodyl, senna, cascora.

(3) Lubricants: dioctyl sodium, sulphosuccinate

(IV) Drugs used in Inflammatory Bowel disease

(1) Anti-inflammatory drugs

(i) Corticosteroids: hydrocortisone, predrisolone suppositaries, enemas, foam, oral prednisolone

(ii) Sulphasalazine

(2) Immuno suppressants: azothioprine

(V) Anti-spasmodics

(1) Muscarinic antagonists: atropine, propantheline, dicyclomine

(2) Directly acting on muscle: mebeverine, alverine

(VI) Anti-diarrhoeal drugs

(1) Morphine-like agents: morphine codeine, opium, diphenoxylate, lopermaide.

(2) Adsorbants: Kaolin, chalk.

(VII) Appetizers

(1) Bitters: Chirata I.P., Gentian I.P.

(2) Alcohol: augment the gastric secretion and act as appetizer.

(3) Miscullancous: insulin, anabolic steroids, vit. B_{12}, buclizine, cyperophetadine etc.

(VIII) Digestants

(1) HCl, (2) Pepsin (3) Pancreatin (4) Bila, Bilesalts & bile acid (5) Taka diastage

(IX) Carminatives

These are used to expel gas from the stomach or the intestines, e.g., cardamom seeds, ginger, fennel seeds, asefoetida, cinnamon bark, cloves, coriander etc., dimethypolysiloxane.

(X) Appetite suppressents *(Anorexients)*

(1) Amphetamine and related compounds (2) Bulk anorexients (Methylcellulose) (3) Miscellaneous (thyroxine, biguanides etc.)

(6) Drugs acting on the kidney, diuretics

[I] Loop agents:	Frusemide, bumetanide, ethacrynic acid
[II] Carbonic Anhydrase Indhibitors:	acetazolamide, minor actions of thiazides and loop agents.
[III] Thiazides:	Chlorothiazide, bendrofluazide, others.
[IV] Aldosterone:	
[V] Potassium sparing diuretics:	spironolactone, amiloride, triamterence.

(7) Chemotherapy

Chemotherapy is defined as the use of chemical compounds in the treatment of infectious diseases, so as to destroy offending parasites or oganisms without damaging the host tissues.

Mechanism of action of Antimicrobial agents

(1) **Interference with cell wall synthesis:** Pencillins, caphalosporins, Bacitracin, vancomycin & cycloserine.

(2) **Damage to the cytoplasmic membrane:** Polymixins, colistin and Polyene antibiotics.

(3) **Inhibition of Protein synthesis and impairment of the function of ribosomes:** Aminoglycosides, Tetracyclines, Chloramphenicol, Macrolide antibiotics and Lincomycin.

(4) **Interfering with the transcription of genetic information on the ribosomes:** Rifampicin.

(5) **Antimetabolite action:** Sulfonamides, Sulfones, PAS, INH, and Trimethoprim.

(I) Sulfonamides

(i) Short acting- Sulfadiazine, Sulfasomidin, Sulfacetamide etc.
(ii) Intermediate acting - Sulfamethoxazole, Sulfaphenazole etc.
(iii) Long acting - Sulfadimethoxine, Sulfamethoxypyridazine.

(II) Nitrofurans: Nitrofurantoin, Furazolidone, Nifuroxime etc.

(III) Nalidixic acid: mainly against gram negative bacteria. Imp. action on Proteus

(IV) Trimethoprim: effective against many bacteria

(V) Pencillins & Antibiotics specific for Gram positive organisms:

(1) Against gram positive- Pencillins, Erythromycin, Lincomycin, oleandomycin, Vancomycin, Novobiocin & Fucidin.

(2) Against gram negative- streptomycin, Kanamycin, Gentamicin, Polymixin B, Colistin, cycloserine

(3) Against both gram positive & negative- Ampicillin, Amoxycilline, Cephalosporins, Rifamycins; Neomycin, Framycetin.

(4) Against gram positive, gram negative, rickettsiae & chlamydia- Tetracyclines & chloramphenicol.

(5) Against acid fast bacilli- streptomycin, cycloserine, viomycin, Karamycin, Rifampici.

(6) Against protozoa- Nystatin, Amphotericin B. Griseofulvin, Pimaricin, Hamycin.

(7) Antimaligrancy- Actinomycin D, Mitomycin, Azascrine

References about karma

1. Sharma J.N., "Ayurvediya Karma Mimamsa". Dept. of D.G., IPGTR, G.A.U.: Jamnagar, M.D. Thesis, 1961.
2. Damodar Pandey; "A study of Grahi Karma", Dept. of D.G., Jamnagar: IPGTR, G.A.U., M.D. Thesis 1961.
3. Trivedi Hemaben; Dadima Twak Ka Krimighna Karma. Dept. of D.G., IPGTR, G.A.U., Jamnagar 1977, M.D. Thesis.
4. Parmar R.M.; Study of Katushigres for its Lekhana Karma in the management of obesity (sthaulya). Dept. of D.G.; IPGTR, G.A.U., Jammagar, 1994, M.D. Thesis.
5. Rao Thimalgin S.; Mutrala Karma with Trina Pancha Moola Kashaya and Pashanabheda. Dept. of D.G., IPGTR, G.A.U. Jamnagar, 1965, M.D. Thesis.
6. Metkar Ashok N.; "Concept of Rakshoghna karma with Antimicrobial activity of Rakshoghna drug". Dept. of D.G., IPGTR, G.A.U. Jamnagar, 1986. M.D. Thesis.
7. Acharya R.N.; A study on Vidarikanda w.s.r. to its Vrishya karma. Dept. of D.G., IPGTR, G.A.U. Jamnagar, 1996, M.D. Thesis.
8. Dongarwar L.A.; A study of Vajeekarana karma of certain Ayurvedic drugs w.s.r. to effect on Sukra Vardhana. Dept. of D.G., IPGTR, G.A.U., Jamnagar; 1987, M.D. Thesis.
9. Nisteswar K. & Seshagiri Rao T.; "Role of Deepaniya and Balya drugs in Therapeutics". Nagarjuna Vol. XXV, No. 5 1982. pp.102-103.
10. Nistewar K. & Seshagiri Rao T.; Implications of certain pharmacological actions delineated in Ayurvedic classics, Nagarjma, Vol. XXVII No.3 pp.67-68.

✵

Chapter-XI

Botanical Classification and Different Groups of Drugs used in Ayurveda

1. Determination of Botanical Classification

The primitive man calssified plants into useful plants, poisonous plants and non-useful plants on the basis of their use. Later, Theopharastus (275 AD) classified plants basing on habit, into herbs, shrubs and trees. Hence he is called as 'Father of Botany', Herbs are again classified as annuals, bienniels and perennials.

John Ray & Carolus Linnaeus (1754) classified plant kingdom into 24 classes based on staminal characters like number of stamens, union and arrangement. He laid down the foundation for the modern concept of taxonamy, hence called as 'father of Taxonamy'.

Adanson suggested that a wide range of characters should be taken as cirteria for classification. With added knowledge but also anatomical features, ecological features, physiological features, embryological features, geographical distribution are being taken into consideration for classification of plants. The scientific studies are also based on the principle of evolutionary development.

'Plant taxonomy' or 'Systematic Botany' is a branch of biological science which is concerned with identification, nomenclature and classification of plants.

A.P. de Condolle was the first taxonomist who introduced the term 'taxonomus' into biological terminology. Carl Von Linnaeus (1707-1778) a Sweedish Scientist adopted "binomial nomenclature" in naming the plants.

The object of classification is to classify the things in such manner that their relationship with regard to their descent from a common ancestry may be brought out. The ultimate object of classification is to arrange plants in such a way as to give us an idea about their origin and evolution from simpler, earlier and more primitive types of more complex, more recent and more advanced types in different periods of earth.

Among various classifications of plants proposed so far, three are the most important, namely artificial, natural and phylogenetic.

(1) Artificial System *(Key classification)*

An artificial systems classifies plants with the help of one or a few characters, primarily with an intention of easy identification of an organism. The classical example of the artificial system is the so called "Sexual system" of Linnaeus, the "Father of Taxonomic Botany and Zoology". He classified plants on the basis of the number and arrangement of sexual parts. It is structured for convenience, using easily observed phenotypic characters and not necessarily indicating phylogenetic relationships.

(2) Natural System

In natural system of classification all the important characters are taken into account and the plants are classified according to their related characters. The system proposed by de Jussieu, de Condolle, Benthom and Hooker can be considered more natural systems of classification with emphasis on the reproductive parts (flowers, fruits and seeds etc).

This is based not only on the characters of reproductive organs and structural relationship but all the other important characters are also taken into consideration and the plants are classified according to their related character. It helps us not only to ascertain the name of a plant but also its relationship and affinities with other plants. All the modern systems of classification are natural.

(3) Phylogenetic System

Phylogenteic system classifies plants according to their evolutionary and genetic relationships. The so called phylogenetic systems were proposed by Eichler, Engler and Prantl, Bessey and Hutchinson etc.

It enables us to find out the ancestors or derivatives of any taxon. Our present day knowledge is insufficient to construct a perfect phylogenetic classification and all present phylogenetic systems are formed by the combination of natural and phylogenetic evidences.

Taxa
↓
Taxonomic Characters

↓	↓	↓
Use of habit and importance to man	Use of many characters as possible to group taxa	Use of many characters possible plus phylogenetic evolutionary interpretation.
↓	↓	↓
Artificial classification	Natural classification	Phylogenetic classification

Objectives of Plant Taxonomy

(i) To inventory the world's flora.

(ii) To provide a method for identification & communication.

(iii) To provide a coherent and universal system of classification.

(iv) To demonstrate the evolutionary implications of plant diversity.

(v) To provide a single Latin 'Scientific' name for every group of plants in the world, both existent and fossil.

Scope of Taxonomy

Plants are grouped into taxonomic hierarchy. Each level of hierarchy is called a 'rank' or 'category' e.g., family, genus, species. A taxonomic group of any rank is called a taxon (plural taxa) e.g., Ranunculaceae, Ranunculus, Ranunculus scleratus.

The basic Rank of hierarchy is the species and so on e.g.

Plant-Kingdom
↓
Divisions
↓
Classes
↓
Order

↓
Families
↓
Genera
↓
Species

Study of systematic botany consists of:

(i) Plant Taxonomy– which establishes the phylogenetic relationships that extent exist naturally between many groups of plants.

(ii) Nomenclature– giving names to all kinds of plants.

Units of Classification

There are certain units of classification viz., (1) Species (2) Genus (3) Family (4) Order (5) Series (6) Sub-classes (7) Classes (8) Sub-divisions (9) Divisions (10) Kingdom.

(1) A Species is an aggregation of individual plants which are so similar that they have descended from a common ancestro. The species is the "basic unit of classification".

(2) A Genous is an assemblage of related species. All species in a genus have more features in common. For example, different species like squamosa, reticulata, muricate etc., belonging to the same genus Annona. They all will have similar floral characters.

(3) The Family is a higher group of closely related genera. For example, the related genera like Annona, Polyalthia, Artabotrys belong to the same family, since they have similar floral structures.

(4) The Order represents the assemblage of related families like Magnoliaceae, Annonaceae are grouped together in the order 'Ranales', Fabaceae & caesalpinaceae etc., in the order 'Rosales'.

(5) A number of closely related orders constitute, *Series*. For example, orders like Ranaks, Parietales, Malvales are grouped under the series Thalamiflorae.

(6) The series with one important uniform character will make **sub-class** e.g., series Thalamiflorae, Disciflorae etc., with polypetalous corolla make-up a sub-class polypetalae.

(7) The sub-classes together constitute a **class** e.g., sub-classes Polypetalae, Gamopetalae, Monochlamydeae together make-up the class 'Dicotyledonae'. These plants have tap-root system, reticulately veined leaves as common features.

(8) Different classes with common features may form *sub-divisions.*

(9) Classes of different plants with some common features are placed under *Division.* e.g., Dicotyledonae & Monocotyledonae are placed under 'Angiospermae', because the seeds are enclosed within fruit.

(10) Kingdom is the highest taxonomic hierarchy with all plants.

2. Groups of Drugs of Plant Origin

(1) Dasa Mula *(Ten Roots)*

Charaka mentioned the 'Dasamulas' described by Sushrita under "Sothahara varga". Sushrita considered Brihat and Laghu Panchamulas together as 'Dasamula'. The constituents are:

(i) Bilva (Aegle marmelos)

(ii) Agnimantha (Clerodendrum phlomidis)

(iii) Syonāka (Oroxylum indicum)

(iv) Pātala (Stereospermum saveolens)

(v) Gambhari (Gmelina arborea)

(vi) Gokshura (Tribulus terrestris)

(vii) Brihati (Solanum indicum)

(viii) Kantakari (Solanum surattens)

(ix) Sali parni (Desmodium gangeticum)

(x) Prisni parni (Uraria picta)

Properties: Tridosha hara, Sotha hara, Swasa hara, Āma pachana.

Indications: Swasa, Sotha, Jwara, Sirahsula, Tandra, Ānaha,

Parswa sula[1].

(2) Pancha Mula: ***(Five Roots)***

(i) Brihat Panchamula: ***(Roots of five trees)***

Brihat Panchamula or Mahat Panchamulas are described seperately by Sushrita along with other groups. The are composed of-

(a) Bilva (Aegle marmelos)

(b) Agnimanthā (Clerodendrum phlomidis)

(c) Gambhāri (Gmelina arborea)

(d) Shyōnāka (Oroxylum indicum)

(e) Pātalā (Stereospermum sauveolens)

Proterties: Tikta-Kashaya-Madhura Rasa, Kapha-Vata hara, Deepana, Swasa hara.

Indications: Swasa-Kasa, Agni mandya, Vāta vyadhi etc[2].

(ii) Laghu Panchamula: ***(Root of five herbs)***

This group contain the following herbs:

(a) Gokshura (Tribulus terrestris)

(b) Brihati (Solanum indicum)

(c) Kantakari (Solanum Surattens)

---

१. (i) पाटलाग्निमन्थश्योनाक बिल्व काश्मर्य कण्टकारिका बृहती शालपर्णी पृश्निपर्णी गोक्षुरा इति दशेमानि श्वयथुहराणि भवन्ति ॥ (च.सू. ४/१३)

(ii) ....अनयोर्दशमूलमुच्यते ॥ गण: श्वासहरो ह्येष कफपित्तानिलापह: । आपस्य पाचनश्चैव सर्वज्वरविनाशन: । (सु.सू. ३८/७०-७१)

(iii) उभाभ्यां पञ्चमूलाभ्यां दशमूलमुदाहृतम् ॥ दशमूलं त्रिदोषघ्नं श्वासकासशिरोरूज: । तन्द्राशोथज्वरानाहपार्श्वपीडाऽरुचीर्हरेत् ॥ (भा.प्र.)

(iv) उभाभ्यां पञ्चमूलाभ्यां दशमूलं त्रिदोषनुत् ॥
तन्द्राकासज्वरश्वासपार्श्वरूक् सशिरोर्तिजित् ।
हिध्मानाहाग्निसादेषु प्रतिश्याये प्रशस्यते ॥ (कै.नि.१/७३-७४)

२. (i) बिल्वाग्निमन्थटुण्टुकपाटला: काश्मर्यश्चेति महत् ॥ (सु.सू. ३८/६८)

(ii) बिल्वा काश्मर्य तर्कारी पाटला टिण्टुकैर्महत् ॥
जयेत्कषायतिक्तोष्णं पञ्चमूलं कफानिलौ । (अ.हृ.सू. १/१६७-१६८)

(iii) श्रीफल: सर्वतोभद्रा पाटला गणकारिका । श्योनाक: पञ्चभिश्चैतै: पञ्चमूलं महन्मतम् ॥
पञ्चमूलं महत् तिक्तं कषायं कफवातनुत् । मधुरं श्वासकासघ्नमुष्णं लघ्वग्निदीपनम् ॥ (भा.प्र.)

(d) Sali parni (Desmodium gangeticum)

(e) Prisni parni (Uraria picta)

Properties: Kashaya-Tika-Madhura Rasa, Vata-Pitta hara, Brimhana, Balya, Anushna virya, Grahi.

Indications: Atisara, Jwara, Swasa, Ashmari[1].

(iii) Kantaka Panchamula: ***(Roots of five thorny plants)***

According to Sushrita the following are the constituents of this group:

(a) Karamarda (Carissa carandas)

(b) Gokshura (Tribulus terrestris)

(c) Sairēyaka (Barleria cristata)

(d) Shatāvari (Asparagus racemosus)

(e) Gridhra Nakhi (Capparis zeylanica)

* **Note:** Some scholars denote Vyaghranakhi as Himsra. But according to syllabus, Himsra is Capparis sepiaria.

Properties: Pittta hara, Sotha hara

Indications: Rakta pitta, Sotha, Prameha, Sukra doshas etc.

(iv) Valli Panchamula: ***(Roots of five climbers)***

These are the roots of five climbers; namely:

(a) Vidari kanda (Pureria tuberosa)

(b) Sariva (Hemidisamus indicus)

(c) Haridra/Rajani (Rubia cardifolia)

(d) Guduchi (Tinospora cordifolia)

(e) Meshasringi (Damia extensa)

---

१. (i) त्रिकण्टकबृहतीद्वयपृथक्पर्ण्यो विदारिगन्धा चेति कनीयः ॥ (सु.सू. ३८/६६)

(ii) कषायतिक्तमधुरं कनीयः पञ्चमूलकम् । वातघ्नं पित्तप्रशमनं बृंहणं बलवर्धनम् ॥ (सु.सू.३८/६७)

(iii) ह्रस्वं बृहत्यंशुमतीद्वयगोक्षुरकैः स्मृतम् ॥ स्वादुपाकरसं नातिशीतोष्णं सर्वदोषजित् । (अ.हृ.सू.६/१६८-१६९)

(iv) शालपर्णी पृश्निपर्णी वार्त्ताकी कण्टकारिका । गोक्षुरः पञ्चभिश्चैतैःकनिष्ठं पञ्चमूलकम् ॥
पञ्चमूलं लघुस्वादु बल्यं पित्तानिलापहम् । नात्युष्णं बृंहणं ग्राही ज्वरश्वासाश्मरीप्रणुत् ॥ (भा.प्र.)
करमर्द-त्रिकण्टक-सैरेयक-शतावरी– गृध्रनख्य इति कण्टकसंज्ञः । (सु.सू. ३८)

Protertics: Pitta hara, Sotha hara

Indications: Rakta pitta, Sotha, Prameha, Sukra doshas etc[1].

(v) Trina Panchamula: ***(Roots of five grasses)***

(a) Kusa
(b) Kāsa
(c) Nala
(d) Darbha
(e) Kandekshu

These five are known as Trina pancha mulas. They are to be used mainly with milk.

Properties: Pitta hara, Mutrala.

Indications: Mutra krichchra, Rakta pitta[2].

(vi) Madhyama Panchamula: ***(Roots of five shrubs)***

(a) Bala (Sida cardifolia)
(b) Punarnava (Boerhavia diffusa)
(c) Eranda (Ricinus communis)
(d) Mudga parni (Phaseolus trilobus)
(e) Masha parni (Teramnus labialis)

Properties: Kapha-Vāta hara, Balya, Vājikarana.

Indications: Vata vyadhis, Sukra dosha, Sosha etc[3].

(vii) Jeevaniya Panchamula: ***(Five roots which acts as tonic)***

(a) Abhiru
(b) Veera
(c) Jeevanti
(d) Jeevaka
(e) Rishabhaka

---

१. (i) विदारी-सारिवा-रजनी-गुडूची-अजशृङ्गी चेति वल्लीसंज्ञ: ॥ (सु.सू. ३८)
(ii) रक्तपित्तहरौ ह्योतौ शोफत्रयविनाशनौ । सर्वमेहहरौ चैव शुक्रदोषविनाशनौ ॥ (सु.सू. ३८)
२. (i) कुश-काश-नल-दर्भ-काण्डेक्षुका चेति तृणसंज्ञक: ॥ (सु.सू. ३८)
(ii) मूत्रदोषविकारं च रक्तपित्तं तथैव च । अन्त्य: प्रयुक्त: क्षीरेण शीघ्रमेव विनाशयेत् ॥ (सु.सू. ३८)
३. बलापुनर्नवैरण्डसूर्पपर्णीद्वयेन तु । मध्यमं कफवातघ्नं नातिपित्तकरं स्मृतम् ॥ (अ.हृ.सू. ६)

Properties: Pitta-Vāta hara, Jeevaniya, Vrishya, Chakchushya.

Indications: Netra rogas, Dhatu kshaya, Sukra doshas etc[1].

(3) Pancha Valkala: ***(Five barks with latex)***

It appears that Chakrapāni described them in his text 'Chakradatta' as Kshiri vrikshas i.e., trees with latex in their bark. They are also known as "Twak panchaka". Narahari quoted them as "Pancha vetasa". They are:

(1) Nyagrodha (Ficus benghalensis)

(2) Udumbara (Ficus glomerata)

(3) Aswatha (Ficus religiosa)

(4) Pārisha (Thevetia populnea)

(5) Plaksha (Ficus lacor)

***Note:** Some scholars considered either Sirisha (Albezzia lebbek) or Vetasa (?) in place of Pārisha. Charaka quoted the following five trees without quoting them as Panchavalkalas in Dina charya context: Vata, Udumbara, Aswatha, Plaksha & Lodhra (Cha.Su.5).

Properies: Kashaya Rasa, Seeta virya, Varnya, Ruksha guna, Sotha hara, Sthanya janana, Sandhana kara, Pitta-Kapha hara, Medo hara, Grahi, Lekhana.

Indications: Yoni vyapath, Vrana, Medo roga (Sthoulya), Visarpa, Sotha, Rakta vikaras, Asthi bhagna, Sthanya kshaya, Atisara etc[2].

** Their leaves are Grahi, Seeta, Kapha-vata hara and Raktadosha hara in nature[3].

---

१. अभीरूवीश जीवन्ती जीवकर्षभकै स्मृतम् । जीवनाख्यं तु चक्षुष्यं वृष्यं पित्तानिलापहम् ॥ (अ.हृ.सू. ६)

२. (i) उदुम्बरो वटोऽश्वत्थो वेतसः प्लक्ष एव च । पञ्चैते क्षीरिणो वृक्षाः संज्ञया समुदाहृताः ॥ (च.द.)

(ii) न्यग्रोधोदुम्बराश्वत्थ पारीषप्लक्षपादपाः । पञ्चैते क्षीरिणो वृक्षास्तेषां त्वक्पञ्चवल्कलम् ॥
(केचित्तु पारीषस्थाने शिरीषं, वेतसं परे वा वदन्तीति विशेषः ॥) (भा.प्र.वटादिवर्गः १४-१५)

(iii) त्वक्पञ्चकं हिमं ग्राहि व्रणशोथविसर्पजित् ॥ (भा.प्र.)

(iv) क्षीरिवृक्षा हिमा वर्ण्या योनिरोगव्रणापहाः । रूक्षाः कषाया मेदोघ्ना विसर्पामयनाशनाः ॥ (भा.प्र.)
शोथपित्तकफास्रघ्नाः स्तन्या भग्नास्थियोजकः । (भा.प्र.)

(v) न्यग्रोधोदुम्बराश्वत्थप्लक्षवेतसवल्कलैः । सर्वैरेकत्रमिलितैः पञ्चवेतसमुच्यते ॥ (रा.नि.)

३. तेषां पत्रं हिमं ग्राहि कफवातास्रनुल्लघु । विष्टम्भाध्मानजित्तिक्तं कषायं लघु लेखनम् ॥ (भा.प्र.)

(4) Pancha Pallava: ***(Five leaves group)***

(i) Āmra (Mangifera indica)

(ii) Jambu (Eugenia gambosa)

(iii) Kapitha

(iv) Beejapura (Citrus medica)

(v) Bilwa (Aegle marmelos)

These five are considered as Pancha pallava by Narahari.

Properties: Vāta-kapha hara, Grahi, Deepana-pāchana.

Indications: Atisāra, Grahani, Gandha karma[1].

(5) Triphala: ***(Three fruits)***

Suśruta mentioned Triphala as a specific gana for the first time. All the Ācharyas described Triphala and their utility. It is often said by traditional Vaidyas that Triphala alone is sufficient to deal with 50% of cases in clinical practice.

This small group comproses of viz.,

(i) Haritaki (Terminalia chebula)

(ii) Āmalaki (Emblica officinalis)

(iii) Vibhitaki (Terminalia bellirica)[2].

These three are also known as 'Phala Traya' or 'Varā'.

It is essential to note that the ratio in which Triphala are to be mixed is not quite clear.

According to Sushrita	: Haritaki	: Āmalaki	: Vibhitaki	(1:1:1)
According to Bhavamishra	: Haritaki	: Vibhitaki	: Āmalaki	(1:1:1)
According to Chakradatta	: -do-	: -do-	: -do-	(1:2:4)
According to Yoga Ratnakara	: -do-	: -do-	: -do-	(1:2:4)
According Madanapala	: -do-	: -do_	: -do-	(3:6:12)

१. आम्रजम्बू कपित्थानां बीजपूरक बिल्वयो: । गन्धकर्मणि सर्वत्र पत्राणि पञ्चपल्लवम् ॥ (रा.नि.)

२. (i) हरीतक्यामलकविभीतकानीति त्रिफला ॥
त्रिफला कफपित्तघ्नी मेहकुष्ठविनाशनी । चक्षुष्या दीपनी चैव विषमज्वरनाशनी ॥(सु.सू.३८/५६-५७)
(ii) पथ्याविभीतधात्रीणां फलै: स्यास्त्रिफला समै: । फलत्रिकं च त्रिफला सा वरा च प्रकीर्तिता ॥
त्रिफला कफपित्तघ्नी मेहकुष्ठहरा सरा । चक्षुष्या दीपनी रूच्या विषमज्वरनाशिनी ॥ (भा.प्र.)
(iii)एका हरीतकीयोज्या द्वौ च योज्यौ विभीतकौ ॥ चत्वार्यामलकान्येत त्रिफलैषा प्रकीर्तिता ।
त्रिफला शोथमेहघ्नी नाशयेद्विषमज्वरान् ॥
दीपनी श्लेष्मपित्तघ्नी कुष्ठहन्त्री रसायनी । सर्पिर्मधुभ्यां भागा: सैव नेत्रामयान्जयेत् ॥ (यो.र.और च.द.)
(iv)हरीतक्यास्त्रयो भागा: शिवा द्वादशभागिका । षड्भागा: स्युर्विभीतस्य त्रिफलेयं प्रकीर्तिता ॥ (म.पा.१/३१)

If the usually accepted 1:2:4 combination is applied to Sushrita's and Bhavamishra's views then the quantity of individual drugs will vary. Therefore, the author advise the young scholars to study whether 1:1:1 or 1:2:4 or 1:4:2 is therape tically effective.

The traditional approach is to accept equal volume or weight of the fruit pulp (dried) i.e., 1:1:1.

Properties: Kapha-Pitta hara, Kushta hara, Prameha hara, Deepana, Chakchushya, Jwara hara, Rasayana.

Indications: Prameha, Kushta, Agni mandya, Netra Roga, Vishama jwara, Sotha, Mala bandha etc.

(6) Trikatu: *(Three Pungents)*

This is also separately discribed by Sushrita. The constituents of this small group are:

(i) Pippali (Piper longum)

(ii) Maricha (Piper nigrum)

(iii) Sunthi (Zingiber officinale)[1].

Properties: Kapha hara, Medo hara, Kushta hara, Deepana, Swasa hara, Ruchyam.

Indications: Prameha, Medo roga (Sthoulya), Kushta, Twak rogas, Agni mandya, Gulma, Peenasa, Swasa-Kāsa, Sleepada, Sula etc.

Trikatu are otherwise called as Vyosha or Tryushana or Katu trika.

(7) Trimada: *(Three inebrients)*

(i) Vidanga (Embelia ribes)

(ii) Mustha (Cyprus rotundus)

(iii) Chitraka (Plumbago zeylanica)

---

१. (i) पिप्पली मरिच शृङ्गवेराणीति त्रिकटुकम् ॥ त्र्यूषणं कफमेदोघ्नं मेहकुष्ठत्वगामयान् ।
निहन्याद्दीपनं गुल्मपीनसाग्न्यल्पतामपि ॥ (सु.सू. ३८/५८-५९)

(ii) विश्वोपकुल्या मरिचं त्रयं त्रिकटु कथ्यते । कटुत्रिकं तु त्रिकटु त्र्यूषणं व्योषमुच्यते ॥
त्र्यूषणं दीपनं हन्ति श्वासकासत्वगामयान् । गुल्ममेहकफस्थौल्य मेदःश्लीपदपीनसान् ॥ (भा.प्र.)

(iii) पिप्पली मरिचं शुण्ठी त्रयमेतद्विमिश्रितम् । त्रिकटु त्र्यूषणं व्योषं कटुत्रिकमथोच्यते ॥
दीपनं रुचिदं वातश्लेष्ममन्दाग्निशूलनुत् ॥ (यो.र.)

Properties: Thikta-katu rasa, Ushna virya, Katu vipaka, Krimi hara, Grahi.

Indications: Krimi, Atisāra, Sthoulya, Pandu etc[1].

(8) Chatūrushana: ***(Four pungents)***

(i) Sunthi

(ii) Pippali

(iii) Maricha

(iv) Pippali mula (Root of long pepper)

Properties: Kapha hara, Medo hara, Swasahara, Agni deepana.

Indications: Swasa-kasa, Gulma, Prameha, Sthoulya, Sleepada.

(9) Pancha Kola:

The five drugs which are used in the quantity of one Kola (5 gm=1/2karsha) each as a group are known as 'Pancha kola'. They are also called as 'PANCHA USHANAS'.

(i) Pippali (Piper longum)

(ii) Pippali mula (Root of Pipper longum)

(iii) Chavya (Piper retrofractum)

(iv) Chitraka (Plumbago zeylanica)

(v) Sunthi (Zingiber officinale)

Properties: Kapha-Vata hara, Deepana, Pachana, Teekshna & Ushna guna, Sula prasamana, Pitta vardhaka.

Indications: Agnimandya, Gulma, Pleeha roga, Udara, Ānaha, Sula[2].

(10) Shdūshana: ***(Six spices)***

The above five drugs i.e., Pancha kolas along with Maricha (Black Pepper) are known as 'Shadushana'.

---

१. विडङ्गमुस्तचित्रैश्च त्रिमदः समुदाहृतः । (रा.नि.)

२. (i) पिप्पली पिप्पलीमूलं चव्यचित्रकनागरैः । पञ्चभिः कोलमात्रं यत् पञ्चकोलं तदुच्यते ॥ (भा.प्र.)

(ii) पञ्चकोलं रसे पाके कटुकं रूक्षकृन्मतम् ।
तीक्ष्णोष्णं पाचनं श्रेष्ठं दीपनं कफवातनुत् । गुल्मप्लीहोदरानाहशूलघ्नं पित्तकोपनम् ॥ (भा.प्र.)

Properties: Kapha-Vata hara, Visha hara, Deepana-Pachana

Indications: Gulma, Ānaha, Sula, Visha rogas, Pleehodara etc[1].

(11) Chāturbeeja: ***(Four seeds)***

(i) Methika (Trigonella foenum-greacum)

(ii) Chandra sura (Lepidium sativum)

(iii) Krishna Jeeraka (Carum carvi)

(iv) Yavanika (Apium graveolens)

Properties: Vāta hara, Deepana-Pachana, Sula hara

Indications: Vata vyadhi, Parswa sula, Kati sula, Ajeerna, Sula, Ādhmana etc[2].

(12) Jeevaniya Gana: ***(Group of nutrients)***

Charaka and Vriddha Vagbhata have mentioned Jeevaniya varga. Sushrita quoted Kākolyadi gana as Jeevaniya. In a different form these are again described under Ashta varga. This Jeevaniya varga consists of : (1) Jeevaka (2) Rishabhaka (3) Meda (4) Mahā Meda (5) Kākoli (6) Ksheera kākoli (7) Mudgaparni (8) Māsha parni (9) Jeevanti (10) Yashti Madhu[3].

Properies: Madhura rasa, Seeta virya, Jeevaniya, Balya, Vāta hara.

Indications: Vata vyadhi, Sosha, Sukra dosha, Kārsya, Ojo kshaya etc.

(13) Ashta Varga: ***(Eight drugs which are tonics)***

Bhava Mishra described the following eight dravyas under Ashta varga.

(i) Jeevaka (ii) Rishabhaka (iii) Meda (iv) Maha Meda (v) Kākoli (vi) Kshira kākoli (vii) Ridhi & (viii) Vriddhi[4].

---

१. पञ्चकोलं समरिचं षडूषणमुदाहृतम् । पञ्चकोलगुणं तत्तु रूक्षमुष्णं विषापहम् ॥ (भा.प्र.)

२. मेथिका चन्द्रशूरश्च कालाजाजी यवानिका । एतच्चतुष्टयं युक्तं चतुर्बीजमिति स्मृतम् ॥
तच्चूर्णं भक्षितं नित्यं निहन्तिपवनामयम् । अजीर्णशूलमाध्मानं पार्श्वशूलं कटिव्यधाम् ॥ (भा.प्र.)

३. जीवकर्षभकौ मेदा महामेदा काकोली क्षीरकाकोली मुद्गपर्णीमाषपर्ण्यौ जीवन्ती मधुकमिति दशेमानि जीवनीयानि भवन्ति ॥ (च.सू. ४)

४. (i) जीवकर्षभकौ मदे काकोल्यौ ऋद्धिवृद्धिके । अष्टवर्गोऽष्टभिद्रव्यैः कथितश्चरकादिभिः ॥ (भा.प्र.)
(ii) अष्टवर्गो हिमः स्वादुर्बृंहणः शुक्रलो गुरुः । भग्नसन्धानकृत् कामबलासबलवर्धनः ॥
वातपित्तास्रतृड्दाहज्वरमेहक्षयापहः । (भा.प्र.)

Vinodalal Sen (in Ayurveda Vijnana) had advocated the substitutes for these eight drugs owing to the contraversy in their identity. The substitutes are:

(a) **Guduchi** for Jeevaka
(b) **Vansalochana** for Rishabhaka
(c) **Aswagandha** for Meda
(d) **Sāriva** for Maha Meda
(e) **Satavari** (2 times) for Kākoli & Kshira Kākoli
(f) **Bala** for Ridhi
(g) **Maha Bala** for Vriddhi.

Properties: Madhura Rasa & Vipaka, Seeta virya, Guru guna, Vrishya, Brimhana, Jeevaniya, Vata-Pitta hara, Kapha vardhana, Daha prasamana, Jwara hara, Sukrala, Balya.

Indications: Sukra-kshaya, Ojo kshaya, Prameha, Asthi bhagna, Vāta roga, Rakta vikara, Trishna, Jwara, Dāha, Kshaya etc.

(14) Trijātaka: *(Three aromatics)*

(i) Twak (Cinnamomum zeylanica)
(ii) Ela (Cinnamomum cardamomum)
(iii) Patra (Cinnamomum zeylanica)

These three are together known as "Trijataka" or "Trisugandhi". Vagbhata quoted them first.

Properties: Katu-Madhura Rasa, Ushna virya, Ruksha-Teekshna guna, Kapha-vāta hara, Vishaghna, Deepana varnya.

Indications: Agni mandya, Visha rogas, Mukha, Durgandha, Sula etc[1].

(15) Chāturjataka: *(Four aromatics)*

The Trijatakas along with Nāga kesara (Mesua ferrca) are called as Chāturjātaka.

They also possess the same properties of Trijataka[2].

---

१. (i) त्वगेलापत्रकैस्तुल्यैस्त्रिसुगन्धि त्रिजातकम् । (भा.प्र.)
(ii) एलावराङ्गपत्रैश्च त्रिसुगन्धि त्रिजातकम् । (कै.नि. ८/१)

२. (i) नागकेसरसंयुक्तं चातुर्जातकमुच्यते ॥ (भा.प्र.)
(ii) त्रिगन्धकं सनागाह्वं चातुर्जातं प्रकीर्तिततम् ॥ (कै.नि. ८/१)
(iii) तद् द्वयं रोचनं रूक्षं तीक्ष्णोष्णं मुखगन्धहृत् । लघुपित्ताग्निकृद्वर्ण्यं कफवातविषापहम् ॥

(16) Pancha Tikta: ***(Five bitters)***

(i) Gudūchi (Tinospora cordifolia)

(ii) Nimba Mūla Twak (Root bark of Azdiridachta indica)

(iii) Vāsa Patra (Leaves of Adhathoda vascica)

(iv) Kantakari Phala (Fruits of Solanum Xanthocarpum)

(v) Patola Patra (Leaves of Tricosanthes dioica)

Properties: Pitta hara, Jwara hara, Swasa hara

Indications: Jwara, Rakta pitta, Kushta, Kasa-Swasa etc[1].

(17) Panchāmla: ***(Five sour substances)***

In Raja Nighantu we come across two groups of Amla dravyas each containing five drugs.

Panchāmla - I

(1) Kola (Zizyphus jujuba)

(2) Dādima (Punica granatum)

(3) Vrikshamla (Garcinia indica)

(4) Chullika

(5) Amla vetasa (Garcinia pedunculata)

Panchāmla - II

(1) Jambira (Citrus lemon)

(2) Naranga (Citrus)

(3) Amla vetasa (Garcinia pedunculata)

(4) Tintidika (Rhus parviflora)

(5) Beejapura (Citrus medica)

Later Rasa Tarangini described about five fruits which are sour in taste. Hence 'Phala Panchamla'. They are:

(i) Amla vetasa

(ii) Jambira

(iii) Matulunga (Beejapura)

(iv) Naranga

(v) Nimbuka (Jambira)

---

१. गुडूची निम्बमूलत्वक् भिषग्माता निदिग्धिका । पटोलपत्रमित्येतत् पञ्चतिक्तं प्रकीर्तितम् ॥ (र.त.)

Properties: Hridya, Deepana-Pachana, Sula Prasamana.

Indications: Hridroga, Trishna, Arsas, Sula[1]

(18) Visha Varga: *(Poisonous plants)*

Medeival texts have mentioned many poisonous plants in Ayurvedic therapeutics. Rasa Tarangini delineated two Sthavara visha (vegetable poisons) groups viz., (i) Vatsanabhadi and (ii) Tindukadi[2].

We come a cross Mahā vishas (major poisonous plants) and Upa vishas (minor poisonous plants) in the literature.

(i) Maha Vishas: They are five in number namely,

(a) Sringika

(b) Kāla kuta

(c) Mustaka

(d) Vatsanabhi

(e) Saktuka

Bhava mishra however mentioned nine drugs under Visha dravyas. They are:

1. Vatsanabhi
2. Hāridraka
3. Saktuka
4. Pradipana
5. Sourashtrika
6. Sringika
7. Kālakuta
8. Hālahala

---

१. (i) कोलदाडिमवृक्षाम्लं चुल्लकी साम्लवेतसा । फलपञ्चाम्लमुद्दिष्टमम्लपञ्चफलं स्मृतम् ॥ (रा.नि.)
(ii) जम्बीरनारङ्गसहाम्लवेतासैः सतिन्तिडीकैश्च सबीजपूरकैः । समांशभागेन तु मेलितैरिदं द्वितीयमुक्तं च फलाम्लपञ्चकम् ॥ (रा.नि.)
(iii) अम्लवेतस जम्बीर लुङ्ग नारङ्ग निम्बुकैः । फलपञ्चाम्लकं ख्यातं कीर्तितश्चाम्लपञ्चकम् ॥ (र.त.)

२. विषं चोपविषं चेति द्विविधं स्थावरं विषम् । प्रथमं वत्मनाभादि द्वितीयं तिन्दुकादिकम् ॥ (र.त.)

9. Brahma Putra[1]

Properties: Vyavayi, Vikasi, Āsukari, Visha hara

Indications: Jangama Visha (animal poisons)

(ii) Upa Vishas: These are seven in number namely,

(a) Arka ksheera

(b) Snuhi ksheera

(c) Langali

(d) Karaveera

(e) Gunja

(f) Ahiphena

(g) Dhattura

Rasa Vagbhata mentioned Upa vishas with a little difference from Bhava Prakasa.

Jayā for Snuhi; Visha tinduka for Ahiphena; and Bhallataka for Gunja[2].

Properties: Uyavayi, Vikasi, Āsukari, Visha hara.

Indications: Jangama Visha, Swāsa-Kāsa.

Charaka emphatically stated that even poison can be used as medicine if selectively administered. In modern medicine also several poisons are being used as medicines[3].

3. Groups of Drugs of Animal Origin

(1) Ksheerashtakam *(Milk of eight animals)*

(i) Hasthi Kshira (Elephant's milk)

(ii) Ushtra kshira (Camel's milk)

---

१. (i) शृङ्गिकं कालकूटश्च मुस्तको वत्सनाभकः । सक्तुकश्चेति योगोऽयं महापञ्चविषाभिदः ॥ (रा.नि.)

(ii) शृङ्गीकं कालकूटश्च वत्सनाभं च सक्तुकम् । मुस्तं च विषवर्गोऽयं स वरः परिकीर्तितः ॥

(र.र.स. १०/८२)

(iii) वत्सनाभः सहारिद्रः सक्तुकश्च प्रदीपनः ।
सौराष्ट्रिकः शृङ्गिकश्च कालकूटस्तथैव च । हालाहलो ब्रह्मपुत्रो-विषभेदा अमी नव ॥ (भा.प्र.)

२. (i) अर्कक्षीरं स्नुहिक्षीरं लाङ्गली करवीरकौ । गुञ्जहिफेनो धत्तूरः सप्तोपविषजातयः ॥ (भा.प्र.)

(ii) लाङ्गली विषमुष्टिश्च करवीरो जया तथा । नीलकः कनकोऽर्कश्च वर्गो ह्युपविषात्मकः ॥

(र.र.स.१०/८४)

३. योगादपि विषं तीक्ष्णं उत्तमं भेषजं भवेत् । भेषजं चापि दुर्युक्तं तीक्ष्णं संपद्यते विषम् ॥ (च.सू. १)

(iii) Aswa kshira (Horse's milk)

(iv) Gokshira (Cow's milk)

(v) Ajā kshira (Goat's milk)

(vi) Avika kshira (Sheep's milk)

(vii) Māhisha kshira (Bufallo's milk)

(viii) Sthanya (Human milk)[1].

General Properties: Balya, Jeevaniya, Medhya, Āyushya, Vrishya, Vata-pitta hara[2].

Common Indications: Prameha, Amla pitta, Vāta rogas

(2) Mutrashtakam: ***(Urine of eight animals)***

(i) Khara mutra (Doney's urine)-useful in Apasmara, Unmada, Graha rogas.

(ii) Ushtra mutra (Camel's urine)-useful in Swasa, Kasa, Arsas.

(iii) Aswa mutra (Horse's urine)-useful in Kushta, Vrana, Visha rogas.

(iv) Gomutra (Cow's urine)-Mudhura, Krimighna, Kushtaghna.

(v) Ajā mutra (Goat's urine)-Kashaya, Madhura, Tridosha hara.

(vi) Avika mutra (Sheep's urine)-Tikta Rasa, Pitta kara, Snigdha

(vii) Mahisha mutra (Bufallo's urine)-useful in Arsas, Sopha, Udara.

(viii) Hasthi mutra (Elephant's urine)-Lavana rasa, Seeta guna, Krimihara, Kushtaghna.

General properties: Ushna-Teekshna-Ruksha gunas, Dipaniya, Krimi hara, Vata hara.

Common indications: Krimi roga, Visha roga, Vāta vyadhi[3]

---

१. (i) गव्यं माहिषमाजं च कारभं स्त्रैणमाविकथ् । एभमैकशफं चेति क्षीराष्टकमिहोच्यते ॥
(ii) अविक्षीरं अजाक्षीरं गोक्षीरं माहिषं च यत् । उष्ट्रीणामथ नागीनां वडवायाः स्त्रियास्तथा ॥

२. प्रायशो मधुरं स्निग्धं शीतं स्तन्यं पयो मतम् । प्रीणनं बृंहणं वृष्यं मेध्यं बल्यं मनस्करम् ॥
जीवनीयं श्रमहरं श्वासकासनिबर्हणम् । हन्ति शोणितपित्तं च सन्धानं विहितस्य च॥
सर्वप्राणभृतां सात्मयं शमनं शोधनं तथा । तृष्णाघ्नं दीपनीयं च श्रेष्ठं क्षीणक्षतेषु च ॥
पाण्डुरोगेऽम्लपित्ते च शोषे गुल्मे तथोदरे । अतीसारे ज्वरे दाहे श्वयथौ च विशेषतः ॥
योनिशुक्रप्रदोषेषु मूत्रेष्वप्रचुरेषु च । पुरीषे ग्रथिते पथ्यं वातपित्तविकारिणाम् ॥
नस्योपलेपावगाहेषु वमनास्थापनेषु च । विरेचने स्नेहने च पयः सर्वत्र युज्यते ॥(च.सू. १/१०७-११२)

३. (i) मूत्रैर्गोजाविमहिषी गजाश्वोष्ट्रखरोद्भवैः मूत्राष्टकमिति प्रोक्तं ।
(ii) अविमूत्रमजामूत्रं गोमूत्रं माहिषं च यत् ॥
हस्तिमूत्रमथोष्ट्रस्य हयस्य च खरस्य च । उष्णं तीक्ष्णयथोऽरूक्षं कटुकं लवणान्वितम् ॥
(च.सू. १/९३-१०४)

(3) Pitta Panchaka: *(Five biles)*

(i) Matsya pitta (Fish bile)

(ii) Gopittam (Cow's bile)

(iii) Aswa pitta (Horse bile)

(iv) Mayura pitta (Peacock's bile)

(v) Manushya pitta (Human bile)

Properties: Ushna, Teekshna Ruksha gunas, Deepaniya, Vishaghna, Krimighna, Mutrala etc.

Indications: Udara, Arsas, Gulma, Kushta, Kilasa, Krimi Pandu etc[1].

4. Groups of Drugs of Mineral Origin

(1) Lavana Panchakam: *(Five salts)*

Sandhava lavana, Souvarcha lavana, Vida lavana, Oudbhida lavana and Samudra lavana are known as Pancha lavanas according to Charaka.The Oudbhida lavana is replaced by Romaka lavana in Rasa tarangini. Some consider Sambara lavana in its place[2].

Properties: Snigdha, Tikshna, Ushna gunas; Deepana, Ubhaya bhaga hara, Sula prasamana, Niruha and Anuvasanopaga etc.

Indications: Gulma, Sula, Udara, Ajeerna, Ānaha, Vāta-roga, Pancha karmas etc.

(2) Kshara Dwaya: *(Two Alkalies)*

Sarja kshara and Yavakshara are together called as "Kshara Dwaya". If Tankara (Borax) is added to these two they are known as "Kshara Traya" (triad of Alkalies).

---

१. पित्तं पञ्चविधं मत्स्यगवाश्वनर बर्हिजम् । (रसार्णवम्)

२. (i) सौवर्चलं सैन्धवं च विडमौद्भिदमेव च ॥
सामुद्रेण सहैतानि पञ्चस्युर्लवणानि च । (च.सू. १/८८-८९)

(ii) सैन्धवञ्चाथ सामुद्रं विडं सौवर्चलं तथा । रोमकञ्चेति विज्ञेयं बुधैर्लवणापञ्चकम् ॥ (र.त. २/३)
स्निग्धान्युष्णानि तीक्ष्णानि दीपनीयतमानि च ॥
आलेपनार्थे युज्यन्ते स्नेहस्वेदविधौ तथा । अधोभागोर्ध्वभागेषु निरूहेष्वनुवासने ॥
अभ्यञ्जने भोजनार्थे शिरसश्च विरेचने ॥ शस्त्रकर्मणि वर्त्यर्थमञ्जनोत्सादनेषु च ॥
अजीर्णानाहयोर्वाते गुल्मे शूले तथोदरे ॥ (च.सू. १/८९-९२)

Properties: Teekshna, Ushna gunas; Ushna veerya, Kapha hara.

Indications: Vrana, Sula, Gulma, Amlapitta, Udara, etc[1].

(3) Kshāra Ashtakam: ***(Eight alkalies)***

(i) Palasa (Butea monosperma)

(ii) Snuhi (Euphorbia nerifolia)

(iii) Apāmarga (Achyranthes aspera)

(iv) Chincha (Tamarindus indicus)

(v) Arka (Calotrapis gigantca)

(vi) Tila Nala (Sesamum indicum stem)

(vii) Sarja Kshara

(viii) Yaya Kshara

The above eight are known as Kshāra Ashtaka.

Properties: Kapha-Vata hara, Sula Prasamana

Indications: Sula, Gulma, Vrana etc[2].

5. Miscellaneous Groups of Drugs

There are many more groups of drugs mentioned in different texts which are not dealt in the CCIM syllabus. Some of them are described here:

(1) Ksheera Traya

(i) Arka (Calotropis gigantea)- for vamana as well as virechana

(ii) Snuhi (Euphorbia nerifolia)- for virechana

(iii) Ashmantaka (Ficus spp.)- for vamana

Some scholars consider vata (Ficus benghalensis) in place of Ashmantaka. In Rasa Taraugini we find the term 'Ksheera Traya' but

---

१. (i) स्वर्जिक्षारो यवक्षारः क्षारद्वयमुदाहृतम् । (र.त. २/६)
(ii) सर्जिकायवशूकश्च क्षारद्वयमुदाहृतम् ॥ (भा.प्र.)
(iii) सौभाग्येन समायुक्तं क्षारत्रिकमुदाहृतम् ॥ (र.त. २/६)

२. (i) पलाशवज्रिशिखरिचिञ्चार्कतिलनालजाः । यवजः सर्जिका चेति क्षाराष्टकमुदाहृतम् ॥ (भा.प्र.)
(ii) सुधापलाशशिखरचिञ्चार्कतिलनालजाः । स्वर्जिका यावशूकश्च क्षाराष्टकमुदाहृतम् ॥ (र.त. २/८)

not in Charaka Samhita[1].

(2) Tri Valkala

(i) Putika- for virechana

(ii) Krishna gandha- for Sotha, Arsas, Vidradhi etc.

(iii) Tilvaka- for virechana

These are mentioned by charaka for Sodhana which are quoted as Trivalkala by Acharya P.V. Sharmaji[2].

(3) Pancha Sūrana

Atyamlaparṇi, Kāṇḍira, Mala kanda, Mana kanda, Surana kanda- these five are called as 'Pancha Surana'. They will be useful in Arsas and Udara[3].

(4) Tri Samam

Haritaki, Sunthi and Guda (jaggary) mixed in equal quantities is known as 'Tri Sama'. They are indicated in Jwara, Agnimandya, Swasa, Kasa[4].

(5) Trikarshika

Sunthi, Ativisha & Musta mixed in the quantity of one Karsha (10gm) each are known as Tri kārshika. They act as grahi, Deepana-Pachana, Jwara hara[5].

(6) Chaturbhadra

Trikarshikas along-with Guduchi are denoted as Chaturbhadras. They are very useful in Bāla Rogas (paediatric conditions). Also act as grahi, jwarahara, sthambhana, Swasa-kasa hara, krimihara. In Chāturbhadra churna Guduchi is replaced with Karkata Sringi.

---

१. (i) वमनेऽश्मन्तकं विद्यात्स्नुहिक्षीरं विरेचने । क्षीरमर्कस्य विज्ञेयं वमने स विरेचने ॥ (च.सू. १)
(ii) रविक्षीरं वटक्षीरं स्नुहिक्षीरं तथैव च । क्षीरत्रयमिति ख्यातं मारणादौ प्रशस्यते ॥ (र.त. २)

२. इमांस्त्रीनपरानाहुर्वृक्षा येषां हितास्त्वचः । पूतीकः कृष्णगन्धा च तिल्वकश्च तथातरुः ॥
विरेचने प्रयोक्तव्यः पूतिकस्तिल्वकस्तथा । कृष्णागन्धा परीसर्पे शोथेष्वर्शःसु चोच्यते ॥
दद्रु विद्रधिगण्डेषु कुष्ठेष्वप्यलजीषु च । (च.सू. १)

३. अत्यम्लपर्णी काण्डीरमालाकन्दद्विशूरणैः । प्रोक्तो भवति योगेऽयं पञ्चशूरणसंज्ञकः ॥ (रा.नि.)

४. हरीतकी नागरं च गुडश्चेति त्रयं समम् । समत्रिकमित्युक्तं निरुक्तं च समत्रयम् ॥ (रा.नि.)

५. नागरातिविषामुस्तात्रयमेतत् त्रिकार्षिकम् । गुडूच्या मिलितं तच्चचातुर्भद्रकमुच्यते ॥ (रा.नि.)

(7) Tri-Madhura

Madhu (honey), ghrita (ghee) and guda (jaggary) are collectively known as 'Tri-Madhuras'. They act as balya, Prinana, Jeevaniya etc[1].

(8) Tri-Kantaka

Brihati, Agnidamani (Kantakari) & Duhsparsa are called as Tri-kantaka[2].

(9) Visha Dwaya

Visha (vatsanabhi)- Aconitum ferox; Ativisha - Aconitum heterophyllum

(10) Sūrpaparṇi Dwaya

Mudga parni.

Masha parni[3]

(11) Ādya Pushpa

(i) Chandana

(ii) Kumkuma

(iii) Hriberam[4].

(12) Pancha Beeja

Chatur beeja + Jyotishmati

(13) Katu Chaturjataka

(i) Twak

(ii) Ela

(iii) Patra

(iv) Maricha

(14) Sugandha Panchaka *(Five aromatic drugs)*

(i) Karpura

(ii) Twak

---

१. ....त्रिमधुरं मधुसर्पिगुडैर्युतम् ॥ (कै.नि.८/२)

२. बृहतीचाग्निदमनीदुःस्पर्शा चेति तु त्रयम् । कण्टकारीत्रयं प्रोक्तं त्रिकण्टं कण्टकत्रयम् ॥ (रा.नि.)

३. Vagbhata

४. Raja Nighantu

(iii) Kankola
(iv) Jatiphala
(v) Lavanga

(15) Maha Sugandha: ***(Major aromatic drugs)***

(i) Chandana
(ii) Agaru
(iii) Kumkuma
(iv) Kasturi
(v) Karpura

(16) Lavana Groups

(i)	Eka Lavana	-	Saindhava lavana.
(ii)	Dwi Lavana	-	Saindhava, Souvarcha lavanas.
(iii)	Tri Lavana	-	Saindhava, Souvarcha & Vida lavanas.
(iv)	Chaturlavana	-	Saindhava, Souvarcha, Vida & Sāmudra lavanas.
(v)	Pancha lavana	-	Already discussed.
(vi)	Shat Lavana	-	Samudra, Saindhava, Vida, Souvarcha, Romaka & Chullika (Navasara).

(17) Sugandhamalaka

Jatamansi, Mura, Sunthi, Mustha, Haridra, Ela, Kushta, Yuthika, Twak, Tagara, Salcya and Āmalak.

(18) Trina Rāja: ***(Trees with leaves at the top)***

Guvāka, Tāla, Hintāla, Kētaki, Brihat vara, Kharjura and Narikela

(19) Kshara Panchaka

Yava, Sarja, Ṭilanala (or Tankana), Palasa and Mushkaka Kshara are called as Pancha Ksharas[1].

(20) Sugandha Triphala

(i) Lavanga
(ii) Jatiphala

१. Rasa Tarangini

(iii) Kramuka[1]

(21) Mahā Triphala

(i) Draksha

(ii) Parushaka

(iii) Kashmarya phala[2]

(22) Pancha Nimba

Nimba patra, mula, Phala, Twak & Pushpa are Pancha Nimbas.

(23) Pancha Garyam

Milk, Curd, Urine, Faeces & ghee obtained from cow are known as Pancha gavyas[3].

---

१. लवङ्गमालतीसस्यक्रमुकैस्त्रिफलाक्वचित् । द्राक्षापरूषकाश्मर्यफलैः क्वापि फलोत्तमा ॥(कै.नि.८/३-४)

२. पञ्चनिम्बं निम्बपत्रफलत्वङ्मूलपुष्पकैः ॥ (कै.नि. ८/९)

३. पञ्चगव्यं गवां क्षीरदधिमूत्रशकृद्घृतैः । (कै.नि. ८/१०)

Chapter - XII

Nomenclature; Soil-types; Collection of Durgs; Preservation Methods and Measurements

1. The Basis of Nomenclature and Synonyms of Drugs in Ayurveda

Actually, these aspects have been studied in XV and XI chapters from Ayurvedic and modern perspectives respectively. In this chapter the concept of Nomenclature proposed by Narahari will be specifically highlighted.

In Rāja Nighantu seven factors are described as the basis of nomenclature of drugs in Ayurveda[1]. They are: Rudhi, Prabhava, Desokti, Lanchana, Upama, Virya and Itarahwa.

(1) Rudhi: *(specific term)*

These names have no specific meaning but are used in certain areas. Hence are called as Rūdhi e.g., Katam kateri (Daruharidra), Pacham pacha (Daruharidra), Kinihi (Apamarga), etc.

However the author could document the root meanings of the above examples. There fore, Rudhi may be a name or synonym proposed by the ancient Acharyas whose root meanings or derivations are not frequently discussed in the texts.

(2) Prabhava: ***(natural power)***

Some of the names are given to herbs on the basis of their therapeutic efficacy or original nature of action. e.g., Kushtaghni (Bakuchi), Dadrughni (Chakramarda), Nidrari (Kirata tikta), Pleehaghna (Rohitaka) etc.

(3) Desokti: ***(place of origin)***

Certain names are given to the plants according to the place of

---

१. नामानि क्वचिदिह रूढित: प्रभावात् दोशोक्तया क्वचिदिहलाञ्छनोपमाभ्यां ।
वीर्येण क्वचिदितराह्वयातिदेशात् द्रव्याणां ध्रुवमिति सप्तथोदितानि ॥ (रा.नि.)

availability. e.g., Vaidehi (Pippali), Magadhi (Maricha), Ramatha (Hingu), Kashmiram (Kumkumam), Malayaja (Sami) etc.

(4) Lanchana: ***(special characters)***

Certain herbs are named on the basis of the special characters e.g., Chitra Tandula (Vidanga), Pancha Raji Phala (Patola), Koshataki etc.

(5) Upama: ***(simile)***

Names of the herbs are also coined as per the similarity of useful part etc., to other objects or animals etc. e.g., Kulira vishana (Karkata Sringi), Kāka jangha (Peristrophe bicalculata), Mayura sikha (Actinopteres radiata), Panchangula (Eranda) etc.

(6) Virya: ***(potency)***

Some of the names will indicate the potency of the herbs e.g., Ushna (Maricha), Seeta (Bala), Ooshana (Sunthi) etc.

(7) Itarahwaya: ***(Miscellaneous)***

Different comparisions may be seen with the nomenclature of herbs. e.g., Sakrahwa (Indra yava), Anala nāme (Chitraka) etc.

It is said that the names of the herbs are known to the saints, forest tribes, shepereds etc. Therefore the local names and identification features of different herbs should be obtained from them only[1]. The physician who will passess knowledge on identity of herbs and their therapeutic utility is only considered to be the best (Tattwa vits).

Dr. K. Nisteswar enumerated the following nomenclature of Ayurvedic herbs basing upon their appearance, nature, parts used, action, characteristics etc. They are:

(1) on the basis weight

Kala	=	Pippali
Akshaphala	=	Vibhitaki

(2) on the basis of nodes

---

१. (i) गोपालास्तापसा व्याधा ये चान्ये वनचारिणः । मूलाहाराश्च ये तेभ्यो भेषजव्यक्तिरिष्यते ॥(सु.सू. ३७)

(ii) तेभ्यः सकाशादुपलभ्य वैद्यः पश्चाच्च शास्त्रेषु विमृश्य बुद्ध्या ।
विकल्पयेत् द्रव्यरसप्रभावान्विपाकवीर्याणि तथा प्रयोगात् ॥ (रा.नि.)

Shadgranthi = Vacha
Satagranthi = Druva

(3) on the basis of historical importance

Koushika = Guggulu
Vibhishana = Nala

(4) on the basis of latex

Peeta dugdha = Swarna ksheeri
Payasya = Ksheera kakoli

(5) on the basis of spines

Deergha kantaka = Babbula
Tikshna kantaka = Ingudi

(6) on the basis of flowers

Peeta pushpa = Atibala
Visha pushpaka = Madanaphala

(7) on the basis of fruits

Kantaphala = Jeemutaka
Sneha phala = Kantakari

(8) on the basis of leaves

Tamra pallava = Rohitaka
Lekhya dala = Tala

(9) on the basis of action on animals

Aswa mara = Kara veera
Kakaghna = Karnanja bheda

2. Division of Different Areas (Desa) & Soils (Bhumi)

Usually the word 'Desa' indicates the area as well as the body of a patient. In this context only the former meaning is preferred[1].

Etymologically *Desa* means a part of the country or geographical area. Similarly, Bhumi means the area which allows different creatures to survive[2].

---

१. (i) तत्र त्रिविध: खलु देशो जाङ्गलोऽनूप: साधारणश्चेति ॥ (च.क. १/८)

२. (i) देश: पुन: द्विविध: भूमिरातुरश्च ॥ (च.वि. ८/९४)

(ii) भूमिदेहप्रभेदेन देशमाहुरिहद्विधा ॥ (अ.हृ.सू. १/२३)

(I) Desa (Area) Divisions

Ancient Ayurvedic texts mention about three types of areas (Desa) depending upon geographical conditions and natural flora of the respective places[1]. They are:

(i) Jāngala (dry areas) - predominant of vata

(ii) Ānūpa (wet areas) - predominant of kapha

(iii) Sādhāraṇa (balanced areas of climate)- predominant of pitta[2].

(i) **Jangala Desa:** Areas with clear sky; possessing trees like Kadara (Acacia fernosiana), Khadira (Acacia catechu), Asana (Pterocarpus marsupium), Aswakarna (Dipterocarpus alatus), Dhava Tinisa, Sallaki (Boswellia serrata), Sala (Dillenia indica), Soma Valka (Acacia), Badari (Z.jujuba), Tinduka (Diospyros montana), Aswatha (F. religiosa), Vata (F. benghalensis), Āmalaka (E. officinalis), Sami (Prosopis specichera), Kakubha (T. arjuna), Simsapa (Dalbergia sissoo) etc.; full of mirages, small ponds here and there with little water; more rocky area; full of stones; birds like Lava, Tittiri, Chakora are abundently seen. The people living in these areas are usually harsh, strong and rough in nature[3].

Charaka considered Jangala desa as the best among the areas. This climate does not allow diseases to spread and good for health.

(ii) **Ānupa Desa:** This area consists of trees like Hintala (date-palm), Tamala (Garcinia sps.), Narikela (Coconut tree), Kadali (Musa paradisiaca) etc., lakes and seas; cool breez; beautiful sea coasts or

---

१. जाङ्गलं वातभूयिष्ठमानूपं तु कफोल्बणम् ॥
साधारणं सममलं त्रिधा भूदेशमादिशेत् । (अ.हृ.सू. १/२३-२४)

२. (i) दिश्यते निर्दिश्यते इति देशः । दिश निर्देशे । भूगोलभागविशेषः । (श.क.द्रु.)
(ii) **भवन्ति** भूतान्यस्यामिति भूमिः । (वाचः)

३. (i) तत्र जाङ्गलः पर्याकाशभूयिष्ठस्तरूभिरपि कदरखदिरसनाश्वकर्णधव तिनिश शल्लकी शाल सोमवल्क बदरी तिन्दुक अश्वत्थ वटआमलकवनगहनोऽनेक शमी ककुभ शिंशपाप्रायः स्थिरशुष्क पवनबल-विधूयमानप्रवृत्त्यस्तरूणविटपः प्रततमृगतृष्णाकूपोपगूढस्तनुखरपरूषसिकताशर्कराबहुलो लावति-त्तिरचकोरानुप्रचित **भूमिभागो** वातपित्तबहुलस्थिरकठिन मनुष्यप्रायो ज्ञेयः ॥ (च.क. १/८)
(ii) अल्पोदकद्रुमो यस्तु प्रवातः प्रचुरातपः । ज्ञेयः स जाङ्गलो देशः स्वल्परोगतमोऽपि च ॥ (च.वि. ३/४७)
(iii) मरूभूमिरारोग्यदेशानां (हिंत)..........। (च.सू. २५)

river banks; full of trees; many flowering plants; swans (Hamsa), sea gulls (Chakravaks) etc. birds. The people living in these areas will be usually delicate, beautiful, gentle in nature[1].

Charaka considered Ānupa desa is not good for health.

(iii) **Sadharana Desa:** Both the above described flora and fauna will be seen in this area. The people living in this area will show average qualities[2].

* **Note:** The division of areas depending upon climatic conditions appear to be more scientific. We often come across tropical diseases which are challenging the medical science today. Most of the areas which are marshy and full of water are suffering from malaria, filariasis etc. Extreme cold climates produce frost bites while extreme hot conditions causes sunstroke. Therefore under standing the climatic conditions will be essential in their management. Even commonly seen respiratory problems like Asthma is 'atopic' as well as 'non-atopic'.

(II) Bhumi (Soil) Divisions

Bhumi or Soil is sub-divided into five or six groups basing upon their Bhutas (elements) or Rasas (tastes) respectively:

(i) classification on the basis of Pancha Bhutas.

(ii) classification on the basis of Rasas.

(i) Division on the basis of Pancha bhutas:

(a) Parthiva Bhumi– full of heavy rocks, greyish or blackish

---

१. (i) अथानूपो हिन्ताल तमाल नारिकेल कदली वनगहनः, सरित्समुद्र पर्यन्तः, शिशिरपवनबहुलो, वञ्जुलवनवानीरोपशोभिततीराभिः सरिद्भिरुपगतभूमिभागः, क्षितिधरनिकुञ्जोपशोभितो, मन्दपवनानुवीजितक्षितिरूहगहनो ऽनेकवनराजीपुष्पित वनगहनभूमिभागः, स्निग्धतरुप्रतानोपगूढो, हंसचक्रवाक-बलाकानन्दीमुख पुण्डरीक कादम्ब मद्गुको यष्टि भृङ्गराज शतपत्र मत्तकोकिलानुनादित तरुणविटपः सुकुमारपुरुषः, पवनकफप्रायो ज्ञेयः। (च.क.१/८)

(ii) प्रचुरोदकवृक्षो यो निवातो दुर्न्तभातपः ।
आनूपो बहुदोपश्च ....॥ (च.वि. ३/४८)

(iii) आनूपोऽहितं देशानां । (च.सू. २५)

२. (i) अनयोरेव द्वयोर्देशयोर्वीरुद्वनस्पतिर्वानस्पत्यशकुनिमृगगणयुतः स्थिरसुकुमारवर्णसंहननोपपन्न-साधारण गुणपुरुषः साधारणो ज्ञेयः ॥ (च.क. १/८)

(ii) समः साधारणो मतः । (च.वि. ३/४८)

coloured soil, and huge trees are present[1].

(b) Āpya Bhumi– Smooth soil, full of water & grass, delicate trees and whitish soil are present[2].

(c) Āgneya Bhumi– different colours of soil, lighter, mixed with plenty of stones, smaller trees are present[3].

(d) Vāyaviya Bhumi– rough and ash-coloured stones, lean and small trees, xerophytes are more seen in this type of soil[4].

(e) Ākasiya Bhumi–sandy, taste-less water, dry trees, trees which grow near rocky mountains are seen and soil is greyish black in colour[5].

(ii) Division on the basis of Rasas

Soil will be of six types on the basis of Rasa i.e.; Madhura Bhumi, Amla Bhumi, Lavana Bhumi, Katu Bhumi, Tikta Bhumi & Kashaya Bhumi. If all the six Rasas are present in a soil it is considered as Sadharana[6].

Ideal Soil for herbs *(Prasasta Bhumi)*

The soil which is devoid of big stones, excessive water, without Valmika (Snake nest); nearer to water tanks, unctuous, smooth, tight, blackish-white or redish soil; and with grass is best for finding quality herbs. Herbs from such soil are only recommended for collection of raw materials[7]

Modern Perspective of Soil Types

There are seven major soil types in India viz., (1) Ferruginous

---

१. अश्मवती स्थिरा गुर्वी श्यामा कृष्णा वा स्थूलवृक्षस्यप्राया स्वगुणभूयिष्ठा । (सु.सू. ३६/३)

२. स्निग्धा शीतलाऽऽसन्नोदका स्निग्धशस्यतृणकोमलवृक्षप्राया शुक्लाऽम्बुगुणभूयिष्ठा । (सु.सू. ३६/३)

३. नानावर्णा लघ्वश्मवती प्रविरलाल्पपाण्डवृक्षप्ररोहाऽग्निभूयिष्ठा । (सु.सू. ३६/३)

४. रूक्षाभस्मरासमवर्णा तनुवृक्षाल्परसकोटरवृक्षप्रायाऽनिलभूयिष्ठा । (सु.सू. ३६/३)

५. मृद्वीसमाश्वभ्रवत्यव्यक्तरसजला सर्वतोऽसारवृक्षा महापवर्ततवृक्षप्राया श्यामाचाकाशगुणभूयिष्ठा ॥ (सु.सू. ३६/३)

६. गन्धवर्णरसोपेता षड्विधाभूमिरिष्यते । तस्माद्भूमिस्वभावेन बीजिनः षड्रसायुताः ॥
अव्यक्तः किल तोयस्य रसो निश्चयनिश्चितः । रसः स एव चाव्यक्तो व्यक्तो भूमिरसाद्भवेत् ॥
सर्वलक्षणसंपन्ना भूमिः साधारणा स्मृता । द्रव्याणि यत्र तत्रेव तद्गुणानि विशेषतः ॥(सु.सू.२६/१२-१४)

७. श्वभ्रशर्कराविषवल्मीकश्मशानाघातनदेवायतनसिकताभिरनुपहताममूषरामभङ्गुरामदूरोदकां स्निग्धां प्ररोहवतीं मृद्वीं स्थिरां समां कृष्णां गौरीं लोहितां वा भूमिमौषधग्रहणाय परीक्षेत ॥ (सु.सू. ३६/२)

gravelly (2) Ferruginous soil (3) Alluvial soil (4) Black soil (5) Medium black soil (6) Deep black soil and (7) Laterite soil.

The moisture holding capacity of different soils will vary from each other:

Nature of the soil		**water holding capacity per kg**
1. Sand	-	25 kg
2. Sandy clay	-	40 kg
3. Strong clay	-	50 kg
4. Cultivated soil	-	52 kg
5. Garden soil	-	81 kg
6. Humus soil	-	190 kg

Different plants will grow in different types of soils and seasons. For example.

1. Aswagandha– sandy loam or light red soils (pH 7-5 to 8). It requires relatively dry season and is a late rainy season (kharif) crop.
2. Yashtimadhu– Loamy soils of light texture are ideal. This crop requires a warm and dry climate.
3. Sarpagandha– It grows on a wide range of soils. Clayey loam or clay containing humus with proper drainage is ideal (pH 8 or above).
4. Vacha– It may be cultivated in any good but fairly moist soil. It comes up well in clayey loams and light alluvial soils of river banks. It grows in tropical to sub-tropical climates.

Botanical regions of India:

From the view point of general vegetation and floristic elements, India is divided into eight botanical regions.

(I) **North-Western Himalaya—** It shows altitudinal zonation. In the foot hills, below 1000 m, such as in the Shiwalik, the forests are of subtropical dry evergreen type having species of Acacia, Olea etc. The lower altitudes have subtropical pine forests, chiefly composed of pinus roxburghii. Between 1500 and 3000 m, there are moist temperate forests of Abies, Quercus, cedrus etc. Above 300 m, the vegetation is of moist alpine scrub type of Betula, Berberis etc.

(II) Eastern Himalya— Eastern Himalayas are richly vegetated, wetter and warmer than western Himalyas. The forests of this region are rich in orchids. The lower slopes of the region have tropical, semi-evergreen type of forests, comprising of Michelia champaka, Litsea etc. Some patches of subtropical broad-leaved hills forest having species of Quercus, Schima are also seen in this portion. The forests are of montane wet or moist temperate type, between the altitudes of 1800 m and 3000 m having species chiefly of Cinnamomum, Mangolia etc. Above the 3000 m, there are moist-alpine scrub forests.

(III) North-Eastern Region— It includes broadly the plain region of Arunachal pradesh and all other seven eastern states. It is rich in orchids and several of them endemic only to this region. The type locality of the only Nepenthes khasiana falls under this region (Maghalaya). It has various kinds of tropical forests. Tropcial moist deciduous forests occur in the state of Meghalaya, Tripura & Mizoram. The dominant medicinal species are Terminalia, Careya etc. Tropical wet evergreen forests comprising species of Dipterocarpus, Prunus, Aquallaria etc; occur in eastern and Southern Asam. Tropical semi evergreen forests comprising species of Terminalia, Michelia etc., occur in the foot hills of Assam. The subtropical pine forests dominated by Pinus kesiya occur in higher elevations in Meghalaya, Manipur and Nagaland. It also has one of the richest bamboo forests in the country.

(IV) Gangetic Plains— The Gangetic plain streches from eastern Rajasthan through U.P. to Bihar and W. Bengal and the region is predominant agricultural belt. The larger part of this region is under tropical dry deciduous forests cover, having species of Anogeissus, Buchnania, Aegle, Melia etc. Some parts have tropical moist deciduous forests of Shorea robusta- mixed with species of Litsea, Mallotus etc. Some tall grasses of the genera like Saccharum, Vetiveria etc., are common in this region.

(V) **Western Region—** This region mainly covers western ghats and arid region of India. The western ghats have tropical moist deciduous and tropical semi-evergreen forests. Species like Dalbergia, Pterocarpus, Terminalia etc., are common in tropical moist deciduous forests. Plants like Grewia, Ficus, Syzygium etc., occur in tropical semi-evergeen forests.

The western arid region has four fairly distinct habitats and climatic conditions, viz.,

(i) sandy plains and dunes- sparse vergetation with Acacia etc.

(ii) gravelly plains- have species of Commiphora, Calotropic, Zizypphus etc.

(iii) rocky habitats- have bushes of Euphorbia and Grewia.

(iv) saline depressions- plants like Salvadora, Tecomela etc., occur.

(VI) The Deccan Plateau— This is the large rather triangle-shaped plateau with its base in the south of the vindhyachal mountains. Large parts of this region are covered by tropical thorny forests of Acacia, Dichrostachys, Strychnos etc.

The northern, central and southern parts of Deccan plateau have tropical dry deciduous forests of Teak intermixed with species of Diospyros, pterocarpus, Aegle, Butea etc. The eastern parts have moist deciduous forests of Bombax, Terminalia, Dalbergia, Madhuca. Tamarindus, Ceiba, Shorea are abundant in north eastern part of the plateau.

(VII) Eastern Peninsular Region— Large areas of this region are under tropical dry deciduous forests or thorny forests. Some northern parts bordering Orissa has moist deciduous forests. Important species are Myristica, Symplocos etc. In Tamil Nadu, the evergreen forests have dominance of species of Diospyros, Litsea, Pterocarpus, Vitex etc. P. santalinus, A. Pyrethrum, C. amboinicus, C. Sappan, S. aromaticum etc. are common in this region.

(VIII) Western Peninsular Region— Tropical wet ever green forests occur in this region. They comprise mainly Mesua, Calophyllum, Dipterocarpus etc.

The higher hills have montane wet sub termperate forests having species of Garcinia, Hydnocarpus, Cinnamomum etc.

The Nilgiris have subtropical broad-leaved hill forests of species of Syzygium, Meliosma etc.

[Chandel K.P.S. et al., "Biodiversity in Medicinal & Aromatic Plants in India- conservation & utilization". New Delhi: ICAR; 1997.]

3. Collection of Drugs and Characteristics of Collected Drugs

The drug grown in the best soil mentioned earlier shall be collected for medicinal usage. Even that herb should have the following characteristics:

(i) not affected by smoke, rain, air or water and

(ii) collected in the respective seasons.

such raw material may be collected and stored in the drug stores[1].

The drug which is obtained from the are where best types of soil is available is only useful for internal administration. It should be free from pests (Krimi), poisons (Visha), weapon (Sastra), severe sunlight (Ātapa), high breeze (Pavana), fire (Dahana), excessive moisture (Toya), diseases (Sambadha) and road sides (Marga). It must have single predominant taste, well developed, strong, deeply rooted in the soil. Such herb grown in the Eastern side should be collected for all medicinal purposes[2].

Sushrita further quoted that the drug which is to be collected and preserved (either new or old) should not loose natural odour, is not spoiled and has not lost the taste etc[3]. Such drug may be collected and preserved for therapeutic utility.

4. Method of Collection of Raw Materials

The person who wants to collect the raw material should follow the ritual procedures, must be clean & neat, should wear white cloths,

---

१. धूमवर्षानिलक्लेदैः सर्वर्तुषु नभिद्रुते । ग्रहयित्वा गृहेन्यस्येद्विधिनौषधसंग्रहम् ॥ (सु.सू. ३८/८०)

२. तस्यां जातमपि कृमिविषशस्त्रातपपवनदहनतोयसंबाधमार्गैरनुपहतमेकरसं पुष्टं पृथ्ववगाढमूलमुदीच्यां चौषधमाददीत ॥ (सु.सू. ३६/२)

३. विगन्धेनापरामृष्टमविपन्नं रसादिभिः ।
नवं द्रव्यं पुराणं वा गृह्णीयाद्दोषवर्जितम् ॥ (सु.सू. ३६/१६)

should perform prayer etc., earlier to collection and he must be fasting overnight. Then the useful part shall be collected either from the East side or North side[1].

Dr. Pushpangadan (Director NBRI, Lucknow) in his address at the Ayurveda 2000 at chennai on 30th January 2000 was mentioning their work which proved that the roots etc., collected from east and north directions do passess more active principles than the parts collected from other directions. This may be because of the earth's magnetic field which is strong in these two directions in India.

Sararngdhara advocates complete mental and physical well-beingness for a person who is about to collect the raw materials. The raw materials available near the valimka, polluted areas, water logged areas, burrial ground, dry and sandy areas, the road sides, infected with pests, burnt or covered with snow etc., are to be avoided[2].

5. Knowledge on Time of Collection of Drugs:

The raw materials used in Ayurveda shall be collected according to part used, season, potency etc., in a specific manner.

(i) Time of collection according to part used

(a) According to Charaka[3]

	Part used		Season
1.	Tender leaves & branches	-	Varsha & Vasanta Ritu (Autumn & spring)
2.	Root of trees which have	-	Greeshma (Summer) for plants

१. मङ्गलाचार: कल्याणवृत्त: शुचि: शुक्लवासा: संपूज्य देवतामग्निमश्विनौ गोब्राह्मणांश्च कृतोपवास: प्राङ्मुखो उदन्मुखो वा गृह्णीयात् ॥ (च.क. १/१०)

२. (i) गृह्णीयात्तानि सुमनाश्शुचि: प्रातस्सुवासरे । आदित्य सम्मुखो मौनी नमस्कृत्य शिवं हृदि ॥
साधारणधराद्रव्यं गृह्णीयादुत्तराश्रितम् । वल्मीक कुत्सितानूपश्मशानोषरमार्गजा: ॥
जन्तुवह्निहिमव्याप्तानौषध्य: कार्य सिद्धिदा: । (श.सं.पू.खं. १)

(ii) अन्येष्वपि प्ररोहन्ति वनेभूपवनेषु च । गृह्णीयात्तानि सुमना: शुचि: प्रात: सुवासरे ॥
आदित्यसम्मुखो मौनी नमस्कृत्य शिवं हृदि । साधारणधराद्रव्यं गृह्णीयादुत्तराश्रितम् ॥
वल्मीककुत्सितानूपश्मशानोषरमार्गजा: जन्तुवह्निहिमव्याप्ता नौषध्य: कार्यसाधिका: ॥
(भा.प्र.पू.खं. ५/१०७-१०९)

३. तेषां शाखापलाशमचिरप्ररूढं वर्षावसन्तयोर्ग्राह्यं ग्राष्मे मूलानि शिशिरे च शीर्णप्ररूढानां, शरदि त्वक्कन्दक्षीराणि, हेमन्ते साराणि, यथर्तु पुष्पफलमिति ....। (च.क. १/१०)

	shed off leaves and regenerating fresh leaves	which are Ushna veerya Sisira (late winter) for plants which are Seeta veerya
3.	Bark, Tubers & latex	- Saradritu (late autumn)
4.	Heart wood or sap wood	- Hemanta (early winter)
5.	Flowers and fruits	- According to their season.

(b) According to Suśruta[1]

1. Roots - Pravrit Ritu (between summer and rainy season)
2. Leaves - Varsha Ritu (during rainy season)
3. Bark - Sarat Ritu (late autumn)
4. Latex - Hemanta Ritu (early winter)
5. Heart wood - Vasanta Ritu (spring)
6. Fruit - Greeshma Ritu (Summer)

(c) According to Narahari[2]

1. Tubers & Rhizomes - Hemanta Ritu
2. Root & Leaves - Sisira Ritu
3. Flower & Fruit - Vasanta Ritu
4. Tender leaves - Greashma Ritu
5. Panchangas - Sarat Ritu

Collection of raw materials according to season

S. N.	Prayojyanga (Part used)	Cha. Ka.1. Chapt.	Su.Sutra.36. Chapt.	Ra.Ni.2. Chapt.
1.	Mula (Roots)	Greeshma, Sisira	Pravrit	Sirira
2.	Palasa (Tender leaves)	Varsha, vasanta	–	Greeshma
3.	Sakha (branches)	Varsha, Vasanta	–	–

१. तत्र केचिदाहुराचार्याः प्रावृड्वर्षशरद्धेमन्तवसन्तग्रीष्मेषु यथा संख्यं मूलपत्रत्वक्क्षीरसारफलान्याददीतेति........। (सु.सू. ३६/५)

२. कन्दं हिमर्तौ शिशिरे च मूलं पुष्प वसन्ते फलदं वदन्ति ।
प्रवालपत्राणि निदाघकालेस्युः पञ्चजातानि शरत्प्रयोगे ॥ (रा.नि.)

4.	Pushpa (flowers)	as per season	–	Vasanta
5.	Twak (Bark)	Sarat	Sarat	–
6.	Ksheera (latex)	Sarat	Hemanta	–
7.	Sara (sap wood)	Hemanta	Vasanta	–
8.	Phala (fruits)	as per season	Greeshma	Vasanta
9.	Kanda (tubers or rhizomes	Sarat	–	Hemanta
10.	Patra (leaves)	–	Varsha	Sisira
11.	Panchanga	–	–	Sarat

(ii) Time of collection according to potency (veerya)

Suśruta while contradicting the view of others regarding collection of raw materials as per the season and prat used, proposed collection as per the potency (veerya)[1].

(a) Soumya oushadha (Seeta Veerya Dravya)- in Soumya Ritu (cold Season) i.e., in varsha, Hemanta & Sisira.

(b) Agneya oushadha (Ushna Veerya Dravya)- in Agneya Ritu (Hot season) i.e., in Sarat, Varsha & Grishma ritus.

Chakrapani also opined that the roots of Ushna veerya dravyas shall be collected in summer (Greeshma) and those of Seeta veerya dravyas in winter (Sisira)[2].

(iii) Collection of drugs as per Area (Desa)

Sarangdhara advocates collections of Agneya dravyas (Ushra virya Dravyas) from Vindhya ranges and Soumya dravyas (Seeta virya Dravyas) from Himalayan ranges[3].

(iv) Collection of drugs as per the soil (Bhumi)

Suśruta described the significance of soil while collecting the drugs for different therapeutic procedures.

---

१. तत्र केचिदाहुराचार्याः....... तत्तु न सम्यक्, सौम्याग्नेयत्त्वाज्जगतः सौम्यान्यौषधानि सौम्येष्वृतुष्वाददीत, आग्नेयान्याग्नेयेषु....। (सु.सू. ३६/५)

२. ....गीष्मे मूलानि शिशिरे वेति कथनेन यान्याग्नेयानि तेषां मूलानि ग्रीष्मे, यानि सौम्यानि तेषां मूलानि शिशिरे, ग्राह्याणीति व्यवस्थां सूचयतिः........। (चक्रपाणि-च.क. १/१०)

३. आग्नेयाविन्ध्यशैलाद्यास्सौम्योहिमगिरिर्मतः । (शा.सं.प्र.खं. १)

(1) Prithvi & Jala prodominant soil– Virechana dravyas (purgatives)[1].

(2) Agni, Akasa & Vayu predominant soil– Vamana dravyas (emet ics)[2].

(3) Both the above soils together– Ubhaya bhagahara dravyas (purgatives & emetics)[3].

(4) Akasa predominent soil– Samana dravyas (drugs used for pallia tive treatment)[4].

(V) Collection of raw materials according to the pharmacological property and season relation

Sarangdhara explained the relation between the collection of drug in a specific season and for specific therapeutic effect depending upon their respective pharmacological properties[5].

(1) Generally for all purposes	-	Sarat Ritu
(2) for Virechana (purgation)	-	Vasanta Ritu
(3) for Vaman (emesis)	-	Vasanta Ritu

6. Collection of Animal Products

When ever animal products are to be collected the following general rules must be followed:

(1) Vayastha (young adults)– for collecting blood, hair, hoofs etc.

(2) Jeernahara (after the food is digested)– for milk, urine and fae-ces etc[6].

7. Collection of Food Materials

Suśruta & Bhavamishra have denoted certain specifications for the collection of food materials also.

---

१. तत्र पृथिव्यम्बुगुणभूयिष्ठायां भूमौ जातानि विरेचनद्रव्याण्याददीत । (सु.सू. ३६/४)

२. अग्न्याकाशमारूतगुणभूयिष्ठांयां वमनद्रव्याणि । (सु.सू. ३६/५)

३. उभयगुणभूयिष्ठायामुभयतो भागानि । (सु.सू. ३६/६)

४. आकाशगुणभूयिष्ठायां संशमनानि, एवं बलवत्तराणि भवन्ति ॥ (सु.सू. ३६/७)

५. शरद्याखिलकार्यार्थं ग्राह्यं रसरसमौषधम् ।
विरेकवमनार्थं च वसन्तान्ते समाहरेत् ॥ (शा.सं.पू.खं. १)

६. जङ्गमानां वय:स्थानां रक्तरोमनखादिकम् ।
क्षीरमूत्रपुरीषाणि जीर्णाहारेषु स हरेत् ॥ (सु.सू. ३६/१७)

(i) **Fruits–** It is advised not to collect the unripen or over-ripen fruits. Fruits which are well ripen shall only be collected from the plants. However Bilwa phala (fruit of Aegel marmelos) may be collected in unripen state only.

Fruits which are not affected by diseases, pests, over-ripen, unseasonal shall not be used[1]. Certain fruits like grapes, myrobalons etc., will be used as dry fruits mainly.

(ii) Leafy Vegetables– Leafy Vegetables which are hard, dry infected by pests, produced in unnatural habitats and which are grown unseasonaly are to be avoided[2].

(iii) Tubers– Immature, unseasonaly harvested, dried and infected tubers should not be used as foods[3].

(iv) **Rice Grains–** The rice grains exposed to cold, hot, air, bugs, animals, water, polluted soil, unsprouting, mixed with other food grains, less potent, very old etc., should not be used[4].

Modern Perspective

Quality of food or drug effects the quality of health and disease. While collecting the naturally occuring foods, one must carefully find out the xenobiotics, aflotoxins and other contaminations/adultrations.

Food usually may have two types of contaminations viz., Microbial and Chemical.

1. Microbial
   - Bacterial
   - Fungal

---

१. फलेषु परपिक्वं यद्गुणवत्तदुदाहृतम्, बिल्वादन्यत्रविज्ञेयमामं तद्धि गुणोत्तरम् ॥
व्याधितं कृमिजुष्टं च पाकातीतमकालजम् वर्जनीयं फलं सर्वमपर्यागतमेवच ।
फलं हिमाग्निदुर्वातव्यालकीटादिदूषितम् । अकालजं कुभूमिजं पाकातीतं न भक्षयेत् ॥ (भा.प्र)

२. कर्कशं परिजीर्णं च कृमिजुष्टमदेशजम् ।
वर्जयेत् पत्रशाकं तद्यदकाल विरोधि च ॥ (सु.सू. ४६)

३. बालं ह्यनार्तवं जीर्णं व्याधितं कृतिभक्षितम् ।
कन्दं विवर्जयेत् सर्वं यो वा सम्यक् न रोहति ॥ (सु.सू. ४६)

४. हिमानलोष्णदुर्वातव्यालालादिदूषितम् । जन्तुजुष्टं जलेमग्नमभूमिमनार्तवम् ॥
अन्यधान्युयुतं हीनवीर्यं जीर्णतयाऽति च धान्यं त्यजेत् ॥ (अ.सं.सू. ७)

2. Chemical
   - Heavy metals
   - Pesticide residues
   - Veterinary drug residues

Since all foods are not of the same quality from a nutritional point of view, man's ability to meet his nutritional needs and maintain good helth depends upon the types and quantity of foodstuffs he is able to include in his diet to satisfy his hunger.

Man has evolved his habitual dietary pattern to maintain good health, perhaps after a good deal of trial and error. Satisfaction of hunger is usually the primary criteria for adequate food intake. But satisfaction of hunger itself is not a safe guide for the selection of proper foods. For sustaining healthy and active life, diets should be planned on sound nutritional principles.

8. Storage of collected raw materials and Drug stores (Bhēshajāgāra)

The collected raw materials are to be preserved and stored in the suitable containers. Then they are kept in the store rooms which are built in air-tight area with plenty of precautions for sanitation. The store house shall be cleaned regularly by ritual methods. It should be free from fire, water, water vapor, smoke, dust, rats and away from cross roads. The drug stores must be completely sterile where the raw materials or drugs are stored[1].

The collected materials may be preserved in cloth, clay pots, planks, conical flasks etc., as per the necessity. Afterwards they are to be preserved in the Bheshajagara (drug stores) in a suitable corner by following all the preservative measures[2].

---

१. गृहीत्वा चानुरूपगुणवद्भाजने संस्थाप्यागारेषु प्रागुदद्वारेषु निवातप्रवातैकदेशेषु नित्यपुष्पोपहारबलिकर्मवत्सु अग्निसलिलोपस्वेदधूमरजोमूषिकचतुष्पदामनभिगमनीयानि स्ववच्छन्नानि शिक्येष्वासज्य स्थापयेत् ॥ तानि च यथा दोषं प्रयुञ्जीत ॥ (च.क. १/११)
*चक्रपाणि:- अनुरूपगुणवद्भाजनस्थानीति अनुरूपगुणवत्ता च भाजनस्य भेषजसमानगुणतयैव । स्ववच्छन्नानीति सम्यक् पिहितानि ॥

२. प्लोतमृद्भाण्डफलकशंकुविन्यस्त भेषजम् ।
प्रशस्तायां दिशि शुचौ भेषजागारमिष्यते ॥ (सु.सू. ३६/१८)

Expiry dates for Ayurvedic preparations

1. Generally preparations will expire after one year.
2. for churna – 2 months
3. for pills and linctus – one year
4. for oils and ghees – 16 months
5. for fermented products – oldest will be the best
6. for decoctions – 6 hours**

Modern perspective collection of crude drugs

Crude drug or raw material includes the subject matter collected naturally from either of the following three sources i.e., vegetable, animal and mineral origin.

(i) vegetable origin – senna leaflets, costus root, turmeric etc.

(ii) animal origin – gall bladder of ox, musk etc

(iii) mineral origin – light kaolin, chalk etc

The crude drugs are complex bodies consisting of several components occuring intimately mixed together. 'Pharmacognosy' is the scientific study of the structural, physical, chemical and sensory characters of crude drugs. It includes also their history, cultivation and collection, and their particulars relating to the treatment they receive during their passage from the producer to the pharmacist.

There are different times and specifications for collection of the raw materials. For example:

(1) To collect the Sandal wood the tree must be grow in arid situations upon poor and stony soil to yield the largest proportion of oil. In yellow Sandal wood a volatile oil is deposited in the heartwood.

(2) Barks are usually collected during spring or early summer, when the sap is rising in the stem and the combium is active and, therefore, more easily torn than at other seasons. If there is a rainy

---

** गुणहीनंभवेद्वर्षादूर्ध्वं तद्रूपमौषधम् । मासद्वयात्तथा चूर्णं हीनवीर्यत्वमानुयात् ॥
हीनत्वं घुटिकालेहौ लभेते वत्सरात्परम् । हीनास्युर्घृततैलाद्याश्चतुर्मासाधिकास्तथा ॥
ओषध्यो लघुपाकास्स्युर्निर्वीर्यावत्सरात्परम् । पुराणास्स्युर्गुणैर्युक्ता आसवा धातवो रसाः॥ (शा.सं.पू.ख.१)

season, it is during that period that the bark is most easily collected, as is done with cinnamon.

(3) Leaves may be collected when the flowers are just begining to expand, or the flowering is just arriving at its height. At this time it is reasonable to assume that the whole plant has arrived at its condition of maximum vigour and that the leaves are in the most healthy state and contain an optimum of the products of the plant's metabolism and therefore should be at this period of their development suited to exert the most desirable therapeutic action. The actual collection should be made, so far as possible, in dry weather, since leaves collected in wet weather deteriorate in quality and are apt to become discoloured during drying.

(4) Flowers must be collected in fine, dry weather, because petals which are damp when gathered become badly discoloured during drying.

(5) Roots and rhizomes are usually collected when their tissues are fully stored with reserve foods, it being assumed that medicinal constituents will be also most abundant at this season.

(6) Galls are collected after the escape of the gall wasp.

It is also important to note that crude drugs frequently exhibit notable features which are quite unrelated to the plants or animals which yield them. This is because of cultivation, collection,packing, marketing etc. stages. Therefore drugs collected from wild plants often differ from those from cultivated plants because of modification resulting from the cultivation itself or from the methods of collection. For example:

(i) Cinnamon from wild trees is a heavy bark with a coarse flavour; that from cultivated plants is in small quills with a more agreeable flavour.

(ii) The root of cultivated aconite is usually collected in the autumn after the stem has died down and hence English root, which is mainly cultivated, consists of plump tubers with a bud at the summit.

9. Collection and Preservation of raw materials on dry and wet basis

Usually all the herbs must be collected a fresh and used in wet state. The exceptions to this rule are: Madhu (honey), Ghrita (ghee), Guda (jaggary), Pippali (long pepper) & Vidanga (embelia seeds)[1].

Certain drugs shall only be used in the wet state as far as possible e.g., Guduchi, Kutaja, Vasa, Kushmanda, Shatavari, Aswagandha, Sahachara, Satapushpa, Prasarini. It is specifically mentioned that these drugs need not be used double quantity though they are being used in wet state[2].(Note:- Generally, wet drugs are advocated in double dose compared to dry drugs[3].

The usual period to consider a drug used when it is dry or old is one year.

Modern Perspective

Drugs are maintained in a sound condition by adopting proper methods of *storage*, and a study of the causes of deterioration enables one to perceive the general principles which must govern conditions of storage. It is clear that *dryness* is the most fundamental requirement, since no living organism can exist or develop without a minimum of moisture; for example, it has been shown that mites are unable to develop in flour if the moisture content is maintained below 11% and that a moisture content below 9% prevents the growth of bacteria and fungi upon cotton-wool.

---

१. (i) सर्वाण्येव चाभिनवानि, अन्यत्र मधुघृतगुडपिप्पलीविडङ्गभ्यः ।
तेषामसंत्तावतिक्रान्तसंवत्सराण्याददीतेति ॥ (सु.सू. ३६/९)
* सर्वाण्येव सक्षीराणि वीर्यवन्ति ।
(ii) विडङ्गं पिप्पली क्षौद्रं सर्पिश्चप्यनवं हितम् ।
शेषमन्यत्त्वभिनवं गृह्णीयाद्दोषवर्जितम् ॥ (सु.सू. ३६/१६)
(iii) नवान्येव हि योज्यानि द्रव्याण्यखिलकर्मसु ।
विना विडङ्गकृष्णाभ्यां गुडधान्याज्यमाक्षिकैः । (शा.सं.पू.खं. १)
२. गुडूची कुटजो वासा कूष्माण्डश्च शतावरी । अश्वगन्धा सहचरौ शतपुष्पा प्रसारिणी ॥
प्रयोक्तव्या सदैवार्द्रा द्विगुणानैव कारयेत् । (शा.सं.पू.खं. १)
३. शुष्कं नवीन द्रव्यं च योज्यं सकल कर्मसु । आर्द्रं च द्विगुणं युंज्यादेष सर्वत्र निश्चयः॥ (शा.सं.पू.खं.)

Next to moisture, light and temperature should be controlled and the access to the drugs or spores and of living organisms must be prevented. These conditions may be satisfied by different means, and the exact method adopted for any given drug may not necessarily be the same in all circumstances. Well closed opaque containers fulfill most of the necessary conditions. A dry atmosphere is maintained by the use of dessicating agent, such as quick lime. The ill effects produced by light can be largely prevented by the use of amberglass bottles.

The fact that a raised temperature facilitates the production of dry atmosphere may lead one to over look the often necessary to store articles in a cool place as well as in a dry atmosphere. A low temperature is also useful to prevent the development of spores and egges which generally speaking, are unable to develop unless the temperature is higher than about 10°C. For this reason cold storage is some form of refrigeration is a valuable means of preventing the development of living organisms in all kinds of drugs. It enables one to store large stocks of substances which are particularly prone to attack.

The raw materials which are to be preserved in wet state may be preserved in the cold storage with the help of refregeration. Similarly those drugs which are to be preserved in dry state may be kept free from moisture and stored in the drug stores. A list of drugs which are to be used in dry and wet states according to Ayurveda is already enumerated above.

10. Measurements

The process of recording length, weight and volume is known as "Manam" (measurement)[1]. Without the measurements we can not prepare the drugs for therapeutics. In different conditions different quantities are advocated. In order to use the drug as per dose or while preparing the compound medicines, we need some or the other measurement. Hence it is very important.

---

१. मीयतेऽनेनेति मानम् । (द्र.गु.नि)

Actually this Mana is not different from 'Parimanam' mentioned under Parādi Guṇas[1]. Knowledge about the Māna (measurement) is very essential for the physician since treatment is directly linked-up with the measurement and assessement of Rasa, Dravya, Doshas, Vyadhi, Bheshaja, Desa, Kāla, Bala etc. Therefore charaka considers that management of diseases is not possible without the knowledge of Māna[2]. Sarangdhara also expressed similar view[3].

As mentioned previously, the usual procedure is to double the quantity of wet drugs compared to those in dry state.

In the Ayurvedic texts two types of measuring systems are famous viz., Kalinga and Magadha[4]. From Amara kosha we get the information regarding three measuring systems viz[5].,

(i) Poutava (weight measurement)

(ii) Druvaya (volume measurement)

(iii) Payya (lenght measurement)

(i) Poutava Mana

(a) Poutava Mana of Charaka[6]

---

१. (i) परिमाणं पुनर्मानम् । (च.सू. २६)
(ii) परिमितिव्यवहारकारणं परिमाणं मानं प्रस्थाढकादि । (योगेन्द्रनाथ:)
(iii) परिमाणं भवेन्मानव्यवहारास्य कारणम् । (कारिकावलि)

२. रसद्रव्यदोष विकारभेषजदेशकालबलशरीरसाराहारसात्म्यसत्त्वप्रकृतिवयसां मानमवहितमनसा यथावज्ज्ञेयं भवति भिषजा, रसादिमानज्ञानायत्तत्वात् क्रियाया:,न ह्यमनज्ञो रसादीनां भिषग् व्याधिनिग्रहसमर्थो भवति । (च.वि. १)

३. न मानेन विना युक्तिर्द्रव्याणां जायते क्वचित् । अत: प्रयोगकार्यार्थं मानमत्रोच्यते मया ।। (शा.सं.पू.खं.१)

४. कालिङ्गं मागधं चैव द्विविधं मानमुच्यते । कालिङ्गान्मागधं श्रेष्ठं एवं मानविदो विदु: ।। च.क.१२, शा.सं.

५. (i) पैतवं द्रुवयं पाय्यमिति मानार्थकं त्रयम् । मानं तुलाङ्गुलिप्रस्थै: ।। (अ.को. २)
(ii) मानं प्रस्थाढकादितुलामेयम् । (चक्रपाणि-च.सू. २६)
(iii) पाय्यं हस्तादिभिर्मानं, द्रवयं कुडवादिभि:, पौतवं तुलया । (वैजयन्ती)

६. जालान्तरगतौर्भानुकरैर्वंशी विलोक्यते । षड्वंश्यस्तुमरीचि: स्यात् षण्मरीच्यस्तु सर्षप: ।।
अष्टौ ते सर्षपा रक्तास्तण्डुलश्चापि तद्द्वयम् । धान्यमाषो भवेदेको धान्यमाषद्वयं यव: ।।
अण्डिकास्ते तु चत्वारस्ताश्चतस्रस्तु माषक: । हेमश्च धान्यकश्चोक्तो भवेच्छाणस्तु ते त्रय: ।।
शाणौ द्वौ द्रंक्षणे विद्यात् कोलं बदरमेव च । विद्याद् द्वौ द्रंक्षणौ कर्ष सुवर्णं चाक्षमेव च ।।
द्वे सुवर्णे पलार्धं स्याच्छुक्तिरष्टमिका तथा । द्वे पलार्धे पलं मुष्टि: प्रकुञ्चोऽथ चतुर्थिका ।।
बिल्वं षोडशिका चाम्रं द्वे पले प्रसृतं विदु: । पलं चतुर्गुणं विद्यादञ्जलि कुडवं तथा ।।
अष्टमानं तु विज्ञेयं कुडवौ द्वौ तु मानिका । चत्वार: कुडवा: प्रस्थश्चतु: प्रस्थमथाढकम् ।।
कंसश्चतुर्गुणो द्रोणश्चार्मणं नल्वणं च तत् । घटस्तु द्विगुण: शूर्पो विज्ञेय: कुम्भ एव च ।।
गोणीं शूर्पद्वयं विद्यात् खारी भारी तथैव च । द्वात्रिंशतं जानीयात् वाहं शूर्पाणि बुद्धिमान् ।।
तुलां शतपलं विद्यात् परिमाणविशारद: । (च.क. १२)

6 Vamsi	=	1 Maricha		
6 Maricha	=	1 Sarshapa		
6 Sarshapa	=	1 Tandula		
2 Tandula	=	1 Dhanya Masha		
2 Dhanyamasha	=	1 Yava (1/2 Ritta)		
4 Yava	=	1 Andika (2 Ratti)		
4 Andika	=	1 Mashaka (8 Ratti)		
3 Mashaka	=	1 Sana (24 Rattis)	=	1/4 Tula
2 Sāṇa	=	1 Kola (48 Rattis)	=	1/2 Tula
2 Kola	=	1 Karsha (96 Rattis)	=	1 Tula
2 Karsha	=	1 Sukti	=	2 Tula
2 Sukti	=	1 Pala	=	4 Tula
2 Pala	=	1 Prasruta	=	8 Tula
2 Prasruta	=	1 Kudava	=	16 Tula
2 Kudava	=	1 Manika	=	32 Tula
2 Manika	=	1 Prastha	=	64 Tula
4 Prashta	=	1 Ādhaka	=	256 Tula
4 Ādhaka	=	1 Droṇa	=	1024 Tula
2 Droṇa	=	1 Surpa	=	2048 Tula
2 Surpa	=	1 Khari	=	4096 Tula
32 Surpa	=	1 Vaha	=	65,536 Tula
100 Pala	=	1 Tulā	=	400 Tula

(b) Poutava Mana of Suśruta

(c) Poutava Mana of Sarangdhara[1]

१. त्रसरेणुर्बुधैः प्रोक्तस्त्रिंशता परमाणुभिः । त्रसरेणुस्तु पर्यायनाम्ना वंशी निगद्यते ॥
जालान्तरगते भानौ यत्सूक्ष्मं दृश्यते रजः । तस्य त्रिंशत्तमो भागः परमाणुः स कथ्यते ॥
जालान्तरगतैः सूर्यकरैर्वंशी विलोक्यते । षड्वंशीभिर्मरीचिः स्यात्ताभिः षड्भिस्तु राजिका ॥
तिसृभी राजिकाभिश्च सर्षपः प्रोच्यते बुधैः । यवोऽष्टसर्वपैः प्रोक्तो गुञ्जा स्याच्चतुष्ठयम् ॥
षड्भिस्तु रक्तिकाभिः स्यान्माषको हेमधान्यकौ । माषैश्चतुर्भिः शाणः स्याद्धरणः स निगद्यते ॥
टंकः स एव कथितस्तद्द्वयं कोल उच्यते । कोलद्वयं च कर्षः स्यात् स प्रोक्तः पाणिमानिका ॥
स्यात् कर्षाभ्यामर्धपलं शुक्तिरष्टमिका तथा । शुक्तिभ्यां च पलं ज्ञेयं मुष्टिराम्रं चतुर्थिका ॥

क्रमशः पृष्ठ ३२० में..........

30 Paramanus	= 1 Vamsi	= 0.035 mg	
6 Vamsi	= 1 Marichi	= 0.21 mg	
3 Marichi	= 1 Rajika	= 1.25 mg	
3 Rajika	= 1Sarshapa	= 4 mg	
8 Sarshapa	= 1 Yava	= 32 mg	
4 Yava	= 1 Gunja or Ratti	= 125 mg	
6 Ratti	= 1 Mashaka	= 750 mg	
1 Mashaka	= 1Sāṇa	= 1/4 Tula = 3 gm	
2 Sāṇa	= 1 Kola	= 1/2 Tula = 6 gm	
2 Kola	= 1 Karsha	= 1 Tula = 12 gm	
2 Karsha	= 1 Sukthi	= 2 Tula = 24 gm	
2 Sukthi	= 1 Pala	= 4 Tula = 48 gm	
2 Pala	= Prasruti	= 8 Tula = 2 Pala = 96 gm	
2 Prasruti	= 1 Kudava	= 16 Tula = 4 Pala = 192 gm	
2 Kudava	= 1 Manika (Sarava)	= 32 Tula = 8 Pala = 384 gm	
2 Sarava	= 1 Prastha	= 64 Tula = 16 Pala = 768 gm	
4 Prastha	= 1 Ādhaka	= 256 Tula = 64 Pala = 3072 gm	
4 Ādhaka	= 1 Drōṇa	= 1024 Tula = 256 Pala = 12.288 kg	
2 Drōṇa	= 1 Surpa	= 2048 Tula = 512 Pala = 24.576 kg	
2 Surpa	= 1 Drōṇi	= 4096 Tula = 1024 Pala = 49.152 kg	
4 Droni	= 1 Khari	= 16384 Tula = 4096 Pala = 196.608 kg	
2000 Pala	= 1 Bhara	= 8000 Tula = 96 kg	
100 Pala	= 1 Tulā	= 400 Tula = 4.8 kg	

पृष्ठ ३१९ से क्रमशः..........

पलाभ्यां प्रसृतिर्ज्ञेया प्रसृतश्च निगद्यते । प्रसृतिभ्यामञ्जलिः स्यात्कुडवोऽर्धशरावकः ॥
अष्टमानं स विज्ञेयः, कुडवाभ्यां च मानिका । शरावोऽष्टपलं तद्वज्ज्ञेयमत्र विचक्षणैः ॥
शरावाभ्यां भवेत् प्रस्थश्चतुःप्रस्थैस्तथाढकम् । चतुर्भिराढकैर्द्रोणः कलशो नल्वणोन्मनौ ॥
द्रोणाभ्यां शूर्पकुम्भौ च चतुःषष्टिशरावका । शूर्पाभ्यां च भवेद् द्रोणो वहो गोणी च सा स्मृता ॥
द्रोणीचतुष्टयं खारी कथिता सूक्ष्मबुद्धिभिः । पलानां द्विसहस्रं च भार एकः प्रकीर्तितः ॥
तुला पलशतं ज्ञेया सर्वत्रैवैष निश्चयः । (शा.सं.सू.खं. १)

Quadruple Formula of Sarngdhara[1]

1 Masha	=	1 Tanka (Sāṇa)
4 Tanka	=	1 Aksha (Karsha)
4 Aksha	=	1 Bilwa (Pala)
4 Bilwa	=	1 Kudava
4 Kudava	=	1 Prastha
4 Prastha	=	1 Ādhaka
4 Ādhaka	=	1 Rāsi (Drona)
4 Rasi	=	1 Droṇi
4 Droṇi	=	1 Khari

Poutava Mana of Suśruta

12 Dhanya Masha	=	1 Suvarna Maha
16 Suvarna Masha	=	1 Suvarna (karsha)
19 Nishpava	=	1 Dharana
2 Dharana	=	1 Karsha

Afterwards the measurements increase by four-folds viz., Pala, Kudava, Prastha, Ādhaka and Drona.

100 Pala	=	1 Tulā
20 Tulā	=	1 Bhara

Note: This measurement is meant for dry drugs. In case of wet drugs double the quantity may be accepted.

(ii) Drivaya Mana of Suśruta

8 Bindus	=	1 Sāṇa
32 Bindus	=	1 Sukti
64 Bindus	=	1 Paṇi Sukti[2]

१. माषटंकाक्षबिल्वानि कुडवः प्रस्थमाढकम् । राशिर्द्रोणी खारिकेति यथोत्तरचतुर्गुणाः ॥ (शा.सं.पू.खं.१) पलकुडवादीनामतो मानं तु व्याख्यास्यामः- तत्र द्वादश धान्यमाषा; मध्यमाः सुवर्णमाषकः, ते षोडश सुवर्णम्, अथवा मध्यमनिष्पावा एकोनविंशतिर्धरणम्, तान्यर्धतृतीयानि कर्षः, ततश्चोर्ध्वं चतुर्गुण-मभिवर्धयन्तः पलकुडवप्रस्थाढकद्रोणा इत्यभिनिष्पद्यन्ते, तुला पलशतं, ताः पुनर्विंशतिर्भारः, शुष्काणामिदं मानं, आर्द्राणां तु द्विगुणमिति ॥ (सु.चि. ३१)

२. तस्य प्रमाणमष्टौ बिन्दवः प्रदेशिनीपर्वद्वयनिःसृताः प्रथम मात्रा, द्वितीया शुक्तिः, तृतीया पाणिशुक्तिः । (सु.चि. ४०)

Note– the quantity of 'Bindu' is fixed as the quantity of any fluid/liquid obtained after inserting index finger upto the second interphalangeal joint (second node)[1].

Usualy we come across 'Anjali' as the measurement used in Ayurvedic tests to denote fluid volumes. Dr. N Anjaneeya Murthy, Professor, Govt. Ayurvedic College, Bellary (Karnataka) had communicated personally that 'Anjali' Pramana is calculated to be about 80-100 ml on average. Body fluids and their quantities are described in Anjalis and Bindus.

(iii) Payya Mana

Payya mana and its utility will be found in the context of Rasa Sastra i.e., Putas mainly. Length of intestines etc., was also mentioned in terms of Hasta and Vyama. Acharya P.V. Sharmaji mentioned the following measurements under this:

12 Angulis	=	1 Bitasti	=	9 inches
21 Angulis	=	1 Aratni	=	161/2 inches
2 Bitasti	=	1 Hastha	=	18 inches
4 Hastha	=	1 Vyama	=	6 feet

Note– One Anguli is the length equivalent to the measurement of width of 8 yavas (8 red wheat) which are joined together with the help of a fine needle.

Magadha & Kalinga Mana

From Yava to Kudava the measurements are specific for kalinga Mana. Afterwards both Magadha and Kālinga Mana are equal. These two can be considered as Poutava Mana.

12 Goura Sarshapa	=	1 Yava
2 Yava	=	1 Gunja

१. (i) प्रदेशिन्युङ्गली पर्वद्वयान्मग्नसमुधृतात् यावत् पतत्यसौ बिन्दुः । (अ.हृ.सू. २०)
(ii) प्रदेशिन्या निमग्ने द्वे पर्वणी निर्गतस्ततः ।
नस्यादिषु तु विज्ञेयो भिषग्भिर्बिन्दुसञ्ज्ञितः ॥
बिन्दुभिश्चाष्टभिःशाणः प्रोक्तश्चैव भिषक्तमैः ।
द्वात्रिंशाद्बिन्दुभिश्चात्रशुक्तिश्चैव निगद्यते ॥
द्वे शुक्ती पाणिशुक्तिश्च नस्यकर्मणि पूजिता । (वृद्धहारीत)

3 Gunja	=	1 Valla
8 Gunja	=	1 Masha
4 Masha	=	1 Sāṇa
6 Masha	=	1 Gadyana
10 Masha	=	1 Karsha
4 Karsha	=	1 Pala
4 Pala	=	1 Kudava

Metric Weights & Measures

Length

10 Millimetres	=	1 Centimetre
10 Centimetres	=	1 Decimetre
10 Decimetres	=	1 Metre
10 Metres	=	1 Dekametre
10 Dekametres	=	1 Hectometre
10 Hectometres	=	1 Kilometre

Volume

1000 Cu centimetres	=	1 Cu decimetre
1000 Cu decimetres	=	1 Cu metre

weight

10 Milligrams	=	1 Cntigram
10 Centigrams	=	1 Decigram
10 Decigrams	=	1 Gram
10 Grams	=	1 Dekagram
10 Dekagrams	=	1 Hectogram
10 Hectrograms	=	1 KILOGRAM
100 Kilograms	=	1 Quintal
10 Quintals	=	1 Metric ton

Capacity

10 Millilitres	=	1 Centilitre
10 Centilitres	=	1 Decilitre

10 Decilitres	=	1 LITRE
10 Litres	=	1 Dekalitre
10 Dekalitres	=	1 Hectolitre
10 Hectolitres	=	1 Kilolitre

Area

1000 Sq. metres	=	1 Are
1000 Are	=	1 Hectare
100 Hectares	=	1 Sq. kilometre

Abbreviations

Kilometre - km	Tonne - t
Meter - m	Quintal - q
Centimetre = cm	Kilogram - kg
Millimetre - mm	Gram - g
Kilolitre - kl	Are - a
Litre - l	Hectare - ha
Millilitre - ml	Centiare - ca

Chapter-XIII

Impurities in Drugs and their Purification Methods

1. Various Impurities of Drugs

Suśruta advocated collection of drugs which are devoid of krimi (pests), Visha (poisoning), Sastra (foreign bodies), Ātapa (affected by sun-light), vayu (affected by wind), Agni (affected by fire), Jala (affected by water) etc[1].

However we often come across drugs consisting of various organic and inorganic impurities.

(i) Organic impurities- plant materials, animal materials, synthetic materials.

(ii) Inorganic impurities- stones, sand, minerals.

These impurities may occur either in *natural form* or sometimes added *artificially*. The artificial impurity is otherwise called as 'Adultration'.

The impurities may be cateorized as physical impurites and chemical impurities also.

It is important to realize that there are several mineral drugs which contain lot of impurities. In Rasa sastra the following types of impurities are usually described:

(i) Naisargika- physically occuring in natural form (Natural).

(ii) Yougika- chemically occuring in natural form (Pysico chemical)

(iii) Oupadhika- chemically occuring in artificial form (purely chemical).

In the context of Dravya guna the herbal drug impurities and purification of their poisonous effects are dealt with.

---

१. तस्यां जातमपि कृमि-विष-शस्त्र-आतप-पवन-दहन-तोयसंबाधमार्गैरनुपहतमेकरसं पुष्टं पृथ्ववगा-ढमूलमुदीच्यां चौषधमादधीत ॥ (सु.सू. ३७)

Impurities

- Physical — e.g., Guggulu, Silajit, Sarjarasa etc., containing stones, sand, sticks etc.
  - Natural
  - Artificial
- Chemical — e.g., Langali, Visha tinduka, Vatsanabhi, Ballataka etc., consisting of poisonous ingredients
  - Natural
  - Artificial

2. Purification Methods of Drugs

The process of removing the impurities from a substance is defined as Sodhana or purification[1].

Sodhana is defined as purification of drugs by using grinding, boiling soaking etc[2].

Sodhana is the process by which the unwanted impurities are removed from a substance and the potency & efficacy are enhanced[3,4].

From the Rasa sastra texts we find two types of purification procedures viz.,

(a) Sāmanya Sodhana: ***(General procedures of purification)***

These are commonly applied to a group of drugs e.g., Amla rasa Bhavana for dhatus and upadhatus.

(b) Visesha Sodhana: ***(Special procedures of Purification)***

These are specially applied to individual drugs belonging to the same group e.g., Triphala kashaya bhavana for Abraka; Nara mutra bhavana for vaikranta etc.

Dr. Nisteswar in his text on Dravyaguna Moulikasidhantalu (Telugu) quoted about eight common procedures of purification. They are: (1) Bhāvana (soaking) (2) Swedana (boiling) (3) Āvapa (mixing) (4) Nirvapa (dipping) (5) Mardana (grinding) (6) Pātana (Distillation

---

१. शोधनं कर्मविज्ञेयं द्रव्यदोषनिवारणम् ।

२. उद्दिष्टैरोषधैः सार्द्धं क्रियते पेषणादिकम् ।
मलविच्छित्तये यत्तु शोधनं तदिहोच्यते ॥ (र.त. २/५२)
* श्रीहरिदत्तशास्त्रीः- आदिपदेन स्वेदनक्षालनादि ग्राह्यम्, मलविच्छित्तये मलनाशाय ।

३. शोधनं दोषहरणं संस्कारश्च बलतेजोऽभिवर्धनम् । (ध.ध.सं.)

४. मुक्तादिष्वविशुद्धेषु न दोषः स्याच्च वस्तुतः । तथाऽपि गुणवृद्धिः स्याच्छोधनेन विशेषतः ॥ (र.चि.)

& Sublimation) (7) Bharjana (Frying) (8) Kshalana (Washing).

Out of these we use Bhāvana, Swedana, Mardana, Bharjana & Kshalana procedures mainly for herbal drugs purification.

(1) Bhavana: ***(Soaking or Trituration)***

The powdered drugs are soaked or triturated in some liquid in a mortar for a specific length of period. This process is known as 'Bhavana'[1].

One of the main aims of Bhavana is to induce certain new qualities in the original drug. The other advantage is that the drug particles are made very finer.

While performing Bhavana, the liquid used should be of sufficient volume to soak the entire powder of the drug. Decoction may be prepared with 1:8 (drug: water) ratio and it must be reduced to 1/8[2].

Charaka mentioned certain Bhavanas for vamama kalpa on the basis of Tridoshas[3]. They are:

(i) Vata doshas - Sura, souviraka, tushodaka, Dhanyamla etc.

(ii) Pitta doshas - Draksha rasa, Madhūka Rasa, Phanita, Kshira etc.

(iii) Kapha doshas - Madhu, Mutra, Kashaya etc[4].

The effect of Bhavana is proved scientifically through certain studies e.g., The crude root of Aconite contains about 1.4% of total alkaloids where as the root treated with cow's urine contains only 1.27%. Soaking with cow's urine and exposure to sunlight have brought about

---

१. यच्चूर्णितस्य धात्वादेर्द्रवैः सम्पेष्य शोषणम् । भावनं तन्मतं विज्ञैर्भावना च निगद्यते ॥ (र.त.२/४९)

२. द्रवेण यावता द्रव्यं चूर्णितं त्वार्द्रतां व्रजेत् । तावानेव द्रवो देयो भिषग्भिर्भावनाविधौ ॥
भावद्रव्यमितः क़्वथ्यो जलमष्टगुणं ततः ।
वस्वंशशोषितः क्वाथो देयः क्वाथेन भावने ॥ (र.त. २/५०-५१)

३. भूयश्चैषां बलाधानं कार्यं स्वरसभावनैः । सुभावितं ह्यल्पमपि द्रव्यं स्याद्बहुकर्मकृत् ॥
स्वरसैस्तुल्यवीर्यैर्वा तस्माद्द्रव्याणि भावयेत् । (च.क. १२/४७)

४. सुरासौवीरकतुषोदकमैरेयमेदकधान्याम्लफलाम्लदध्याम्लादिभिर्वाते ।
मृद्वीकामलकमधुमधूकपरूषकफलफाणितक्षीरादिभिश्च पित्ते ।
श्लेष्माणि तु मधुमूत्रकषायादिभिर्भावितान्यालोडितानि च इत्युर्द्दशः ।
तं विस्तरेण द्रव्य-देह-दोष-सात्म्यादीनि प्रविभज्य व्याख्यास्यामः ॥ (च.क. १/१२)
*चक्रपाणिः- संक्षेपेण मदनफलादीनां वातादिभेदेन भावनालोडनद्रव्याण्याहतानि च यथा दोषं प्रयुञ्जीतेत्यादि ।.....द्रव्य-देश-दोष-सात्म्यादीनीत्यत्र आदिशब्देन प्रकृतिबलादीनां ग्रहणम् ।

a partial change in the toxic alkaloids aconite and pseudoaconite into a far less poisonous substnaces benzyl-aconine and veratroyl aconine respectively [Kirtikar & Basu; Indian Medicinal Plants vol. I].

Examples of Bhavana

1. Trituration of Bakuchi (Psoralia corylifolia) in ginger juice for 3-7 days.
2. Soaking Vatsanabhi (Aconitum ferox) in cow's urine for 7 days and exposing to sun-light.
3. Guggulu (Commiphora mukul) is triturated in Triphala kashaya.
4. Āmalaki (Emblica officinalis) is triturated in its own juice to enhance the properties.

(2) Swedana: *(Boiling)*

Boiling the drug by suspending in liquids with the help of Dola yantra (a special apparatus for boiling) is known as 'Swedana'[1].

It is known that the poisonous effect of brucine may be brought down by treating with protein. Hence nux-vomica seeds are boiled in milk in Dolayantra to detoxify it.

It is specifically mentioned that only the Badara kashta (wood from zyzyphus jujuba) shall be used for Swedana process.

Examples of Swedana

1. Boiling Guggulu in milk or Triphala kashaya.
2. Nux-vomica seeds are boiled in milk.
3. Gunja seeds are boiled in milk

(3) Āvāpa: *(Mixing)*

When liquified metals are pored into another liquid it is known as Āvapa[2]. This procedure is usually utilized in Rasa sastra.

---

१. (i) दोलायन्त्रे स्थापयित्वा द्रव्यं क्षारैरम्लैरोषधैर्वा कषायैः ।
एकत्या यत्स्यात्पाचनं स्वेदनं तत् प्राज्ञैरूक्तं दोषशैथिल्यकारि ॥ (र.त. २/४६) स्व.
(ii) क्षाराम्लैरोषधैर्वापि दोलायन्त्रे स्थितस्य हि । पाचनं स्वेदनाख्यं स्यान्मलशैथिल्यकारकम् ॥ (र.र.स.)

२. (i) द्रव्यान्तरविनिक्षेपो द्रुते वङ्गादिके तु यः । क्रियते स प्रतीवाप आवापश्च निगद्यते ॥ (र.त. २/३९)
(ii) द्रुते द्रव्यान्तरक्षेपो लोहाद्ये क्रियते हि यः । स आवापः प्रतीवापस्तदेवाच्छादनं मतम् ॥ (र.र.स.)

e.g.: Vanga or Naga (tin or lead) is liquified by heating and then pored into Nirgundi Swarasa or Jayanti Swarasa.

(4) Nirvāpa: ***(Dipping)***

The metallic drugs are heated red hot and then suddenly dipped into various liquids. This process is called as 'Nirvapa'[1]. This is also used mainly in Rasa Sastra. e.g.: heated copper leaves dipped into Amla dravyas

[N.B.:– This process is different from 'Dhālana' since lohas are heated only but not melted.]

(5) Mardana: ***(Grinding)***

Grinding the drugs in a mortar is known as Mardana[2]. Usually grinding is avdised in clockwise direction only. About 50 ^{0}C temperature is possible during grinding continuously and it may result in certain changes in the drug.

Some times Mardana can be done for single herbal drug or group of herbal drugs or a group of herbo-mineral drugs or mineral drugs alone.

(i) single herbal drug– Guggulu to be pounded for 1 lakh times.

(ii) group of herbal drugs– Triphala guggulu.

(iii) group of herbo-mineral drugs– Arogyavardhini Vati, Chandraprabha vati etc.

(iv) group of mineral drugs– Maha Vangeswara rasa.

(v) single mineral drug– pounding gandhaka (Sulfur).

(6) Pātanam: ***(Distillation & Sublimation)***

Originally this process is used for mineral drugs alone. Hence sublimation will be suitable and equivalent term. In this process Mercury, Sulphur and other metallic drugs are mixed and heated in valuka yantra. Therefore sublimation occurs[3].

---

१. (i) तप्तस्याप्सु विनिक्षेपः निर्वापः स्नपनं च तत् । (र.र.स.)
(ii) धात्वादेर्वह्नितप्तस्य जलादौ यन्निषेचनम् ।
स निर्वापः स्मृतश्चापि निषेकः स्नपनञ्च तत् ॥ (र.त. २/४०)

२. क्षाराद्यैरोषधैर्वा यत् खल्वे द्रव्यस्य पेषणम् । तन्मर्दनं बुधैः प्रोक्तं बहिर्मलनिवृत्तये ॥ (र.त. ५/५४)

३. उक्तौषधैरसवरस्य विमर्दितस्य यन्त्राहितस्य यदिहोर्ध्वमधश्च तिर्यक् ।
निष्कासनं तदिह पातनसंज्ञामुक्तं वङ्गादिदोषयुगलं शमयत्यनल्पम् ॥ (र.त. ५/६९)

Sublimation is the process of conversion of a solid directly into vapour, and subsequent condensation, without melting.

This patana is of three types again viz.,

(i) Urdwa patana (sublimation)

(ii) Adho patana (sublimation)

(iii) Tiryak patana (distillation)

However Tiryak patana is mainly useful for herbal drugs since Arka preperations (i.e., distillates) are prepared through this process. This is otherwise known as distillation in chemistry.

Distillation is the process of converting a liquid into vapour, condensing the vapour, and collecting the condensed liquid or distillate.

It is used to seperated mixtures of liquids of different boiling points or for seperating a pure liquid from a non-volatile constituent. It is also used in the seperation of isotopes.

Examples of distillates:

(i) Trijatakadi Arka

(ii) Ajamoda Arka etc.

(7) Bharjanam: *(Frying)*

Frying the drug material in the pan with or without other substance or medium is known as Bharjana. This can by dry or wet.

Dry frying– Pippali (long pepper) is fried as it is before powdering it.

Wet frying– Hingu (asefoetida) is fried in ghee[1].

(8) Kshalanam: *(Washing)*

Washing the drugs to remove physical impurities like mud, stones, dust etc., is known as 'Kshalanam'. e.g.: Tubers like Vidari kanda, Musali kanda, Shatavari are washed to remove the mud.

A part from the above there are other methods like exposing to sun-light, shade drying, exposing to moon light etc., which are used for Sodhana. At the outset Sodhana removes impurities and detoxification is also done.

१. चूर्णेषु भर्जितं हिङ्गुं देयं नोत्क्लेदकृद्भवेत् । (शा.सं.म.खं.६/२)

Some Examples for Sodhana

(a) Ahiphena: *(Papaver somniferum)*

(i) Opium is soaked or triturated in ginger juice for 21 times (Yo.Ra.)

(ii) Mardana for one day in cow's ghee (D.M.S.)

(iii) Opium is first dissolved into water and the solution is filtered through a double layered cloth. Later enitre water is evaporated and purified opium is obtained (Ra.Sa.).

(b) Karaveera: *(Thevetia peruviana)*

Its root is cut into small pieces and made as a packet in a piece of cloth. Then it is subjected to swedana for 3-6 hours (Ra.Chi.).

(c) Guggulu: *(Commiphora mukul)*

(i) Equal parts of Triphala and Guduchi are pounded into corase powder and 8 parts of water is added to it to prepare decoction which is half reduced. In this decoction guggulu is subjected to Swedana.

(ii) Swedana in Gokshira (cow's milk).

(d) Gunja: *(Abrus prceatarius)*

Its seeds are subjected to swedana in Kanjika or milk.

(e) Jaya pala: *(Croton tiglium)*

(i) The seeds are dehusked and the germinating bud is also removed. Then they are kept in cow-dung for 3 days. Afterwards soaked in hot water in a mortar. Finally the seeds are soaked in lime juice. (Sa.Sam.)[1].

(ii) The seeds are dehusked by soaking in water for 24 hours. Then swedana is performed in 16 parts of milk (Yo.Ra.)

[**Note:** To touch the seeds with hands, ghee must be applied earlier.]

(f) Dhattura: *(Datura metel)*

Its seeds are subjected to swedana in cow's milk for 3 hours and then washed with hot water.

---

१. जैपालं रहितं त्वगङ्कुररसज्ञाभिर्मलेमहिषे निक्षिप्तं त्र्यहमुष्णतोयविमलं खल्वे सवासोऽर्दितम् ।
लिप्तं नूतनखर्परेषु विगतस्नेहं रजः संनिभं निम्बूकाम्बुविभावितं च बहुशः शुद्धं गुणाढ्यं भवेत् ॥
(शा.सं.म.खं. १२)

(g) Bākuchi: ***(Psoralia corylifolia)***

The seeds are soaked in ginger juice for 7-21 times.

(h) Bhallataka: ***(Semicarpus anacardium)***

(i) The ripen marking nuts are poured into water and the floating ones are picked up and stored amidst of brick powder for 5-7 days. [This method will be more useful while preparing Bhallataka decoction].

(ii) Its seeds are subjected to swedana in a solution prepared with cow-dung 1 part and water 4 parts for 12 hours. Afterwards swedana is again done in cow's urine and cow's milk for 12 hours each.

(i) Bhanga: ***(Cannabis sativa)***

(i) Its leaves are boiled in water at first and then dried (Ra.Sa.)

(ii) Its leaves are fried in ghee on light heat.

(j) Rakta chitraka: ***(plumbago rosea)***

Its root is soaked in lime water.

(k) Rasanjana: ***(berberis aristata)***

It is powdered and soaked in water for one day. Then the solution is filtered. The filtrate is gradually evaporated to obtain pure Rasanjana.

(l) Lasuna: ***(Alium sativum)***

The outer coat of bulb is removed and pounded into paste. This paste is triturated in butter milk (Takra) for 3 days. Every day butter milk should be changed and dried under shade.

(m) Langali: ***(Gloriosa superba)***

The tuber is cut into pieces and soaked in cow's urine for one day. Later it is shade dried (Ra. cha.)

(n) Vatsanabha: ***(Aconitum ferox)***

(i) Swedana in cow's milk for three hours (Ya. Ra.)

(ii) Swedana in goat's milk for 3 hours (Sa. Sam.)[1]

---

१. (i) खण्डीकृत्य विषं वस्त्रपरिबद्धं तु दोलया ॥
अजापयसि संस्विन्नं यामतः शुद्धिमाप्नुयात् ।
अजादुग्धाभावतस्तु गव्यक्षीरेण शोधयेत् ॥ (शा.सं.म.खं. १२/२९३-२९४)

(ii) विषं तु खण्डशः कृत्वा वस्त्रखण्डेन बन्धयेत् । गोमूत्रमध्ये निक्षिप्य स्थापयेदातपे त्र्यहम् ॥
गोमूत्रं च प्रदातव्यं नूतनं प्रत्यहं बुधैः । त्र्यहेऽतीते समुद्धृत्य शोषयेन्मृदु पेषयेत् ॥
शुद्ध्यत्येवं विषं तच्च योग्यं भवति चार्तिजित् । (शा.सं.म.खं. १२/२९१-२९३)

(iii) Swedana in Gomutra for 3 days. Every day the cow's urine must be changed.

(o) Visha tinduka: ***(Strychnos nux-vomika)***

(i) Seeds are dehusked and soaked in cow's urine for 7 days. Later swedana is done in cow's milk (Ra.Sa.)

(ii) Seeds are subjected to sweda for 3 hours in cow's milk. After wards they are dehusked and fried in ghee.

(p) Snuhi ksheera: ***(Euphorbia nerifolia)***

One part of tamarind leaf juice and four parts of latex of Snuhi are mixed and dried in sun-light.

Some of the modern methods of Purification

(i) Washing ***(Kshalana)***– Many of the impurities in a drug can be washed through a flow of water.

(ii) Sifting ***(Chālana)***– Sifting means to seperate the impurities with the help of a sieve.

(iii) Elutriation ***(Vilayana)***– The seperation of insoluble particles from finer ones by deconting the fluid.

(iv) Lixiviation ***(Ksharana)***– Seperation of soluble from insoluble substances by washing and filtration.

(v) Percolation ***(Parisravana)***– Filtration or the process of exhausting virtues of a drug of powdered composition by filtering a liquid solvent through it.

(vi) Maceration ***(Sura vilayana)***– The process of softening a solid by steeping in fluid.

(vii) Dialysis ***(Prithakkarana)***– The passage of a soluble through a membrane or a process in which a liquid to be purified or studied is enclosed in a thin, membranous sack and exposed to water or any other solvent which continually circulates or changes outside the sack. Diffusible substances pass through the membrane, but colloidal material does not.

(viii) Despumation ***(Nirmalikarana)***– Seperation of froth or scum from a liquid is known as despumation.

(ix) Boiling *(Swedana)*– Boiling water destroys organic impurities or boiling toughens and hardens albumen in eggs or boiling toughens fibrin and dissolves in meat or boiling bursts starch granules or boiling softens cellulose in cearls and vegetables.

(x) Sublimation *(Pātana)*--To convert a solid into a vapour and condense it against without liquefying to purify it.

(xi) Discolouration *(Vivarnikarana)*– Any change from an initial colour possessed by any material.

(xii) Grinding *(Mardana)*– To reduce the larger particles into powder or to Grind them with other materials.

(xiii) Dipping *(Nirvapana)*– To plemge a solid material into a liquid medium.

3. Knowledge of Adultration

When ever a drug is scarcely available or rare in occurance, the tendency of man is to replace it by other similar material. This is known as adultration. Some times the abnormal cost of the drug may also result in adultration with cheaper and similar substance.

In the ancient classics we come across some of the artificially prepared drugs. Chakra pani quoted about the sahaja (natural) and kritrima (artificial) viryas. The kritrima virya indicates towards the concept of active principles of modern times.

We also come across artificially prepared karpura and kasturi in Raja Nighantu. Between 16-17th AD some of the Ayurvedic texts discussed in detail about the substitutes. Though substitution is also considered as part of adultration today, the intention of Acharyas was to provide some equally potent drugs in the absence of original drugs.

Gradually, the commercial out look and disruption in traditional and ethical practice of Ayurveda have affected the system and today adultration and substandard medicinal preparations have become the bane of Ayurveda. Hence the slogan of 'drug standardization'.

Food Adultration

This is not only related to intentional addition or substitution or abstraction of substance which adversely affect the nature, substance and quality of foods but also their incidental contamination during the period of growth, harvesting, storage, processing, transportation and distribution.

These aspects are covered by 'Prevention of food Adultration Act' in India. Some of the examples of food adultration are:

(i) Honey is artificially prepared by using sugar or jaggery, sunset yellow and invest sugar.

(ii) Metanyl yellow or tartarin colour are added as artificial colours for vegetable oils.

(iii) The commonly adultrated food spice is turmeric. Metanyl yellow is often used to adultrate it. It causes severe cyanosis in man and nephrotoxicity in other animals.

(iv) Sodium bicarbonate is used as neutralizer while transporting the milk is injurious to health.

(v) Detergent, sugar, water and little quantity of milk etc., are used to prepare synthetic milk.

(vi) Lead oxide (plumbum) is used to adultrate chilly powder.

(vii) Argemone oil is used to adultrate vegetable oils.

(viii) Artificial sweetening agents like Rhodamine B, Dulcin etc. are dangerous and carcinogenic.

(ix) Unwanted and excessive quantites of spraying of D.D.T. resulted in dangerous proportions of DDT in milk among 40% of the milk samples collected and studied by NIN, Hyderabad in one of their studies.

(x) Cajanus indicus (thur dal) is adultrated with highy neurotoxic lathyrus sativa.

To find out the adultration of honey, it is to be mixed with 3 to 4 parts of alcohol. If it forms turbid mixture then it is pure honey. Another method is to mix Resorcinol and HCl. Then this mixture is added to the ether extract of honey. If it turns red, the honey will be considered impure and artificial.

- Food contamination
  - Microbial
    - Bacterial
    - Fungal
  - Chemical
    - Heavy metals
    - Pesticidal residues
    - Veterinary drug residues

Drug Adultration

In general, adultration of crude drug occur when a drug is scarce or when the price of a drug is normally high, though there may be no scarcity.

The adultrant must be some material which is both cheap and available in fairly large amount.

While examining powdered materials it is more specially colour and general texture of the powder which are more important than external macroscopical resemblance. Hence the adulterant may be any kind of material, not necessarily belonging to the same morphological group as that of the genuine drug e.g., powdered guaiacum wood is used to adultrate nux-vomica; dextrin to adultrate powdered ipecacuanha.

Methods of Adultration

(1) Manufacture of substitutes– Materials are artificially manufactured so as to simulate the general form and appearance of various drugs. e.g., bass wood is cut in to pieces and used as adulterant for Nutmegs; powdered chicory is used to adultrate coffee powder.

(2) Substitution of inferior commercial varieties– Some of the cheaper substitutes are used in place of original drugs e.g., Arabian senna, obovate senna and provence senna (cassiaauriculata) have been used to adultrate original senna.

(3) Substitution of exhausted drugs– Some commodities are used in very large amounts for the manufacture of preparations after which the vegetable residue retains very much the appearance of the original material e.g., bitterness of exhausted gentian is restored by adding Aloes to it; removal of volatile oils from cloves, caraway & fennel.

(4) Substitution of superficially similar but cheaper natural substances– Usually they have no relation to the genuine article e.g., leaves of Ailanthus species are substituted for belladona, senna mint etc.; clove stalks and mother cloves are often mixed with cloves.

(5) Addition of worthless heavy materials– The less costly and heavier weight materials are added to the original drug e.g., pieces of limestone are found in asefoetida; lead shot has occured in pieces of opium.

(6) Addition of synthetic principles to fortify inferior products with the drug e.g., addition of citral to the oil of lemon.

(7) The presence of adventitious matter naturally occuring with the drug, if in excessive amount, also constitutes an adultration e.g., Guggulu resin containing stores & sticks etc.

(8) For powdered materials, generally powdered waste products of a suitable colour and density are used e.g.: powdered olive stones are added to drugs like powdered liquorice or pepper.

Methods of detection of Adultration

The processes used fall into two main sections, viz., observations and experiments which (i) establish the identity of the adulterant, and (ii) those which determine the quantity of the drug.

(1) To establish the identity

a. Gross morphology:	e.g.: Europion dill or Caraway containing Indian dill; Indian senna pods substituted for Alexandrian pods are differentiated by definite morphological features.
b. Histology & Microscopical morphology	e.g.: Rhubarb and ginger are characterised by their non-lignified vessels, varieties of Aloes by the presence or absence of crystals of aloin.
c. Microscopical Linear: Measurements	diameter of starch grains, lenght of stomata of leaves etc.
d. Solubilities:	Specific behaviour of solvents will help in identifying many oils, oleo-resins etc.
e. Qualitative Chemi-: cal Tests	These are colour tests etc., which are specific for certain substances.
f. Physical Constants:	Specific gravity, viscocity, optical rotation etc.
g. UV Light:	Flourescent constitnents can be identified by exposing the powder or cut surface to UV light.

(2) To establish the quality

(a) Assay for alkaloids, glycosides, resin, volatile oil etc.

(b) Yield to solvents.

(c) Ash content.

(d) Crude fibre.

(e) Quantitative Microscopy.

4. Knowledge of Synthetic Drugs

The artificially prepared drugs from the component elements or simpler materials which are not obtained directly from natural sources. These are called as Synthetic Drugs e.g. Synthetic pencilline.

Though large scale synthetic herbal drug processing is not known, different fractions and extractions are being prepared by using the natural products and they need some mentioning here.

The following medicinal products are derived from herbs

1.	Ajmalicine	- Vinca rosea root
2.	Atropine	- Hyoscyamus muticus leaves
3.	Berberine	- Berberis bark
4.	Brucine	- Nuxvomica
5.	Colčhicine	- Gloriosa superba root & seeds
6.	Curcumin	- Curcuma longa rhizome
7.	Digoxine	- Digitalis lanata leaf
8.	Glycyrrhetinic Acid	- Liquorice root
9.	Ephedrine	- Ephedra spp. stems
10.	Hyoscyamine	- Hyoscyamus muticis leaf
11.	L-Dopa	- Mucuna pruriens seeds
12.	Peruvoside	- Thevetia peraviana seeds
13.	Psoralene	- Psorelia corylifolia seeds
14.	Quinine & Quinidine	- Cinchona bark
15.	Reserpine	- Rauwolfia serpentina root
16.	Sennoside	- Senna leaves

17. Strychnine - Nux vomica seeds
18. Tannic acid - Chebula fruit cortex
19. Valepotriates - Valaerian Wellichi root
20. Vinblastine & Vincristine - Vinca rosea leaf
21. Coumarin - Melilot spp.
22. Gossypol - Cotton seed
23. Artimissinin - Artemisia annua
24. Physostigmine - Physostigma venenosum (calabar beans)
25. Pilocarpine - Pilocarpus jaborandi leaf.

The above ingredients are otherwise known as the 'active principles' of the respective herbs. They will be extracted by different methods:

(i) Aqueous extracts: (a) Decoction
(b) Infusion
(c) Maceration

(ii) Tinctures
(iii) Fluid extracts
(iv) Thin extracts
(v) Thick or Viscous extracts
(vi) Dry extracts or Extracts sicca
(vii) Oily Drug Extracts or Olea Medicata
(viii) Oleoresin

There are several active ingredients in a drug. The important ones which are extracted or seperated from the original herb and used. Some of them are delineated here.

(1) Alkaloids— They are complex substances which basic or alkali-like and possess physiological activity. They may be defined as organic nitrogenous substances of plant origin. A true alkaloid has a nitrogen atom as a part of heterocyclic system and has a complex molecular structure e.g., nicotine, coniine, spartein, berberine etc.

The alkaloids are fairly soluble in organic solvents like chloroform, ether, alcohol and benzene. These alkaloids are present in different parts: seeds (strychnine), roots (reserpine), bark (kurchin), leaves (Datura), fruits (Pepper) etc.

The alkaloids are three types namely

(i) True alkaloids– Toxic and wide range of activity is seen e.g., colchine, morphine, emetine etc.

(ii) Proto-alkaloids– They are simple amines e.g. mescaline, ephedrine etc.

(iii) Pseudo-alkaloids– not derived from amino acid precursors e.g., steroidal alkaloids (conessine) and purines (caffeine).

(2) **Gycosides—** They are compounds which give rise to one or more sugar (glycone) and a compound which is not a sugar (aglycone or genin) on hydrolysis.

When the sugar formed is dextrose (glucose), the glycoside is referred as *glucoside* e.g., salicin. The glycosides yielding rhamnase are called rhamnosides.

They are soluble in water and alcohol, but insoluble in other organic salvents like petroleum ether, solvent ether, chloroform CCl_4 etc. The glycosoide are of different types:

(i) Steroidal glycosides

(ii) Flavonoid glycosides

(iii) Anthacene glycosides

(iv) Cyanophoric glycosides

(v) Triterpenic glycosides

(vi) Alcohol glycosides

(vii) Lactone glycosides

(viii) Isothiocyanate glucoside

(ix) Saponin glycoside.

(3) **Saponins—** They are highly complex glycosides, e.g., Quillalia, Sarsaparilla and Senega have their medicinal properties due to the saponins they contain. Saponins from colloidal solution in water

gave a soaplike froth on shaking. They may cause haemolysis of RBCs, even at great dilution. Most of them are highly toxic when injected into the body, much less so when taken orally.

(4) Tannins and Phenols— Tannins are complex phenolic compounds which are soluble in water and have an astringent and bitter taste. They belong to two main groups:

(i) Phlobatannins– derived from dihydric catechol. They yield phlobaphenes on heating which are soluble in water. e.g., krameria and Hamamelis.

(ii) Pyrogallol tannins– They are derived from trihydric phenol pyrogallol. There are further categorized as

(a) ellagitannins– yielding ellagic acid on hydrolysis

(b) gallitannins– yielding a sugar & gallic acid.

Tannins are soluble in water and have an astringent taste.

A considerable number of plant substances are phenolic compounds e.g. the anthaquinone derivatives, morphine and the resinotannols.

Tannins may also be classified as three groups viz.

(i) Hydrolysable Tannins

(ii) Condensed Tannins

(iii) Pseudotannins

(5) Volatile oils— They are the flavouring constituents which evaporate on exposure to ordinary temperature. They may be colourless liquids or crystalline or amorphous solids. They are soluble in water, but highly soluble in ether alcohol and other organic solvents.

They are present in flower petals (Saffron), fruits (Fennel), bark (cinnamomum) etc.

Volatiles are the mixture of monoterpenes and sesquiterpenes. All the volatile oils are of vegetable origin (flavonoids or terpenoids etc).

(c) Resins, Gum-resins and oleo-resins

Resins are solid or semisolid plant exudates formed in schizogenous or schizolysigenous ducts or cavities. They are complex mixtures of compounds like resin alcohols, resin acids, resino tannols (resinophenols), esters and vesenes. They are classified as:

(i) **Balsams–** resinous substances containing large quantities of benzoic or connamic acids either free or in combination of their esters.

(ii) **Oleoresins–** resins occuring with volatile oil. e.g. Turpentine, Capsicum, Ginger etc.

(iii) **Gum-resins–** resine found in combination with gum. e.g. asafoetida, Gambage & Myrrh.

(iv) **Oleo-gum-resins–** gum and volatile oil both are present in resin.

(v) **Glycoresins–** resins occuring in combination with glycosides e.g. Ipomea, Jalap, Podophyllum etc.

✸

Chapter - XIV

Ideal Drug; Parts used; Drug combinations; Incompatible drugs; Posology; Anupana (vehicle); Times of drug administration; Routs or drug Administration & prescription writing

1. Qualities of Ideal Drug

An ideal drug should have four qualities according to Charaka[1]. They are:

(a) Bahuta (plenty in availability)

(b) Yogyata (must be eligible for medicament)

(c) Aneka vidha kalpana (should be available in various forms)

(d) Sampat (should possess all the properties/qualities)

Suśruta stated that the high quality drug will be that which is born in fertile land, collected properly, used in appropriate dose, pleasant to mind, possessing pleasant smell-colour-taste, able to destroy the diseases, devoid of side-effects and administered as per time schedule. All there qualities will make a drug highly effective[2].

Vagbhata just followed Charaka's view and accepted four qualities viz., Bahu kalpa (many forms), Bahu Guna (many qualities), Sampanna (full of ingredients) and Yogya (eligible for medicaments)[3].

In another context charaka quoted that the material which cures a disease or condition and provides health is called as oushadha (medicine)[4].

---

१. बहुतातत्रयोग्यत्वमनेकविधकल्पना । संपच्चेति चतुष्कोयं द्रव्याणां गुण उच्यते ॥ (च.सू. ९)

२. प्रशस्तदेशेसंभूतं प्रशस्तेऽहनि चोद्धृतम् । युक्तमात्रं मनस्कान्तं गन्धवर्णरसान्वितम् ॥
दोषघ्नमग्लानिकरमविकारि विपर्यये । समीक्ष्य दत्तं काले च भेषजं पाद उच्यते ॥(सु.सू.३४/२२-२३)
(समीक्ष्य दत्तं यद्भेषजं तद्गुणावहम् ॥) (भा.प्र.पू.खं.५.प्र.१०४-१०५)

३. बहुकल्पं बहुगुणं संपन्नं योग्यमौषधम् । (अ.सं.सू. १. अ.हृ.सू. १)

४. तदेव युक्तं भैषज्यं यदारोग्याय कल्पते । (च.सू.१)

Bhava mishra defined Oushadha as the measure by which the doctor cures the disease[1].

However one should remember that even the best drug requires careful handling. Charaka concluded that a deadly poison can be used as medicine or the vice versa may also be possible. Proper and improper handling are the reasons for the above results respectively[2].

In modern pharmacology and ideal drug must have the following properties:

(i) easily available

(ii) abundently available

(iii) cheaper in cost

(iv) less side effects

(v) maximum therapeutic efficiency

2. Formulation of Compound Drugs

The general concept of preparation of different medicines is to use the drugs of similar potency for a particular purpose[3]. e.g., Vamana kalpa, Virechana kalpa etc.

When drugs of equal potency or equal efficacy are used, their therapeutic effect can be seen even in very low doses. When drugs of opposite qualities or potency used together, their therapeutic effect is reduced and becomes less effective. Therefore the medicaments are to be prepared after carefully assessing combined effect, time effect, analytical approach and modification of original qualities[4].

Drugs with different potencies are sometimes utilized but their final effect only is considered in that combination e.g., Agrvadi taila dravyas, Chandanadi taila dravyas.

---

१. वैद्यो व्याधिहरेद्येन तद्रव्यं प्रोक्तमौषधम् ।
तद्यादृश्यमवश्यं स्याद्रोगघ्नं तादृशंब्रुवे ।। (भा.प्र.पू.खं.५ प्र. १०३)

२. योगादपि विषं तीक्ष्णं उत्तमं भेषजं भवेत् । भेषजंचापि दुर्युक्तं तीक्ष्णं संपद्यते विषम् ।। (च.सू. १)

३. अधिकं तुल्य वीर्ये हि क्रियासामर्थ्यमिष्यते ।। (च.क. १२/४५)

४. अल्पस्यापि महार्थत्वं प्रभूतस्याल्पकर्मताम् ।
कुर्यात् संयोग विश्लेषकालसंस्कारयुक्तिभिः ।। (च.क.१२/४८)

Usually the first drug in a compound drug is used to denote that formulation e.g. Hingwashtaka churna, Talisadi churna, Vidarigandhadi gana etc[1].

Vagbhata mentioned that it will be very difficult to identify the mixed doshas and dushyas in a particular condition. The collective behaviour of combinations and permutations of doshas are very complicated to know. There fore those complicated conditions may be treated on the basis of samyoga, samskara, desa, kala etc[2].

When ever different opposite properties are combining in a combination the most powerful will over come the others[3].

These are three types of drug combinatios which we come across in Ayurvedic texts:

(a) Herbal (b) Mineral and (c) Herbo-mineral

As already mentioned Samyoga means the combination of two or more than two drugs[4]. However the incompatibility of drugs and other aspects must be considered before formulating new combinations. We do not have the scientific validity of various combinations that are seen as patent drugs in today's herbal trade.

Basis of drug combinations in Ayurveda

1. According to the main drug	-	Aswagandha lehya, Brahmi Rasayan etc.
2. According to inventor's name	-	Bhaskara lavana churna, Agastya-haritaki Rasayan etc.
3. Similarity with a particular item	-	Rasa parpati, Kajjali, etc.
4. On the basis of its main action	-	Swasa kuthara, Rechaka vati etc.
5. On the basis of quanity of main ingredient	-	Kamsa haritaki, Ashta katwara taila, Hingu triguna taila etc.

---

१. यदौषधं तु प्रथमं यस्य योगस्य कथ्यते । तन्नम्नैव स योगो हिं कथ्यतेऽत्र विनिश्चय: ॥ (शा.सं.पू.खं.१)

२. न हि विषमविकृति समवेतानां नानात्मकानां परस्परोपगृहीतानां चान्यैश्च
विकल्पनैर्विकल्पितानामवयव प्रभावानुमानेन समुदायप्रभावतत्त्वमद्यवसितुं शक्यम् ।
तथाविधे हि समुदाये समुदय प्रभावमेवोपलभ्य व्याध्यौषधप्रभावतत्त्वमवगच्छेत् । (अ.सं.सू. २३)

३. विरुद्धगुण संयोगे भूयोऽल्पसां हि जीयते । (अ.हृ.सू.)

४. संयोगस्तु द्वयोर्बहूनां वा द्रव्याणां संहतीभाव: स विशेषमारभते यं पुनर्नैकैकशो
द्रव्याण्यारभन्ते; तद्यथा मधुसर्पिषो:, मधुमत्स्यपयसां च । (च.वि.१)

6. According to the processing - Choushashta prahara pippali, Yakrita pippali, Puta pakwa vishama jwarantaka louha etc.

Some hints on herbal formulations in drug industry:

(i) Number of herbal ingredients– This must be kept to a minimum subject to efficacy and safety of the formulation. In western countries, the trend is

(a) 50% formulations - Single herb
(b) 25% formulations - Two herbs
(c) 15% formulations - Three herbs
(d) 10% formulations - More than three herbs

(ii) Herbal ingredients selection– This should be done after study of relevant literature of the herbs said to be useful in the type of formulation intended. Formulator, based on his literature survey or experience.

(iii) Dosages– should be minimum therapeutic as given in any standard pharmacopocia or scientific work relating to drugs of reputed authors or a scientific study, or in scientific journals of repute connected with herbs.

(iv) Safety and efficacy of formulation– Before a formulation is marketed, it must be subjected to pharmacological, toxicological and clinical tests to ensure its safety and efficacy.

(v) Category of formulations– Should be decided after consideration of the type of product and market.

The author feel it necessary to look into the validity of most of the patent formulations. For examples, Gymnema sylvestre may be hypoglycaemic when used alone. In combination its utility is very less in classical books.

3. The parts used in Herbal Medicine

Useful parts of Plants:

Various parts of the plants are used in therapeutics. Even the properties and effects will vary from one part of the plant to another e.g.

Pippali Pippalimula; Gunja beeja- Gunja mula; Kadali kanda-Kadali phala etc.

Charaka quoted the following among the oudbhida gana. They are all different useful parts of the plants. They include:

(1) Mula (root) (2) Twak (bark) (3) Sāra (heart wood) (4) Niryasa (resin or gum-resin) (5) Nāla (tubes) (6) Swarasa (Juice) (7) Pallava (tender leaves) (8) Kshara (alkalies) (9) Ksheera (latex) (10) Phala (fruit) (11) Pushpa (flower) (12) Bhasma (ash) (13) Taila (oil) (14) Kantaka (spines/thorns) (15) Patra (leaf) (16) Sunga (terminal budgs) (17) Kanda (tubers and rhizomes) (18) Praroha (climbers)[1]

Sarangdhara provided certain examples for the useful parts[2]:

1. Twak (bark)	-	Nyagrodha (Banyan trcet) etc.
2. Sāra (heart wood)	-	Beejaka (Pterocarpus morsupium) etc.
3. Patra (leaves)	-	Talisa (Taxus buccata) etc.
4. Phala (Fruit)	-	Triphala (Three myrobalons) etc.
5. Pushpa (Flower)	-	Dhataki (Woodfordia fruiticosa) etc.
6. Ksheera (Latex)	-	Snuhi (Euphorbia nerifolia) etc
7. Sākha (Stem)	-	Guduchi (Tinospora cardifolia) etc.
8. Niryasa (Resin)	-	Hingu (Ferula asefoetida) etc

Kaiyadeva defined the following as the 'Panchangas' and 'Dasangas' (five parts and ten parts)[3]:

(a) Pushpa (flower) (b) Phala (fruit) (c) Twak (bark) (d) Mula (root) and (e) Patra (leaf)- these five are Panchangas. The above five along with - (&) Sāra (heart wood) (g) Niryasa (resin or gum) (h) Sakha (Stem) (i) Sunga (terminal bud) and (j) Kshira (latex)- are known as Dasangas.

---

१. मूलत्वक्सारनिर्यासनालस्वरसपल्लवा: । क्षारा: क्षीरं फलं पुष्पं भस्मतैलानि कण्टका: ॥
पत्राणि शुङ्गा कन्दाश्च प्ररोहाश्चौद्भिदो गण: । (च.सू. १/७३-७४)

२. न्यग्रोधादेस्त्वचो ग्राह्यास्सारं स्याद्बीजकादित: । तालीसादेश्च पत्राणि फलंस्यत्रिफलादित: ॥
धातक्यादेश्च पुष्पाणि स्नुह्यादेक्षीरमाहरेत् । शाखां गुडूचिकादेस्तु निर्यासं रामठादित: ॥ (शा.सं.पू.खं.१)

३. पञ्चाङ्गञ्च तरो: पुष्प फलत्वङ् मूलपत्रकै: । दशाङ्गं सार निर्यास शाखा शुङ्गपयोऽन्वितै: ॥
क्वचिच्छाखापय:स्थाने वृन्तकण्टौ प्रकीर्तितौ । (कै.नि. ८/७-८)

The general rule is that if the root is very big in size then the root bark is to be collected. If the root is small and minute then entire root may be collected[1-2].

Charaka categorized drugs on the basis of useful part[3].

(a) Mulini - 16 drugs
(b) Phalini - 19 drugs
(c) Sodhana - 6 drugs

(a) Mulini– Hastidanti, Haimavati (Vacha), Trivrit, Shyama, Snuhi, Saptala, Sweta, Apamarga, Gavakshi, Jyotishmati, Bimbi, Sanapushpi, Vishanika (Sarkata sringi), Aja gandha, Dravanti & Kshirini.

(b) Phala & Mula– Snuhi, Arka, Asmantaka

(c) Twak– Putika, Krishna gandha, Tilvaka

Sushrita advocated fruit as useful part from Vidari gandhadi gana to Kovidaradi gana. From kovidarādi gaṇa onwards root is the useful part[4].

Useful parts of Animals

The following have been mentioned as Jangama dravyas by charaka. They are used medicinaly for various purposes[5].

(i) Madhu (honey), (ii) Gorasa (milk products etc.) (iii) Pitta (bile) (iv) Vasa (lard) (v) Majja (bone marrow) (vi) Rakta (blood) (vii) Mamsa

---

१. अतिस्थूलजटायास्युस्तासां ग्राह्यान्त्यस्त्वचो बुधैः ।
गृह्णीयात्सूक्ष्ममूलानि सकलान्यपि बुद्धिमान् । (शा.सं.पू.खं.१)

२. महान्ति येषां मूलानि काष्ठगर्भाणि सर्वतः ।
तेषां तु वल्कलं ग्राह्यं ह्रस्वमूलानि सर्वशः ॥ (भा.प्र.पू.खं.५प्र./१११-११२)

३. मूलिन्यः षोडशैकोना फलिन्यो विंशतिः स्मृताः ॥
महास्नेहांश्च चत्वारः पञ्चैव लवणानि च ।.........
....शोधनार्थाश्च षड् वृक्षाः पुनर्वसुनिदर्शिताः । (च.सू. १/७४-७६)
*चक्रपाणिः- मूलं प्रशस्ततमं यासां ता मूलिन्यः, एवं फलिन्योऽपि ।

४. तत्र कोविदारपूर्वाणां फलानि, कोविदारादीनां मूलानि । (सु.सू. ४१)

५. न्यग्रोधादेस्त्वचो ग्राह्याः सारस्याद्बीजकादितः । तालीसादेश्च पत्राणि फलंस्यात्रिफलादितः ॥
क्वचिन्मूलं क्वचित्कन्दः क्वचित्पत्रं क्वचित्फलम् । क्वचित्पुष्पं क्वचित्सर्वं क्वचित्सारः क्वचित्त्वचः ॥
चित्रकं सूरणं, निम्बो, वासा च त्रिफला क्रमात् । धातकी कण्टकारी च खदिरः क्षीरपादपः ॥
क्वचिन्निम्बस्य गृह्णीयात्पत्राभावे त्वचामपि ।
बालं फलं तु बिल्वस्य पक्वमारग्वधस्य च ॥ (भा.प्र.पू.खं.५प्र./११३-११६)

(meat) (viii) Vit (faeces) (ix) Mutra (unine) (x) Varcha (xi) Sukra (semen) (xii) Asthi (bone) (xiii) Snayu (ligament) (xiv) Sunga (horns) (xv) Nakha (nails) (xvi) Khura (hoofs)[1].

4. Combination of drugs and Incompatibility

Different combinations of drugs have been discussed in the previous pages. Here certain examples are provided.

(1) Herbals

(i) Single– Pushkara mula churna, Āmalaki churna, Yashti churna etc.

(ii) Compound

Two–	Punarnava dwayam, Balā dwayam etc.
Three–	Triphala, Trikatu etc
Four–	Chaturjataka, Chaturbhodra etc.
Five–	Panchakola, Pancha mula etc
Six–	Shadushana, Shadanga paniya etc.
Seven–	Rasna saptaka kwatha etc.
Eight–	Punarnavashtaka kwatha etc.
Ten–	Dasamula kwatha, etc
Many–	Avipattikara churna, Pushyanuga churna etc.

(2) Minerals

(i) Bhasmas- Swarna, Loha, Abhraka etc.

(ii) Khalviya Yogas- Kajjali, Tarakeswara rasa etc.

(iii) Kupi pakwa rasa- Rasa Sindura, Makara dhwaja etc.

(3) Herbo-minerals

(i) Churnas- Navayasa churna, Bhaskara Lavana churna etc.

(ii) Vati- Chandraprabha vati, Saptamrita loha etc

(iii) Guggulu- Maha yoga raja guggulu, Simhanada guggulu etc.

(iv) Lehyas- Gandhaka Rasayana etc.

(v) Ghrita- Nārasimha ghrita, Jātyadi ghrita etc.

(vi) Āsavas- Lohāsava, Kumaryasava etc.

---

१. मधूनि गोरसाः पित्तं वसा मज्जाऽसृगामिषम् । विट् मूत्र वर्च रेतोऽस्थि स्नायु शुङ्ग नखाः खुराः ॥
जङ्गमेभ्यः प्रयुज्यन्ते केशा लोमानि रोचनाः । (च.सू.१)

Among these compound preparations some of them are 'mixtures' and some are 'compound drugs'. For examples the churnas and gutikās are mixtures while Kwathas, Āsavas, Lehyas etc., may form compounds.

Incompatibility *(Viruddhatwam)*

Āhara includes both foods and drugs. Some of these substances will stimulate the doshas and activate them towards pathological state. Therefore they become harmful to the body tissues and systems. These are all known as Viruddha dravyas or Ahita dravyas[1]. The same is known as incompatibility in modern science.

Incompatibility is the state which renders admixture of remedies unsuitable through chemical action, insolubility or formation of poisonous compounds. In other words, it is the quality of not being mixed without chemical changes, or without antagonizing the action of ingredients in a compound.

Physiological incompatibility is a condition in which one or more substances in a mixture have a different physiological action than other substances in the mixture.

These Viuddha dravyas neither can act as Samana nor as Sodhana. But they possess qualities which are opposite to tissues (dhatus). Viruddhatwa occurs as one of the potent qualities which are opposite to one another. It does not occur in the case of ordinary qualities. The reason for viruddhatwa may be either Vishamatwa, Samatwa, Vishama-Samatwa, Samskara, Matra, Desa, Kala, Samyoga, Swabhava etc.

Hemadri clarified that Samana and Sodhana does not fall under viruddha category. This is because Sodhana will expel the vitiated

---

१. (i) यत् किञ्चिद्दोषमास्राव्य (दोषमुत्क्लेश्य) न निर्हरति कायतः ।
आहारजातं तत् सर्वं अहितायोपपद्यते । (च.सू. २६/८५)
*चक्रपाणि:- आह्रियत इत्याहारो भेषजमपि ।
(ii) शरीरधातु विरोधं कुर्वन्तीति वैरोधिका: । (चक्रपाणि-च.सू. २६/८०)
(iii) उत्क्लेश्य दोषान्न हरेद्द्रव्यं यत्तत्समासतः । विरुद्धं तद्धि धातूनां प्रत्यनीकतया स्थितम् ॥
बलिनां मिथो गुणानां विषमतया समतयाप्युभताऽपि ।
संस्मारादिवशादपि भवति निसर्गादपि विरोधः ॥ (अ.सं.९अ.)
(iv) यत्किञ्चिद्दोषमुत्क्लेश्य न हरेत्तत्समासतः ॥
विरुद्धम् ....। (अ.हृ.सू.७/४५-४६)

doshas completely. On the other hand Samana dravyas will subside the vitiated doshas without expulsion. But viruddha dravya does not have either of these qualities. It can only vitiate the dhatus[1].

He further described that Viruddhatwa may act as slow poisoning (chronic poisoning). Certain viruddha dravyas however may lead to death immediately also[2].

The incompatibilites (viruddhatwa) may be of different types. It may occur due to opposite qualities, improper drug combinations, unwanted modcifications in original qualities; due to effect of area, time and dose. Some time even natural incompatibility may also be seen[3].

Different types of Viruddhatwa

Charaka mentioned 18 types of viruddhatwa for Āhara (food) and oushadha (drugs) dravyas. They are[4]:

(1) Dēsa Viruddha: ***(Incompatibility dependent on area)***

As per the area certain substance may not be used in that area e.g. usage of Ruksha, Tikshna dravyas in Jangala desa; usage of snigdha, Seeta dravyas in Ānupa desa[5].

(2) Kāla viruddha: ***(Incompatibility dependent on time)***

According to season certain substances are fore bidden e.g. using Seeta, Ruksha dravyas in winter; using hot and pungent materials in summer[6].

---

१. यत्किञ्चिद्द्रव्यं दोषमुत्क्लेशयति न तु निर्हरति, तत्सर्वं विरुद्धम् । शोधनमप्युत्क्लेशयति परं निर्हरति, शमनमपि न निर्हरति' परं नोत्क्लेशयति, इति न तयोर्विरुद्धत्वम् । (हेमाद्रि-अ.हृ.सू.७)

२. "विरुद्धमपि चाहारं विद्याद्विषगरोपमम् ।" कस्यचिद्विरूद्धाहारस्य विषवत्सद्योमारकत्वात्कस्यचित् गरवत्कालान्तरनाशकत्वाद्रोगजनकत्वाच्चोपमानद्वयमुक्तम् । (हेमाद्रि-अ.हृ.सू.७)

३. देहधातुप्रत्यनीकभूतानि द्रव्याणि देहधातुभिर्विरोधमापद्यन्ते; परस्परगुणविरुद्धानि कानिचित्, कानिचित् संयोगात् , संस्कारादपराणि, देशकालमात्रादिभिश्चापराणि, तथा स्वभावादपराणि ॥(च.सू. २६/८१)
*चक्रपाणि:-विरोधश्च विरुद्धगुणत्वे सत्यपि क्वचिदेव द्रव्यप्रभावाद्भवति; तेन षड्रसाहारोपयोगे मधुराम्लयोर्विरुद्धशीतोष्णवीर्यविरोधो नोद्भावनीय: ।

४. यच्चापि देश-काल-अग्नि-मात्रा—सात्म्य-अनिलादिभि: । संस्कारतो-वीर्यतश्च-कोष्ठ-अवस्था-क्रमैरपि ॥
परहािर-उपचाराभ्यां-पाकात्-संयोगतोऽपि च ।
विरुद्धं तच्च न हितं हृत्-संपत् विधिभिश्च यत् ॥ (च.सू. २६/८६-८७)

५. विरुद्धं देशतस्तावद्रूक्षतीक्ष्णादि धन्वति । आनूपे स्निग्धशीतादि भेषजं यन्निषेव्यते ॥(च.सू. २६/८८)

६. कालतोऽपि विरुद्धं यच्छीतरूक्षादिसेवनम् ।
शीते काले, तथोष्णे च कुटकोष्णादिसेवनम् ॥ (च.सू.२६/८९)

(3) Agni viruddha: ***(Incompatibility dependent on digestion)***

Consuming food drug without assessing the digestive function (Agni) e.g. over eating when there is Agni Mandya etc[1].

(4) Matra viruddha: ***(Incompatibility dependent on dose)***

Certain substances can not be mixed and used in equal quantities e.g. honey and ghee should not be used in equal quantities (by volume)[2].

(5) Sātmya viruddha: ***(Incompatibility dependent on habit)***

When an individual is habituated to a particular types of food and exercise, advising opposite food etc., will lead to incompatibility e.g. the person who is habituated to pungent and hot substances consuming sweet and cold substances[3].

(6) Dosha viruddha: ***(Incompatibility dependent on humors)***

When the food or drugs which aggravate respective doshas are used against contraindications e.g. in Vata prakriti or Vata vriddhi or Vata roga, usage of foods and drugs aggravating Vata etc[4].

(7) Samskara viruddha: ***(Incompatibility dependent on procedures)***

Certain procedures of coocking etc., will bring about incompatibility e.g. peacock meat should not be fried in castor oil and by using a lead rod for roasting it[5].

(8) Virya viruddha: ***(Incompatibility dependent on potency)***

Two different potencies should not be mixed directly e.g. one Ushna virya and one Seeta virya dravya mixed and used together[6].

(9) Koshta viruddha: ***(Incompatibility dependent on GIT)***

The administration of drug must be in accordance to the condition

---

१. विरुद्धमनले तद्वदन्नपानं चतुर्विधे । (च.सू. २६/९०)
२. मधुसर्पि: समघृतं मात्रया तद्विरूध्यते ॥ (च.सू. २६/९०)
३. कटुकोष्णादिसात्म्यस्य स्वादुशीतादिसेवनम् ।यत्तत् सात्म्यविरुद्धं तु ....॥ (च.सू. २६/९१)
४. ....विरुद्धंत्वनिलादिभि: ॥ या समानगुणाभ्यासविरुद्धानौषधक्रिया । (च.सू. २६/९१-९२)
५. संस्कारतो विरुद्धं तद्यद्भोज्यं विषवद्भवेत् ॥
एरण्डसीसकासक्तं शिखिमांसं यथैव हि । (च.सू.२६/९२-९४)
६. विरुद्धं वीर्यतो ज्ञेयं वीर्यत: शीतलात्मकम् ॥
तत् संयोज्योष्णवीर्येण द्रव्येण सह सेव्यते । (च.सू. २६/९३-९४)

of Koshta (GIT). e.g., using a mild laxative in chronic and severe constipation; using drastic purgative in mild constipation[1].

(10) Avasthā viruddha: ***(Incompatibility dependent on condition)***

Using substances or advising exercises etc., irrespective of condition of the individual e.g., administering Vata varddhaka dravyas to a severely exhausted person; advising Kapha vardhaka food to individual who is sleepy and lazy etc[2].

(11) Krama viruddha: ***(Incompatibility dependent on behaviour)***

Violation of certain physiological behaviours may lead to incompatibility e.g. forcefully suppressing natural urges while eating (i.e., not evacuating bowels and bladder before food) etc[3].

(12) Parihāra viruddha: ***(Incompatibility dependent on parihara)***

After a particular diet certain things are to be avoided inorder to avoid incompatibility. If that is not avoided it leads to incompatibility e.g., after consuming pork, hot water should not be taken[4].

(13) Upachara viruddha: ***(Incompatibility dependent on upahara)***

After a particular diet certain things are advised to be consumed in order to vaoid incompatibility. If that is not followed it may lead to in compatibility e.g., after consuming ghee hot water should be taken instead if cold water is taken it amounts to Upahara viruddha[5].

[**Note:** There is only minute difference between Parihara and Upahara viruddha. Former one deals with the fore bidden things after consuming a particular diet etc. While later deals with opposite procedure after a particular diet is taken.]

---

१. क्रूरकोष्ठस्य चात्यल्पं मन्दवीर्यमभेदनम् ॥ मृदुकोष्ठस्य गुरू च भेदनीयं तथा बहु ।
एतत् कोष्ठ विरुद्धं तु ....॥ (च.सू. २६/९४-९५)

२. ....विरुद्धं स्यादवस्थया ॥
श्रमव्यवायव्यायामसक्तस्यानिलकोपनम् ।
निद्रालसस्यालस्य भोजनं श्लेष्मकोपनम् ॥ (च.सू.२६/९५-९६)

३. यच्चानुत्सृज्य विण्मूत्रं भुङ्क्ते यश्चाबुभुक्षितः ।
तच्च क्रमविरुद्धं यस्याद्यच्चातिक्षुद्वशानुगः ॥ (च.सू.२६/९७)

४. परिहारविरुद्धं च वराहादीन्निषेव्य यत् । सेवेतोष्णं................................॥ (च.सू. २६/९८)

५. ....घृतादीश्चं पीत्वा शीतं निषेवते ॥ (च.सू. २६/९८)

(14) Pāka viruddha: ***(Incompatibility while coocking)***

Certain wrong procedures in coocking may lead to incompatibility e.g.: under coocked rice or over roasted rice etc[1].

(15) Samyoga viruddha: ***(Incompatibility of combinations)***

Certain combinations may result in incompatibility e.g. combination of milk and sour substances[2].

(16) Hrit viruddha: ***(Incompatibility of mind or heart)***

Things which are not pleasant to the mind or things which are not good for heart. e.g. phobia towards pasticular sights, objects etc[3].

(17) Sampat viruddha: ***(Incompatibility dependent on quality)***

If a substance will have opposite taste etc., than its original taste etc., then it is known as Sampat Viruddha. In this the original qualities of a substance will be found indifferent[4].

(18) Vidhi viruddha: ***(Incompatibility dependent on eating procedure)***

There are certain restrictions imposed over the procedure of eating e.g.: one should not eat alone; one should not laugh or speak while eating etc[5].

Charaka delineated certain exceptions where incompatibility does not affect individuals:

(i) due to habitual usage (Sātmya) (ii) due to little quantity (Alpata) (iii) due to good appetite (Deeptagni) (iv) due to young age (Taruna) (v) due to oleation (Sneha) (vi) due to regular exercise (Vyayma)[6].

Diseases caused by incompatibility

Impotency (Shandya), blindness (Andhya), herpes (Visarpa), ascites (Dakodara), erysepalas (Visphota), Schizophrenia (Unmada),

---

१. विरुद्धंपाकतश्चापि दुष्टदुर्दारूसाधितम् । अपक्वतण्डुलात्यर्थपक्वदग्धं च यद्भवेत् ॥ (च.सू. २६/९९)

२. संयोगतो विरुद्धं तद्यथाऽम्लं पयसा सह । (च.सू. २६/१००)

३. अमनोरुचितं यच्च हृद्विरूद्धं तदुच्यते ॥ (च.सू. २६/१००)

४. संपद्विरुद्धं तद्विद्यादसंजातरसं तु यत् । अतिक्रान्तरसं वाऽपि विपन्नरसमेव वा ॥ (च.सू. २६/१००)

५. ज्ञेयं विधिविरुद्धं तु भुज्यते निभृते न यत् । तदेवं विधमन्नं स्याद्विरुद्धमुपयोजितम् ॥ (च.सू. १६/१०२)

६. सात्म्यतोऽल्पतया, वाऽपि दीप्ताग्नेस्तरुणस्य च ।
स्नेहव्यायामबलिनो विरुद्धं वितथं भवेत् ॥ (च.सू. २६/१०६)

fistula-in-ano (Bhagandara), Syncope (Murcha), stupor (Mada), flatulance (Ādhmāna), throat pain (Gala graha), anaemia (Pandu), autoimmunity (Āma visha), leucoderma (Kilasa), skin diseases (Kushta), malabsorption syndromes (Grahani), edema and inflammation (Sotha), hyperacidity (Amlapitta), fever (Jwara), rhinitis (Peenasa), heriditary problems (Santana dosha) and death (Mrityu) ultimately may result due to incompatibility[1].

5. Posology: *(Oushadha Mātrā)*

(i) **Posology** is a Greek word meaning that– Posos = how much and logos = a study.

Posology is the branch of scientific study dealing with dosage.

(ii) **Dose** is originated from a Greek word *Dosis* meaning that "the amount of medicinal preparation to be taken at one time". There are different terms used for dose–

(a) *Divided dose* Fractional portions administered at short intervals.

(b) *Lethal dose*– A fatal dose

(c) *Maximum dose*– Largest dose that is safe to adminis- .ter.

(d) *Minimum dose*– Smallest dose that will be effective.

(iii) **Dosage** is the amount of medicine to be administered to a patient at one time.

(1) For children under 1 year (Freid's Rule)

$$\frac{\text{Age in months}}{150} \times \text{Adult dose} = \text{child's dose}$$

e.g. If the adult dose of morphine sulphate is 250 mg, then the dose for a 8 month old child will be

१. षाण्ढ्यान्ध्यवीसर्पदकोदराणां विस्फोटकोन्मादभगन्दराणाम् ।
मूर्च्छामदाध्मानगलग्रहाणां पाण्ड्वामयस्यामविषस्य चैव ॥
किलासकुष्ठग्रहणीगदानां शोथाम्लपित्त ज्वरपीनसानाम् ।
सन्तानदोषस्य तथैव मृत्योर्विरुद्धमन्नं प्रवदन्ति हेतुम् ॥ (च.सू. २६/१०२)

8/150 x 250 = 13.33 mg.

(2) For children from 1-12 years (Young's formula)

$$\frac{\text{Age in years}}{\text{Age+12}} \times \text{Adult dose} = \text{child's dose}$$

e.g. If the adult dose of morphine sulphate is 250 mg, then the dose for a 4 year old child will be 4/4+12 x 25- = 62.5 mg

(3) For childern Cow ling's Rule Adult dose x Age+1/24

Dilling's formula Adult dose x Age/20

The median Effective Dose or ED_{50}

This is the dose (mg/kg) which produces a described response in 50% of the total population.

The median Lethal Dose or LD_{50}

This is the dose (mg/kg) which produces death to 50% of the total population.

Concept of Dosage in Ayurveda

(1) Oushadha Matra: *(Dosage of drugs)*

Sarangdhara clearly stated that there is no specific dose for every one. To decide the dose individually, Kala-Agni-Vayah-Bala-Prakriti-Dosha-Desa are to be considered. Then only the dose is finalized[1].

He further mentioned the following dosage as per the age:

Child	1st month	125 mg (Ratti)
	2nd month to 1 year	an increase of 125 gm every month upto one year i.e., 250 gm to 1.5 gm.
	1 year to 16 year	Add one gm (1 Masha) each year i.e., at 16 years 16.5 gm dosage.
	16 to 70 years	Same dose.

There after dose is to be reduced back to the dosage of a infant in

१. स्थितिर्नास्त्येव मात्रायाः कालमग्निं वयो बलम् ।।
प्रकृतिं दोषदेशौ च दृष्ट्वा मात्रां प्रकल्पयेत् । (शा.सं.प्र.खं. १/३७-३८)

as decreasing order after 70 years and upto 80 years[1].

The details of dosage according to Sarngdhar are as following:

1st month - 125 mg	11th month - 1375 mg	12 year - 12.5 gm
2nd month- 250 mg	1 year - 1500 mg	13 " - 13.5 gm
3rd " - 375 mg	2 " - 2.5 gm	14 " - 14.5 gm
4th " - 500 mg	3 " - 3.5 gm	15 " - 15.5 gm
5th " - 625 mg	4 " - 4.5 gm	16 " to - 16. gm Kalka or Churna
	5 " - 5.5 gm	70 year
6th " - 750 mg	6" - 6.5 gm	71 years - 64-66 ml Kashaya
	7" - 7.5 gm	
7th " - 875 mg	8 " - 6.5 gm	71 years - 15.5 gm
8th " - 1000 mg (1gm)	9 " - 9.5 gm	72 " - 14.5 gm
		73 " - 13.5 gm
		74 " - 12.5 gm
9th " - 1125 mg	10 " - 10.5 gm	75 " - 11.5 gm
10th " - 1250 mg	11 " - 11.5 gm	76 years - 10.5 gm
		77 " - 9.5 gm
		78 " - 8.5 gm
		79 " - 7.5 gm
		80 " - 6.5 gm

[***Note:** These dosages are meant for kalka and churna. For kashaya preparations 4 times the above dosage is recommended.]

---

१. बालस्य प्रथमेमासि देया भेषजरक्तिका ।। अवलेहीकृतैकैव क्षीरक्षौद्रसिताघृतैः ।
वर्धयेत्तावदेकैकां यावद्भवति वत्सरः ।।
माषैवृद्धिस्तदूर्ध्वं स्याद्यावत्षोडशवत्सरः । ततः स्थिरा भवेत्तावद्यावद्वर्षाणि सप्ततिः ।।
ततो बालकवन्मात्रा ह्रासनीया: शनैः शनैः ।
मात्रेयं कल्कचूर्णानां कषायाणां चतुर्गुणा ।। (शा.सं.पू.खं. ६/१४-१७)

Kashyapa advocated the following dosage for paediatric uses:

(i) Navajata Sisu (neonate)– Vidanga phala tulya (equal to the weight of Embelia ribes fruit)

(ii) After wards the above dose is gradvally increased as the maximum dose should not exced the weight of Āmalaki (Amla fruit).

In Khila Sthan he mentioned another dosage pattern for children (Ka.Sam.Khila.Sthana 77-86).

(1) Immediately after birth (before 5 days)	-	Badari phala beeja tulya (weight equal to that of the seed of Zizuphus fruit)
(2) 5-10 days	-	slightly increased dose.
(3) 10-20 days	-	Equal to half of the Zizyphus friut
(4) 1 month	-	Equal to Zizyphus fruit
(5) 1-2 months	-	$1\frac{1}{2}$ Zizyphus fruits quantity.
(6) 3 months	-	2 " " "
(7) 4 months	-	Equal to dry Amla fruit quantity
(8) 5-6 months	-	Equal to Amla fruit
(9) 7-8 months	-	More than Amla fruit

Charaka quoted that the drug given to a child must be of low potency and its quantity as well as frequency of administration must be less (cha.chi. 30/282).

Sushrita Advised the following dosage patterns as per the age groups of children: (su.sa. 10/43)

(a) Ksheerapa (1 year)	-	one pinch
(b) Ksheerannada (2 years)	-	equal to Zizyphus seed quantity
(c) Annāda (Above 2 years)	-	equal to Zizyphus fruit quantity.

***Note:** This dose shall be increased as per the age of the individual throughout life. Only after 70 years the dose may be reduced.

Importance of fixation of specific dose

Deciding the dosage of a drug plays an important role in the treatment. Dosage must be decided on the basis of vyadhi bala, Agni bala and Rogi bala. If the drug is used on excessive quantity or with more potency in less severe pathological status, then the original disease may be subsided but the excessive quantity of drug remained in the body may lead to other complications. Similary if a drug is used when the enzymatic activity is dorment, then it is not metabolized properly and leads to reduction of appetite or digestion (Ajeerna) and constipation (vishtambha). If a very potent drug is administed to a weak person who can not tolerate the severity of the drug it may lead to complications again. Even larger doses of a common drug may also produce Glani (weakness), Murcha (syncope) and Mada (stupor). There fore the drug must be used in proper dose[1].

Dosage of Sodhana dravyas

(1) Vamana Dravya: *(Emetics)*

(i) Many Acharyas considered Mushti Pramaana (first full) as the dosage of Vamana dravya

(ii) Dalhana considered that churna (powder) should be given in Prakuncha or Pala mātra (40gm). This is Madhyama matra (medium dose) for emesis[2].

(iii) If Kalka (paste), churna (powder) or Avaleha (linctus) are to be used then:

3 pala (120 gm)	-	maximum (Uttama)
2 pala (80 gm)	-	average (Madhyama)
1 pala (40 gm)	-	minimum (Alpa)

१. तत्र सर्वाण्येवौषधानि व्याध्यग्निपुरुषबलान्यभिसमीक्ष्य विदध्यात् । तत्र, व्याधिबलादधिकमौषधमुपयुक्तं तमुपशम्य व्याधिं व्याधिमन्यमावहन्ति; अग्निबलादधिकमजीर्णं विष्टभ्य वा पच्यते; पुरुषबलादधिकं ग्लानिमूर्च्छामदानावहति संशमनम्; एवं संशोधनमतिपातयति । हीनमेभ्यो दत्तमकिञ्चित्करं भवति । तस्मात् सममेव विदध्यात् ॥
रोगे शोधनसाध्ये तु यो भवेद्दोषदुर्बलः । तस्मै दद्याद्भिषक् प्राज्ञो दोषप्रच्यावनं मृदु ॥
चले दोषे मृदौ कोष्ठे नेक्षेतात्र बलं नृणाम् । अव्याधिदुर्बलस्यापि शोधनं हि तदा भवेत् ॥
स्वयं प्रवृत्तदोषस्य मृदुकोष्ठस्य शोधनम् । भवेदल्पबलस्यापि प्रयुक्तं व्याधिनाशनम् ॥
व्याध्यादिषु तु मध्येषु क्वाथस्याञ्जलिरिष्यते ।
बिडालपदकं चूर्णं देयः कल्कोऽक्षसंमितः ॥ (सु.सू. ३९/१०-१४)

२. चूर्णप्रकुञ्चं पुनरस्य मध्यमा मात्रा; प्रकुञ्चः पलं, 'मुष्टिः' इत्येके । ....अन्तर्नखमुष्टिमिति नखानां मध्ये मुष्टिर्न तु पारिभाषिका पलाभिधाना, अन्तर्नखमुष्टिं यष्टीमधुककषाये आतुरं पाययेदिति संबन्धः॥ (डल्हण)

(iv) If liquids (Drava dravyas) are to be used then

9 Prastha - maximum (Uttama)

6 Prastha - Average (Madhyama)

3 Prastha - Minimum (Alpa)

(2) Virechana Dravya: *(Purgatives)*

	Usual dose	for Kashaya	for Kalka & Churna
Maximum (Uttama)	4 prastha	2 pala (80 ml)	4 karsha (1 pala)
Average (Madhyama)	3 prastha	1 pala (40 ml)	2 karsha
Minimum (Alpa)	2 prastha	1/2 pala (20 ml)	1 karsha

(3) Vasthi Dravya: *(Enemata)*

According to age Niruha Vasthi dosage

1 year	-	$\frac{1}{2}$ Prasrita	(4 Tula)	-	(40 ml)
2 "	-	1 Prasruta	(8 Tula)	-	80 ml
3 "	-	$1\frac{1}{2}$ "	(12 ")	-	120 ml
4 "	-	2 "	(16 ")	-	160 ml
5 "	-	2.5 "	(20 ")	-	200 ml
6 "	-	3 "	(24 ")	-	240 ml
7 "	-	3.5 "	(28 ")	-	280 ml
8 "	-	4 "	(32 ")	-	320 ml
9 "	-	4.5 "	(36 ")	-	360 ml
10 "	-	5 "	(40 ")	-	400 ml
11 "	-	5.5 "	(44 ")	-	440 ml
12 "	-	6 "	(48 ")	-	480 ml
13 "	-	7 "	(56 ")	-	560 ml
14 "	-	8 "	(64 ")	-	640 ml
15. "	-	9 "	(72 ")	-	720 ml
16 "	-	10 "	(80 ")	-	800 ml
17 "	-	11 "	(88 ")	-	880 ml
18 "	-	12 "	(96 ")	-	960 ml
19-70 year	-	12 "	(96 ")	-	960 ml
Above 70 year	-	10 "	(80 ")	-	800 ml

* **Note:** The Maximum dose is 12 Prasrita (960 ml).

Usual dose of Kashaya Vathi

Maximum (Uttama)	-	12 Prasrita	(96 Tula) -	960 ml
Average (Madhyama)	-	8 " "	(64 Tula) -	640 ml
Minimum (Alpa)	-	4 " "	(48 Tula) -	480 ml

Usual dose of Sneha Vasthi

Maximum (Uttama)	-	24 Tula (240 ml)	-	Sneha vasthi
Average (Madhyama)	-	12 Tula (120 ml)	-	Anuvasana vasthi
Minimum (Alpa)	-	6 Tula (60 ml)	-	Mātra vasthi

(4) Nasya Dravya: ***(nasal drops)***

(i) Sneha Nasya	- Alpa (Minimum)	-	8 drops (8 Bindus)
	Madhyama (Average)	-	16 " (Sukti)
	Uttama (Maximum)	-	32 " (Pani Sukti)
(ii) Sodhana Nasya	- Alpa (Minimum)	-	4 drops
	Madhyama (Average)	-	6 "
	Uttama (Maximum)	-	8 "

[***Note:** This type of Nasya shall be used once in 3 days.]

(iii) Marsa Nasya	- Alpa (Minimum)	-	10 drops
	Madhyama (Average)	-	8 "
	Uttama (Maximum)	-	6 "

(iv) Prati-Marsa Nasya - 2 drops every day.

(5) Sneha Karma: ***(Internal oleation)***

Uttama Mātra	-	digested in 24 hrs.
Madhyama Mātra	-	digested in 12 hrs.
Alpa Mātra	-	digested in 6 hrs.
Hrasiyasi Mātra	-	test dose.

The fat may be given for 7 days in the following dose:

1st day	-	20-30 ml
2nd "	-	50-60 ml
3rd "	-	75-90 ml
4th "	-	100-120 ml

5th "	-	125-150 ml
6th "	-	150-180 ml
7th "	-	175-210 ml

Dosage of Samana Dravyas

(1)	Swarasa (fresh juice)	-	$^1/_2$ Pala i.e., 20 ml
(2)	Kalka (paste)	-	1 Karsha i.e., 10 gm
(3)	Kwatha (decoction)	-	1-2 Palas i.e., 40-80 ml
(4)	Churna (powder)	-	1 Karsha i.e., 10 gm
(5)	Asava & Arishta (fermented products)	-	1-4 Pala i.e., 40-160 ml.
(6)	Lehya (linctus)	-	1 Karsha i.e., 10 gm
(7)	Vati (tablets)	-	1 Masha i.e., 1 gm

[***Note:** The dose for vati may vary in certain circumstances e.g. Sanjivani vati in a size of abrus seed (125 mg); Agni tundi vati in a size of black pepper etc]

(2) Āhara Matra: ***(Dosage of food materials)***

Charaka advised that diet to be taken in appropriate quantity. The quantity of food is again depended upon Agni bala (digestive power)[1].

In this context Chakrapani clarified that Āhara matra (quantity of food) is three types viz., Uttama, Madhyama & Alpa depending upon the corresponding Agni bala. But oushadha matra (dosage of drugs) is based upon Vyadhi bala (severity of disease) and Ātura bala (strenght of the patient). Vyayama matra (amount of exercies) on the other hand depends upon Srama (tiredness), Klama (fatique) etc., which are produced by Dosha kshaya or Agni vriddhi. In this way the amount of Āhara, Vihara, Oushadha are discussed by Chakrapani.

---

१. मात्राशी स्यात् । आहारमात्रा पुनरग्निबलापेक्षिणी ॥ (च.सू. ५/३)
*चक्रपाणि- अग्नेर्बलमुत्कृष्टं मध्यमल्पं वाऽपेक्ष्योत्कृष्टा मध्याऽल्पा वा मात्रा भवतीत्यग्निबलापेक्षिणी । पुनः शब्दो भेषजादिमात्रां व्यायाममात्रां च व्यावर्तयति; तेन न सर्वमात्रा ऽग्निबलापेक्षणी; यतो भेषजमात्रा व्याध्यातुरबलापेक्षिणी व्यवस्थापितव्या । यदि वा पुनः शब्दः पौनः पुन्ये, तेनाहारमात्रा पुनः पुनरग्निबलमपेक्षते ।

Charaka described that the quantity of food shall be fixed according to each individual's capacity[1]. He again stated that the total quantity of food may be divided into two groups:

(i) Sarvagraha - total quantity of food to be taken.

(ii) Parigraha - quantity of each individual item to be taken in diet

Here Chakrapani elaborated the individual quantities of dietary ingredients for the first time.

(a) Anna (Rice) - 1 kudava/4pala (160 gm)

(b) Supa (Dal) - 1 pala (40 gm)

(c) Mamsa (curry or meat) - 2 pala (80 gm)

From the above description it is very clear that the 'Trividha kukshiyam' concept is not vague. The total quantity os solids amount to 280 gm according to the above caliculation. Equal amount of water is also allowed (i.e., 280 ml). This is the balanced diet according to Ayurveda.

(6) Vehicle *(Anupana)*

It is observed by the author that many students and teachers (apart from genrral public) are thinking that Anupana is meant for the administration of drugs. But on review of classical literature this openion is found to be incorrect.

The concept of Anupana is originally proposed for proper period of Sārngdhara only we find the references about Anupana for drugs. In the light of the author's detailed study on Anupana concept it will be really interesting to know about Anupana (Vehicle or Adjuvent).

The term vehicle is derived from the Latin word 'Vehiculum' meaning that "which carries". It is a substance used as a medium for the administration of medicine, as syrup in liquid preparations.

The term Adjuvent is also dervied from 'Adjuvans' in Latin meaning that "to aid". It is that which assists or a drug added to a prescrip-

---

१. यावद्ध्यशनमशितमनुपहत्य प्रकृतिं यथाकालं जरां गच्छति तावदस्य मात्राप्रमाणं वेदितव्यं भवति।। (च.सू. ५/४)

tion to hasten or increase the action of a principal ingredient. It can also be called as 'synergist'.

Different meanings have been given for the word 'Anupana' in the texts. Acharya P.V. Sharmaji defined it as the liquid medium used along with a drug[1]. However the original meaning of Anupana from ancient classics do not match with his descriptions. Dalhana very emphatically stated that Anupana means the liquid which is consumed after the diet is taken[2].

Adhamalla and Narahari have defined Anupana as the vehicle used after administering the drug[3].

Anupana for food

The medium which is dissimilar to food but not opposite to the qualities of tissues is known as Anupana. Some of the important Anupanas are - Āsava (ferments), Jala (water), Ksheera (milk) etc[4].

If Anupana is used after food the following benifits will be seen- Tarpana, Preenana, Oorjaskara, Brimhana, Tripti, Pachana, digestion, Mridutva, Kledana, Jarana, easy and complete digestion. Anupana will immediately provide nourishment to the individual, helps in easy digestion and enhances strength and age[5].

Anupana according to disease condition[6].

Vata rogas-snigdha & ushna padarthas

---

१. अनु सह पश्चात् वा पीयते इति अनुपानम् । (द्र.गु.वि. Vol. I)

२. अन्नादनु पश्चात् पीयत इत्यनुपानम् । (डल्हण-सु.सू. ४६/४१९)

३. (i) अनुपानमिति- 'अनु' पश्चात् पानं । (आढमल्लः- शा.सं.म.खं. ८/४)

(ii) अनुपानं- औषधाङ्ग पेयविशेषे । तच्च औषधपानान्तरं विलम्ब्य प्रयोज्यं, रात्तौ पुनः पाचनमेव व्यवस्थेयम्। "विलम्ब्या च क्रमाणमेतदीरितं रात्रौ पुनः पाचनमेतद्रचिरे"- इति रा.नि.व.०२०-१ (वैद्यकशब्दसिन्धुः)

४. यदाहारगुणैः पानं विपरीतं तदिष्ये । अन्नानुपानं धातूनां दृष्टं यन्न विरोधि च ॥ (च.सू. २७/३१९)

५. अथानुपानकर्मगुणान् प्रवक्ष्यामः- अनुपानं तर्पयति, प्रीणयति, ऊर्जयति, बृंहयति, पर्याप्तिमभिनिर्वर्तयति, भुक्तमवसादयति, अन्नसंघातं भिनत्ति, मार्दवमापादयति, क्लेदयति, जरयति, सुखपरिणामितामाशुव्यवायिवां चाहारस्योपजनयतीति॥

अनुपानं हितं युक्तं तर्पयत्याशु मानवम् ।
सुखं पचति चाहारमायुषे च बलाय च ॥ (च.सू.२७/३२५-३२६)

६. अतः सर्वानुपानान्युपदेक्ष्यामः............। (सु.सू. ४६/४१९-४४२)

Pitta rogas - Madhura & Seetala padarthas

Kapha rogas - Ruksha & Ushna padarthas

Kshaya (Dhatu kshaya) - Mamsa rasa (soups)

Exhausted by various reasons - Ksheera (milk)

Krisa (lean persons) - Sura (beverage)

Sthula (obese individual) - Madhu (honey)

Agnimandya (loss of appetite) etc - Madya (alcohol)

Contraindication for Arupana after food

Anupana can not be given to persons suffering from E.N.T. & ophthalmic problems, Hikka (hicough), Swasa (dyspnoea), kasa (cough), singers, dancers, students who read for a long time, Urah kshata (haemothorax etc)[1].

Vriddha Vagbhata considered water as the best vehicle as it is responsible for tastes and maintanance of life[2]. Laghu Vagbhata also discussed Anupana elaborately[3].

Anupāna for drugs

The concept of Anupana for drugs can be traced from the references of Sarngdhara and the Commentator on his work Adhamalla. Afterwards Lolambarajiya etc., texts have mentioned different Anupanas.

Sarngdhara quoted about the quantity of Anupana for Churnas (powders), Avaleha (linctus), Gutika (tablets & pills), kalka (paste) etc., according to the disease[4]. For example

Vata Roga	-	3 Pala (120 ml)
Pitta Roga	-	2 Pala (80 ml)
Kapha Roga	-	1 Pala (40 ml)

१. नोर्ध्वाङ्गमारूताविष्टा न हिक्काश्वासकासिनः । न गीतभाष्याध्ययनप्रसक्ता नोरसि क्षताः ॥
पिबेयुरूदकं भुक्त्वा तद्धि कण्ठोरसि स्थितम् ।
स्नेहमाहारजं हत्वा भूयो दोषाय कल्पते ॥ (च.सू. २७/३२७-३२८)

२. अनुपानं तु सलिलमेव श्रेष्ठं सर्वरसयोनित्वात्सर्वभूतसात्म्यत्वाज्जीवनादिगुणयोगाच्च। (अ.सं.सू. १०)

३. अनुपानं करोत्युर्जां तृप्तिं व्याप्तिं दृढाङ्गताम् ॥
अन्नसंघातशैथिल्य विक्लित्ति जरणानि च । (अ.हृ.सू. ८)

४. चूर्णावलेहगुटिकाकल्कानामनुपानकम् । वातपित्तकफातङ्के त्रेध्वेकपलमाहरेत ॥ (शा.सं.म.खं. ६/४)

In this context Adhamalla defined that any liquid medium which is used after administering the drug or alongwith the drug is known as Anupāna[1].

The Anupana is claimed to distribute the drug throughout the body within no time. It spreads like oil drop on water i.e., spreads in all directions fastly[2].

The drug will be reaching all the parts of the body by two effects of Anupana (i) Anupana Bala (strength of the vehicle) and (ii) Anupana Sakti (potency of the vehicle)[3].

We come across various references of Anupana for individual compound preparations in sarangadhara Sauhita and other texts. Some of them are:

(i) milk, ghee etc., for Avalehas[4].

(ii) Khadira and Asana kashaya for Pancha Nimba churna.

(iii) Sura (beverage) in case of Ādhmana (flatulance) while administering Nārayṇa churna.

(iv) For Loha Rasayana Triphala Kwatha and Guduchi Sattwa are the vehicles.

There are several examples for Anupana in Lolamba Rajiya (Sad vaidya Jeevanam)[5].

---

१. अनुपानमिति । अनुपश्चात्पानमौषधभक्षणोपरि यत्पीतं तदनुपानमित्यर्थः ।
........अनुक्तेष्वनुपानेषु जलानुपानं प्रशस्तम् । (आढमल्लः- शा.सं.म.खं. ६/४)

२. यथातैलं जले क्षिप्तं क्षणेनैव प्रसर्पति । अनुपानबलादङ्गे तथा सर्पति भेषजम् ॥ (शा.सं.म.खं. ६/५)

३. (i) अथानुपानस्य प्रयोजनं निर्देष्टुमाह यथेति ।
भिषजा संस्कृतं द्रव्यं तथा अङ्गेषु प्रसर्पति, कुतः? अनुपानबलादनुपानशक्तितः।(आढमल्लः ६/५)
(ii) अनुपानं प्रयोक्तव्यं देखकालाद्यपेक्षया इति ।
अनुपानमिति 'अनु पश्चात् पानं' । (आढमल्लः शा.सं.म.खं. ८/४)

४. (i) अवलेहे दुग्धादिर्यथायोग्यमनुपानम् । (वाचस्पति-शा.सं.म.खं. ८/४)
(ii) अनुपानान्याह- खदिरासनतोयेनेति । (आढमल्लः-शा.सं.म.खं. ३/१४२)
(iii) दद्याद्युक्तानुपानेनेति । युक्तानुपानमत्रैव कथ्यते तद्यथा-आध्माने सुरादिभिरिति ।
(iv) अनुपाने वराक्वाथं त्रिफलाक्वाथम्, छिन्नासत्त्वं गुडूचीसत्त्वं ।

५. (i) शूले हिङ्गुघृतान्वितम् ।
(ii) मधुयुता कृष्णा पुराणज्वरे ।
(iii) वाते साज्यरसोनकः ।
(iv) श्वसनके क्षौद्रान्वितं त्र्यूषणम् ।

क्रमशः पृष्ठ ३६१ में............

(1) Asefoetida (Hingu) and ghee (ghrita) in abdominal spasm (Sula).

(2) Honey (Madhu) and long pepper (Pippali) in Purana jwara (PUO).

(3) Ghee and Garlic (Lasuna) in Vāta vyadhis.

(4) Honey and Trikatu (Black pepper, long pepper & Ginger) in Swasanaka jwara (pneumonic fever)

(5) Chitraka leaf and Maricha in Seeta jwara.

(6) Triphala & sugar in Prameha (urinary tract diseases).

(7) Honey, Ginger and water for Sannipata rogas.

(8) Musta and Parpataka in fever.

(9) Takra (Butter milk) in Grahani (Mal-absorption syndromes)

(10) Gold (swarna) in visha rogas (poisoning cases)

[**Note:** The author is of the openion that 'Hema' is not gold but Dhattura in this context.]

(11) Lāja in vomiting (chardi)

(12) Kutaja (H. antidysenterica) in diarrhoea.

(13) Vāsa in Rakta pitta (haemorrhages)

(14) Chitra mula in Arsas (haemorrhoids)

[**Note:** Anala is the synonyms used for Bhallataka also Bhallatak may be the suitable example for this]

(15) Vidanga (E. ribes) in Krimi roga (worm infestations etc).

पृष्ठ ३६० से क्रमशः........

(v) शीते व्यांलतादलं समरिचम् ।

(vi) मेहे वरासोपला ।

(vii) दोषाणां त्रितयेऽनुपानमुचितं सक्षौद्रमार्द्रोदकम् ।

(viii) घनपर्पाटकं ज्वरे ।

(ix) ग्रहण्यां मथितम् ।

(x) हेम विषे ।

(xi) वमिषु लाजा ।

(xii) कुटजो अतिसृतौ ।

(xiii) वृषो अस्रपित्ते ।

(xiv) गुदकीलेषु अनलः ।

(xv) कृमी कृमिघ्नम् ।

(लोलम्बराजीयम्)

7. Times of drug administration

Different Acharyas have mentioned different drug administering times. The times of drug administration is a very important aspect since they are dependent up on the diurnal variations in the three humors (vata-pitta-kapha) both in the physiological and pathological state. The following types of drug administration timings are mentioned in the classics of Ayurveda[1].

Charaka (च.चि. ३०)	Suśruta (सु.उ. ६४)	V.Vagbhata (अ.सं.सू. २३)	L. Vagbhata (अ.हृ.सू. १३)	Sarngdhara (शा.सं.पू.खं. २)
1. Bhaktādi-I	1. Abhaktam	1. Abhaktam	1. Anannam	1. Suryodaya
2. Bhaktadi-II	2. Pragbh-aktam	2. Pragbh-aktam	2. Annadi	2. Divasa bhojana
3. Madhye bhakta	4. Madhye-bhakta	3. Madhya bhakta	3. Madhya bhakta	3. Sayam bhojana
4. Pratah Pas-chat bhakta	3. Adhobh-akta	4. Adhobh-akta	4. Pratah Anta bhakta	4. Muhur-muhu
5. Sayam Pas-chat bhakta	6. Antara bhakta	6. Ānantara-bhakta	11. Sayam Anta bhakta	5. Nisi -
6. Muhurmu-huh	8. Muhurmu-huh	8. Muhurmuhu	7. Muhuh	-
7. Sāmudgam	7. Sāmudgam	7. Sāmudgam	9. Sāmudga	
8. Bhakta Sayakta	6. Sabhak-tam	5. Sama bha-kta	8. Sānnam	-
9. Grāsam	9. Grāsam	9. Sagrāsam	6. Grase-Grase	-
10. Grāsānt-aram	10. Grasant-aram	10. Grasan-tara	5. Kavalan-tara	-
-	-	11.Nisi	10. Nisi	-

१. (i) भैषज्यकालो भक्तादौ मध्ये पश्चान्मुहुर्मुहुः ।
सामुद्गं भक्तसंयुक्तं ग्रासे ग्रासान्तरे दश ॥ (च.चि. ३०/२९८)

(ii) तत्राभक्तं, प्राग्भक्तं, अधोभक्तं, मध्येभक्तं, अन्तरभक्तं, सभक्तं, सामुद्गं, मुहुर्मुहुः, ग्रासं, ग्रासान्तरं चेति दशौषधकालाः ॥ (सु.उ. ६४/६५)

(iii) आतुरावस्थासु तु कालाकाल संज्ञा । तद्यथा अस्यामवस्थायामस्यौषधस्य-कालोऽकालो वा । नह्यप्राप्तातीतकालमौषधं यौगिकं भवति, तस्यत्वेकादशधाऽवचारणम् । तद्यथा-अभक्तं, प्राग्भक्तं, मध्यभक्तं, अधोभक्तं, समभक्तं, अनन्तरभक्तं, सामुद्गं, मुहुर्मुहुः, सग्रासं, ग्रासान्तरं, निशि च ॥ (अ.स.सू. २३)

क्रमशः पृष्ठ ३६३ में........

Adhamalla divided sarngdhara's five timings into 11 types namely, (1) Suryodaya (2) Bhojanagra (3) Bhojana Misra (4) Bhojana Madhya (5) Bhojananta (6) Bhojana Purvantam (7) Grasa (Bhaktadi) (8) Grasantara (Bhakta Madhya) (9) Bhaktānta (10) Vāram vāram (Muhurmuhuh) (11) Nisi. He sub-divided the 10th oushadha sevana kala into two viz., Sānnam and Nirannam.

Among different views, the times of adminstration are almost similar except that charaka and Suśruta did not mention 'Nisi' (11th Kāla).

As a general rules Sargdhara advised drug administration in the morning[1]. It appears that except multiple administrations like. Grasantara, Muhurmuhu etc. the drug administration may be done at once according to the disease condition. Most of the drugs are herbal compounds which are composed of polymolecular herbal compounds in raw-form. It will definitely take some time for absorption and metabolism of these molecules. Therefore are advised to use one bulk dose once in a day e.g. Kalka 10 gm (1 karsha), Kashaya 50-100ml etc. We do not come across the concept of divided doses in these contexts. Therefore further study is very essential. Sarngdhara's school of thought:

(i) First time

When there is pitta prakopa to perform Virechana, when there is Kapha prakopa to terform Vamana and to perform Lekhana karma the drug shall be administered early in the morning[2].

पृष्ठ ३६२ से क्रमशः............'

(iv) युञ्ज्यादनन्नमन्नादौ मध्येऽन्ते कवलान्तरे ।
ग्रासे ग्रासे महुः सान्नं सामुद्गं निशि चौषधम् ॥ (अ.हृ.सू. १३/३७)

(v) ज्ञेयः पञ्चविधः कालो भैषज्यग्रहणे नृणाम् ।
किञ्चित्सूर्योदये जाते तथा दिवसभोजने ॥
सायन्तने भोजने च महुश्चापि तथा निशि । (शा.सं.पू.खं. २/२-३)

१. भैषज्यमभ्यवहरेत्प्रभाते प्रायशो बुधः ।
कषायांश्च विशेषेण तत्र भेदस्तु दर्शितः ॥ (शा.सं.पू.खं. २/१)

२. प्रायः पित्तकफोद्रेके विरेकवमनार्थयोः ॥
लेखानार्थं च भैषज्यं प्रभाते तत्समाहरेत् ।
एवं स्यात्प्रथमः कालो भैषज्यग्रहणे नृणाम् ॥ (शा.सं.पू.खं. २/३-४)

(ii) Second time

(a) In Apāna vāta vitiation drug may be given before meals.

(b) In Aruchi along with food the drug should be administered.

(c) In Samana vāta vitiation and in Agni mandya drug is given middle of the meals (Madhya bhojana).

(d) In Vyana vāta vitiation drug may be given after meals.

(e) In Hikka, Ākshepaka, Kampa Vāta drug may be used just before completion of meals[1].

(iii) Third time

(a) In Udāna Vāta vitiation and in Swarabhanga, drug may be administered along with food or at different times while taking the food (Grasa or Grasantara).

(b) In Prana Vāta vitiation drug is used after the night meals[2].

(iv) Fourth time

(a) Drug is to be repeated several times (Muhurmuhuh) in Trishna, Hikka, Kasa, Swasa, Visha rogas.

(b) In these conditions the drug may be given along with the food[3].

(v) Fifth time

The drug may be administered at night in E.N.T. ophthalmological disorders, for Lekhana, for Brimhana, for Pāchana and for Samana[4].

Adhamalla provided detailed explanation on these five timings. He is of the openion that these timings are not applicable for emergency conditions. The *First Kāla* is at sun-rise (early morning) and is

---

१. भैषज्यं विगुणेऽपाने भोजनाग्रे प्रशस्यते । अरूचौ चित्रभोज्यैश्च मिश्रं रूचिरमाहरेत् ॥
समानवाते विगुणे मन्देऽग्रावग्निदीपनम् । दद्याद्भोजनमध्ये च भैषज्यं कुशलो भिषक् ॥
व्यानकोपे च भैषज्यं भोजनान्ते समाहरेत् । हिक्काक्षेपकम्पेषु पूर्वमन्ते च भोजनात् ॥
एवं द्वितीयकालश्च प्रोक्तो भेषजकर्मणि । (शा.सं.पू.खं. २/५-८)

२. उदाने कुपिते वाते स्वरभङ्गादिकारिणि ॥ ग्रासे ग्रासान्तरे देयं भैषज्यं सांध्यभोजने ।
प्राणे प्रदुष्टे सांध्यस्य भुक्तस्यान्ते च दीयते ॥
औषधं प्रायशो धीरै: कालोऽयं स्यात्तृतीयक: । (शा.सं.पू.खं. २/८-१०)

३. महुर्मुहुश्च तृट्छर्दिहिक्काश्वासगरेषु च ॥
सान्नं च भेषजं दद्यादिति कालश्चतुर्थक: । (शा.सं.पू.खं. २/१०-११)

४. ऊर्ध्वजत्रुविकारेषु लेखने बृंहणे तथा ॥ पाचनं शमनं देयमनन्नं भेषजं निशि ।
इति पञ्चमकाल: स्यात् प्रोक्तो भैषज्यकर्मणि ॥ (शा.सं.पू.खं. २/११-१२)

mainly useful for the administration of Kashayas etc. The *Second Kāla* is around morning meals (lunch time) time. It is agian five types viz., Bhojanāgra, Bhojanamisra, Bhojana Madhya, Bhojananta & Bhojana purvanta. *Third Kāla* is near the evening meals time or dinner time. It is again three types viz., Grasa, Grasantara, Bhaktanata, *Fourth Kāla* is said to be repeated administration which is of two types viz., Sānnam & Nirannam. *Fifth Kāla* is at night (Nisi). Thus 11 timings are described by Ādhamalla.

The drug must be administered to an individual after careful evaluation of timing and condition of the disease. Then only the drug will be able to restore complete health[1].

The timings of administration are made on the basis of disease conditions and condition of the patient. For example, in Jwara Āmavastha Langhana is indicated and Nirāmāvastha Kwathas are indicated. If the drug is not administerd even according to the condition of the patient, it will be wasted even if it is administerd as per the time indicated[2].

(1) Abhaktam: ***(on empty stomach)***

In Vyana vata vitiation drug may be given in the early morning on empty stomach. Abhaktam will enhance the potency of the drug i.e., the drug acts quickly and efficiently. When administered on empty stomach the drug will subside aggravated kapha. As food interferes with the drug fatiqueness (Glani) will not develop[3].

Abhaktam should not be used for children, old age people, women, weak individuals etc.

---

१. अतोऽभियुक्तस्सततं सर्वमालोच्य सर्वधा ॥
तथा युञ्जीतभैषज्यमारोग्याय यथा ध्रुवम् । (अ.हृ.सू. २२/७२-७३)

२. आतुरावस्थासु तु याः कालाः भागाः ताः कालाः काल संज्ञाः । यथा ज्वरस्य सामावस्थायां लङ्घनपेयादिः निरामावस्थायां क्वाथादिः, निरामावस्थायां पयः पानादिरिति एष ह्युभयोऽपि कालः भेषजयोग्यत्वमापादयति । (इन्दुकरः-.सं.सू. २३)

३. (i) व्याने तु प्रातरशितं................॥ (च.चि.३०/२९९)
(ii) तत्राभक्तं तु यत् केवलमेवौषधमुपयुज्यते ॥
वीर्याधिकं भवति भेषजमन्नहीनं हन्यत्तथाऽऽमयसंशयमाशु चैव ।
तद्बालवृद्धवनितामृदवस्तु पीत्वा ग्लानिं परां समुपयान्ति बलक्षयं च । (स.उ. ६४/६६-६७)

क्रमशः पृष्ठ ३६६ में.......

Indukara defined it as the quantity of drug which is not combined with food in the body. This time shall be used only if the over night food is completely digested. After the drug is completely digested/metabolized then only food may be consumed.

(2) Pragbhaktam *(Before meals)*

In Apana vata vitiation drug may be given after food. It is used before meals. It is useful in diseases of lower limbs and in lean or weak pessons. The drug will be digested very easily if administered during this time.

The time of administration is specially suitable for old age people, children, lean persons etc[1].

(3) Madhya Bhaktam *(Middle of the meals)*

This time is used for administration of durg when the Samana Vata is vitiated. The drug is given in the middle of the meals (i.e., along with food). It is also helpful in conditions like Koshta gata rogas, Pitta rogas, diseases of head and neck. This time of administration is responsible for increasing the strength of the body[2].

(4) Adhobhaktam *(after meals)*

The drug administered after food is known as Ādhobhaktam. It is

---

पृष्ठ ३६५ से क्रमश:.......

(iii) तत्राभक्तं नामकेवलमौषधम् । तन्निरन्त्रोपयोगादति वीर्यं कफोद्रेके
विमुक्तामाशयस्रोता: प्रातर्बलवानु-पयुञ्जीत । इतरस्तु प्राग्भक्तादिकम् ॥
अन्नसंसर्गेण हि तन्नातिग्लानिकरं भवति ॥ (अ.सं.सू. २३)

(iv) कफोद्रेके गदेऽनन्त्रं बलिनो रोगरोगिणो: । (अ.हृ.सू. १३/३८)

१. (i) अपाने विगुणे पूर्वं..........। (च.चि. ३०/२९९)

(ii) प्राग्भक्तं नाम यत् प्राग्भक्तस्योपयुज्यते ॥
शीघ्रं विपाकमुपयाति बलं न हिंस्यादन्नावृतं न च मुहुर्वदनान्निरेति ।
प्राग्भक्तसेवितमथौषधमेतदेव दद्याच्च वृद्ध शिशुभीरूकृशाङ्गनाभ्य: ॥ (सु.उ. ६४/६८-६९)

(iii) प्राग्भक्तं नाम यदनन्तरं भक्तं । तदपानानिलवकृतावध: कायस्य च बलाधानार्थम्
तद्गतेषु च व्याधिषु प्रशमनाय कृशीकरणं च योज्यम् ॥ (अ.सं.सू. २३)

(iv) अन्नादौ विगुणेऽपाने ....। (अ.हृ.सू.१३/३८)

२. (i) ....समाने मध्यभोजनम् । (च.चि.३०/२९९)

(ii) मध्येभक्तं नाम-यन्मध्ये भक्तस्य पीयते ॥

क्रमश: पृष्ठ ३६७ में........

used in morning in the vitiation of Vyana vata till the aggravated dosha is subsided. In Udana vata vitiation it is utilized in the evening. In order to strengthen the head and to cure the diseases of head & neek it is useful. This time of administration is helpful in inereasing body weight[1].

Charaka quoted it for Udana vata vikaras.

(5) Sama bhaktam *(along with food)*

In this the drug is administered along with easily digestible food. Charaka and Sushrita have stated that the drug shall be used along with food. While vagbhata is of the openion that drug may be coocked along with the food even. It is useful to children, who can not tolerate severity of drugs, who have aversion to drugs etc. It is very useful in systemic diseases. It acts as Hridya, strengthens mind, acts as appetizer etc[2].

(6) Ānantara bhaktam *(after digestion of morning food)*

If drug is administered in the afternoon after the morning food is digested, it is known as Ānantra bhakta. Again food will be given in the evening after the drug is digested/metabolized.

पृष्ठ ३६६ से क्रमशः.......

पीतं यदन्नमुपयुज्यत तदूर्ध्वकाये हन्ताद्गदान् बहुविधाश्चं बलं ददाति ।
मध्ये तु पीतमहन्त्यविसारिभावाद्ये मध्यदेहमभिभूय भवन्ति रोगाः ॥ (सु.उ. ६४/७१-७२)

(iii) मध्यभक्तं मध्येभक्तस्य तत्समानालि विकृतौ कोष्ठगतेषु च व्याधिषु पैत्तिकेषु च ॥(अ.सं.सू. २३)

(iv) ......समाने मध्य इष्यते । (अ.हृ.सू. १३/३८)

१. (i) ...... उदाने भोजनोत्तरम् । (च.चि. ३०/२९९)

(ii) अधोभक्तं नाम-यदधो भक्तस्येति ॥ (सु.उ. ६४/७०)

(iii) अध्योभक्तं भक्तादनन्तरम् । तत्तु व्यानविकृतौ प्रातराशान्तमुदान विकृतौ पुनः सायमाशान्तं पूर्वकायस्य च बलाधानार्थं तद्गदेषु च श्लेष्मिकेषु च प्रशमाय स्थूलीरणं च । (अ.सं.सू. २३)

(iv) व्यानेनऽन्ते प्रातराशस्य, सायमाशस्य तूत्तरे । (अ.हृ.सू. १३/३९)

२. (i) ......लघुनाऽन्नेन संयुतम् ।
संभोज्यं त्वौषधं भोज्यैर्विचित्रैररूचौ हितम् । (च.चि. ३०/३०१)

(ii) सभक्तं नाम-यत् सहभक्तेन ॥
पथ्यं सभक्तमबलाबलयोर्हिनित्यं तद्दोषिणामपि तथा शिशुवृद्धयोश्च ।
हृद्यं मनोबलकरं त्वथ दीपनं च पथ्यं सदा भवति चान्तरभक्तकं यत् ॥ (सु.उ. ६४/७४-७५)

(iii) समभक्तं (सभक्तं) यदन्नेन समं साधितं पश्चादासमालोडितम् ।
तद्बालेषु सुकमारेष्वौषधद्वेषिष्वरूचौ सर्वाङ्गेषु । (अ.सं.सू. २३)

(iv) योज्यं संभोज्य भैषज्यं भोज्यैश्चित्रैररोचके ॥ (अ.हृ.सू. १३/४०)

Similarly drug can be administered in the morning after the over night dinner is digested completely. This should be followed by lunch once the drug is totally digested. This can also be considered as Ānantara bhakta.

This time is used for person with good appetite and in vyana vata vitiation.

Though Charaka did not mention this, Chakrapani while commenting on Sāmudga delineated about Ānantarabhakta[1].

(7) Sāmudgam *(before and after meals)*

This is mainly mentioned for persons suffering from Hikka (hicough). In this drug is administered at the begining of and end of the meals. Pachana drugs, Lehyas, Churnas which are laghu in nature are administered in this method, especially in Hikka, Kampa Vata, Ākshepaka Vata, Ūrdhwa and Adho gata doshas[2].

8. Muhurmuhu *(repeated administration)*

In Swasa, Kasa, Hikka, Chardi, Visha rogas and Trishna the drug is to be administered repeatedly for several times. This refeated usage is known as Muhurmuhu.

It is essential under the above conditions since they aggravate and disappear quite frequently. At the same time their recurrence is also frequent. Hence repeated administration of drug is advised[3].

---

१. (i) अनन्तरभक्तं यत्पूर्वाह्णभक्ते ज़ीर्णे मध्याह्ने भेषजमुपयुज्यते तस्मिंश्च जीर्णे पुनरपराह्ण भोजनम् । एतेन रात्रिर्व्याख्याता । तद्दीप्ताग्नेर्व्यानजेष्वामयेषु । (अ.सं.सू. २३)
(ii) अन्तराभक्तं नाम-यदन्तरा पीयते पूर्वापरयोर्भक्तयो: ॥ (सु.उ. ६४/७३)
(iii) अन्तराभक्तं नाम यदन्नेन संयोगात् संस्काराद्वा तद्विमिश्रितं भुज्यते । (चक्रपाणि-च.चि. ३०/२९८)

२. (i) सामुद्गं हिक्किने देयं............। (च.चि. ३०/३०१)
(ii) सामुद्गं नाम-यद्भक्तस्यादावन्ते च पीयते ॥
दोषे द्विधा प्रविसृते तु सामुद्गसंज्ञमाद्यन्तयोर्यदशनस्य निषेव्यते तु । (सु.उ. ६४/७६-७७)
(iii) सामुद्गं यावदन्ते च भुक्तस्य ॥ तत्तु लघ्वन्नपानयुक्तं पाचनावलेहचूर्णादि हिध्मायां कम्पाक्षेपयोरूर्ध्वाध: संश्रये च दोषे । (अ.सं.सू. २३)
(iv) कम्पाक्षेपकहिध्मासु सामुद्गं लघुभोजनात् । (अ.हृ.सू.१३/४१)

३. (i) श्वासकासपिपासासु त्ववचार्यं मुहुर्मुहु: ॥ (च.चि. ३०/३००)
(ii) मुहुर्मुहुर्नाम-सभक्तमभक्तं वा यदौषधं मुहुर्मुहुरूपयुज्यते ॥
श्वासे मुहुर्मुहुरतिप्रसृते च कासे हिक्कावमीषु स वदन्त्युपयोज्यमेतत् । (सु.उ. ६४/७८-७९)

क्रमश: पृष्ठ ३६९ में............

9,10 Sagrāsa, Grāsāntara *(along with food bolus or in between)*

The drug which will be administered along with rice or meals is known as 'Sagrasam'. Drug which is given in between two rice bolus while taking meals is called as 'Grasantara'. These two are otherwise termed as 'Kavala' and 'Kavalantara'.

It is mainly helpful in Prana vata vitiation. It is also utilized to administer churnas, Avalehas etc., which will improve appetite. Vajikarana drugs (aphrodisiacs) shall be used as 'Sagrasa'. Drugs for heart diseases may be administered as 'grasantara'.

Grasantara is also useful while performing vamana, Dhuma and to cure swasa, kasa etc[1].

11. Nisi *(bed time administation of drug)*

Drugs for Vamana and Dhauma will be used at bed time i.e., at night time. E.N.T. and ophthalmological conditions will be treated during this time. However Charaka and Sushrita did not mention it[2].

In this way all the Oushadha sevana Kalas are described according to various authors. Among the above while administering drug to a patient who is thirsty or who consumed plenty of chilled water or who had indigestion or who is hungry or who is weak, Abhakta is contra-indicated. During other times also, the things which are not good for

---

पृष्ठ ३६८ से क्रमशः..........

(iii) मुहुर्मुहुस्तु पुनः पुनर्भुक्ते यदभुक्ते वा ।
तच्छ्वासकास हिध्मा तृट् छर्दिषु विषनिमित्तेषु च विकारेषु ॥ (अ.सं.सू. २३)

(iv) मुहुर्मुहुर्विषच्छर्दिहिध्मातृट्श्वासकासिषु । (अ.हृ.सू. १३/४०)

१. (i) वायौ प्राणे प्रदुष्टे तु ग्रासग्रासान्तरिष्यते । (च.सू. ३०/३००)

(ii) ग्रासं तु- यत्पिण्डव्यामिश्रम् ॥
ग्रासान्तरं तु यद्ग्रासान्तरेषु ॥
ग्रासेषु चूर्णमबलाग्निषु दीपनीयं वाजीकरणमपि तु योजयितुं यतेत ।
ग्रासान्तरेषु वितरेद्वमनीयधूमान् श्वासादिषु प्रथितदृष्टगुणांश्च लेहान् ॥ (सु.उ. ६४/८०-८२)

(iii) सग्रासं यद् ग्राससंपृक्तं ग्रासान्तरं यद् ग्रासयोर्मध्ये । द्वयमप्येतत्प्राणानिलविकृतौ । तथा सग्रासं चूर्णलेहवटकादिकमग्निदीपनं वाजीकरणानि चोपयुञ्जीत । ग्रासान्तरं हृद्रोगे ......। (अ.सं.सू. २३)

(iv) ग्रासग्रासान्तयोः प्राणे प्रदुष्टे मातरिश्वनि । (अ.हृ.सू. १३/३९)

२. (i) ....वमनं धूमं च जत्रूर्ध्वामयेषु तु निशायाम् । (अ.सं.सू. २३)

(ii) ऊर्ध्वजत्रुविकारेषु स्वप्नकाले प्रशस्यते ॥ (अ.हृ.सू. १३/४१)

heart, which are incompatible, which are corrosive, which are exothermic, which have pungent odour and which are used in large quantities are all contra-indications[1].

In another context Vagbhata stated that Kāla Avastha (time) and Vyadhi Avastha (disease status) are both required to be assessed for proper administration of medicine[2].

Modern View on times of drug Administration[3]

When a madicine is given is as important as what medicine is given, according to speakers at an American Medical Association-sponsored media briefing, "Chronotherapeutics: Synchronizing Drug Therapies with Body Rhythms".

The tenets of chronobiology-the study of biological rhythms- are still unfamiliar to most physicians, a recent Gallup poll shows: 'Chronobiologists say that predictable variations in bodily functions during the day, week month and year alters severity of disease symptoms, results of diagnostic tests, and effects of drugs and other therapy.

Growing evidence that timed dosing substantially improves treatment out comes will bring chronobiology into mainstream medical practice.

Behaviour & Circadian Rhythms

In a Canadian study, for example, 118 children with acute lymphoblastic leukaemia in remission took a daily maintenance dose of mercaptopurine at home. Their parents are told to give the drug when convenient but consistently at the treatment. Treated between 1976 and 1984 and followed up until 1991, the children who took their medicine in the evening are three times less likely to relapse than those who took it in the morning (Chronobiol Int. 1993; 10:201-204).

---

१. तत्राद्ये काले तृषित: पीतशीताम्बुरजीर्णोक्षुधित: क्षामश्च भेषजं वर्जयेत् ।
शेषेषुवाऽहृद्यमसात्म्यमति तीक्ष्णोग्रगन्धं भूरिमात्रं चेति ॥ (अ.सं.सू. २३)

२. क्षणादिर्व्याध्यवस्थाकालो भेषजयोगकृत् । (अ.हृ.सू. १/२४)

३. Lynne Lamberg; "Time of Day Medicine Dose Is Taken May Boost Its Efficacy, cut Toxicity". JAMA-India, July 1996, vol. 19, No.4 p.258-259

Circadian rhythms in every pathway said for drug metabolism alter pharmacokinetics and drug effects across the day said Gaston Labreque, Ph D. Professor of pharmacy at Laval University of Quebec. Behaviour may add other time elements. The childern in the leukemia study, he noted, also drank more milk in the morning than they did in the evening, daily rhythm although obviously not a biological one. An interaction with milk, Labreque suggested, may have further altered the efficacy of 6 MP.

Homeostasis and Chronobiology

Educating physicians to recognize biological rhythms and seperate them from extrinsic behaviour is critical to the widespread application of chronotherapeutics. Medical schools still teach homoeostasis, that is, the body is constant in time, said Michael H. Smolensky, Ph.D., a professor in the school of public Health at the Health Sciences centre of the University of Texas-Houston and press breifing moderator. "They are not teaching chronobiology".

When Harvard Medical school physiologist walter canon, MD, devised his steady-state hypothesis in 1925, it took a pint of blood to do research, Smolensky said. It's no surprise that multiple measurements were not made during the day. "There are set points for the regulation of temperature, blood pressure, cell division, and other bodily functions, all these set points vary across the day, often markedly".

The survey of Gallup proved that only 49% of primary care physicians were familiar with chronobiology. About half the physicians seldom or never considered chronobiology when making diagnostic decisions or treatment recommendations. When read a list that included heart attacks. asthma attacks, angina, migraine headaches, and other disorders with prominent circadian patterns, the majority named-often incorrectly- a specific time of day when there maladies are most likely to occur.

Effects on Hypertension

Behaviour and body rhythms combine to leave many hypertensives without medication when they need it most (William B. White, M.D., Chief of the section of HTN & VCD at the Univ. of connecticut Health centre in Farmington).

B.P. rises about 20% immediately after awakening in the morning. The first hour or two after arising are the peak hours of M.I, haemorrhagic strokes, thromlotic infarctions, and Myocardial ischaemia. Yet people often do not take their medicine until after they have dressed and had breakfast. Furthermore, many currently available anti-hypertensive drugs take a few hours to kick in and work for only 18 to 20 hours.

Though efforts are on for fast-acting and long-acting drugs, once-a-day medication are'nt necessarily chronotherapeutics. "Giving medicine once a day in the morning was okay because B.P. is higher during the day".

Medications that are already main-stay of treatment for numerous disorders also may be more effective and less toxic if properly timed. Delivering the right drug at the right time, also may lower costs of medical care by reducing physician and hospital visits for acute flare-ups.

Other Timely Treatment

Some highlights of the new approach include the following, which apply to day-active people. (For night workers or rotating-shift workers, changes in time of dosage should be keyed to the individual's sleep/ wake schedule).

***Asthma—** Oral steroids give better control when given at 3 PM instead of in the morning . Giving theophylline once a day around 6 or 7 PM with dinner rather than in equal devided doses throughout the day yields a peak level between 3 and 5 AM, when asthma attacks are most frequent. Not all theophyllines, however, are formulated for once-a-day dosing.

***Arthritis—** Non steroidal anti-inflammatory drugs relieve the morning pain of RA better if taken late at night. They work better for evening in OA pain if taken around noon.

***Peptic ulcers—** H_2-recepter blockers (cimetidine or famotidine) are as effective or more effective for ulcer healing when given once a day around 6 or 7 PM with the evening meal than twice a day. The reason is that circadian rhythm in stomach acidity peaks in the evening and later at night.

***Mood Disorders—** Deprivation of sleep in latter half of the night and timed exposure to day light-intensity artificial light, although still experimental therapies, may ease depression premenstrually or during menopause, and benefit both women and men with seasonal and other mood disorders.

Chronotherapeutics, although a leap forward from the familiar 3 or 4 times a day prescription, may herald things to come. The next step is "chronobiotics" i.e.; " Smart drugs" that act only when needed. Also on the horizon are drugs to fix broken biological clocks, perhaps a factor in all illness, in the opinion of some physicians.

The above studies from modern system of medicine will further emphasize the need for the recognition of times of administration as mentioned in the ancient medicine.

(8) Routs of drug Administration

Routs of administration is an important aspect in clinical practice. It is known that different drugs will act at different sites of action. On the other hand different drugs will need different routs of administration to prove their efficacy in the given conditions.

The routs of administration have been explained in the Ayurvedic texts:[1]

1. Āsya (orally given)	- used in Āmasaya rogas (gastric & duodenal diseases).
2. Nasya (nasal administration)	- used in Siro rogas (E.N.T. & eye diseases etc).
3. Guda (enemata)	- used in Pakwasaya rogas (diseases of large intestines).

१. (i) आस्यादामशयस्थान् हि रोगान् नस्त: शिरोगतान् ।
गुदात् पक्वाशयस्थांश्च हन्त्याशु दत्तमौषधम् ॥
शरीरावयवोत्थेषु विसर्पपिडकादिषु ।
यथादेशं प्रदेहादि शमनं स्याद्विशेषत: ॥ (च.चि. ३०/२९४-२९५)
(ii) हन्त्याशु युक्तं वक्त्रेण द्रव्यमामाशयान्मलान् ।
घ्राणेन चोर्ध्वजत्रूत्थान्, पक्वाधानाद्गुदेन च । (अ.सं.सू. २१)और (अ.हृ.सू. १३/३०-३१)

4. Pradeha (exteral applications) - used in generalized infections (Visarpa, Pitikas etc).

Vagbhata explained the reasons for selecting a specific rout and time for administering of a drug. He says the circulating doshas will get vitiated and those morbid doshas which remain in specific those morbid doshas which remain in specific places will lead to pathological condition of those sites. Therefore the site of disease or phothology must be well understood. Accordingly drug may be administered[1].

Sites of Drug absorption:

S.N.	**Āsaya**	**Dosha**	**Properties of Drugs to be Absorbed**
1.	Āmasaya	Kapha	Snigdha (lipid soluble); Seeta (non-ion ized); Guru (heavy in mol. wt.)
2.	Grahani	Pitta	Snigdha (lipid soluble); Ushna (ion ized); Laghu (lighter in mol. wt.).
3.	Pakwāsaya	Vāta	Ruksha (water soluble), Seeta (non-ion ized); Laghu (smaller in mol.size).

The mode of action of a drug in relation with the state of Samprapti

S.N.	**Rasa Panchaka**	**Site of action**	**State of Pathogenesis**
1.	Rasa & Vipaka	Koshta	Chaya & Prakopa.
2.	Guna	Rasa Samvahana	Prasara
3.	Virya & Prabhava	Dushyas & Srotas	Sthana Samsraya & Vyakti

e.g. In Atisara vata is the main dosha and Purisha is the dushya. Purisha vaha srotas is the srotas involved. Ati pravritti is the type of Srotodushti. In this condition, Sunthi (dry ginger) acts on vata, Bhanga (cannabis) acts on Purisha and Ahiphena (opium) acts on purisha vaha srotas. These three drugs prevent the samprapti at different leavels and cure Atisāra (diarrhoeal disorders).

A drug may act either Dosha-Dushya Sammurchana (the combination of vitiated humors and tissues) or on the Srotas (organ system):

---

१. प्रविसृतो हि दोषः स्थानमातङ्कायाधितिष्ठन् मूर्धादीन् वा दूस्तरो भवति ।
ततश्च स्थानविशेषेण भेषजविशेषः पर्येषितव्यः॥ (अ.सं.सू. २३)

(i) If the effect of the drug is on cell membrane that may be com pared to the action of drug on Srotas.

(ii) If the drug acts outside the cell (extracellular) it can be considered as effect on Poshaka dhatu.

(iii) If it is inside the cell (intracellular) the effect is on Poshya dhatu.

(iv) If the effect of the drug is on the cell metabolism, then it shall be considered as the effect on dhatwagni.

Considering these factors the time and rout of administration discussed elaborately in the previous pages may be used in clinical practice.

Modern view on Routs of Drug Administration

(1) Oral or Enteral route— It is the most commonly used rout because of its sefety, convenience and economic. More over the complications involved in parenteral rout may be avoided. It has some disadvantages also.

(a) the onset of drug action is tardy.

(b) irritant and unpalatable drugs can not be given.

(c) not useful in diarrhoea and vomiting, unconcious or uncoopera tive patient.

(d) Some drugs will be destroyed by digestive juices when used through this rout e.g. insulin.

(e) absorption of certain drugs is irregular or negligible.

Through this rout the drugs are usually administered in the form of capsules, tablets, powders, syrups etc.

(2) Enteric coated pills and tablets— Some times, pills and tablets are coated with cellulose- acetate-phthalate, gluten and anionic copolymers of methacrylic acid and its esters. These substances resist the acidic gastric juice, action and permit disintegration in the intestinal alkaline juices.

(3) Enemata— Administration of a medicament in a liquid from into the rectum is called enema. It is two types:

(i) Evacuant enema: e.g. soap water enema. It is used to remove the faecal matter and flatus. About 600 ml will be given as enema.

(ii) Retention enema: The fluid containing drug is retained in the rectum to facilitate drug absorption e.g. prednisolone enema is ulcerative colitis, paraldehyde enema to produce basal anaesthesia. About 100-200 ml will be given as enema.

(4) Sub-lingual administration— Rapid onset of absorption and quick termination of the drug effect will be seen. e.g. Sarbitrate is administered sub-lingually in angival attacks.

(5) Local application— Dusting powder, application of paste, lotion, drops, ointment or plaster is used for its action at the site of application.

Local application may also be: bougie for urethra, pessary for vagina and suppository for vagina and rectum.

(6) Parenteral route— Routes of administration other than the alimentary tract are called parenteral. Its advantages are:

(i) drug can be administered even in unconcious state.

(ii) more helpful in diarrhoea & vomiting.

(iii) drug is not affected by alimentary juices and liver enzymes.

(iv) drugs causing gastric irritation or drugs which are not absorbed in small intestine can be administered.

(v) rapid action and accurate dose are ensured.

The parenteral roots are:

(a) Inhalation:

Drugs may be administered as solid particles (in nebulizers) either in solution form or in vapour form.

(b) Injections:

(i) Intradermal- given into layers of skin e.g. B.C.G. vaceine.

(ii) Subcutaneous- only non-irritant substances are injected by this rout e.g. insuline administation.

This can act as 'depot' therapy e.g. steroid hormone implants.

In paediatric practice, saline is often given by this rout in large quantities. This procedure is known as 'hypodermoclysis'.

(iii) Intramuscular- mild irritants, suspensions and colloids can be given by this route. I.M. absorption is usually faster than oral absorption but diazepam, hydrocortisone, digoxin etc., are more slowly absorbed (on I.M.) compared to oral route.

(iv) Intravenous- drugs given directly into vein produce rapid action, and the desired blood concentration.

(v) Intra-arterial- This is used in diagnostic studies e.g. angiograms and in the treatment of peripheral vascular disorders. Certain cancer drugs are given by this route. Drug administration produces a sudden high concentration in arterial blood and is harmful locally ordamaging to tissues supplied by the artery.

(vi) Intrathecal- this administration involves introduction of drugs such as spinal aneasthetics into the subarachnoid space. These drugs act directly on CNS.

(vii) Intraperitoneal- this route is useful in infants for giving fluids like glucose saline.

(viii) Intramedullary- Introduction of a drug into the bone marrow. This route is now rarely used.

(ix) Intra-articular- certain drugs are administered directly into a joint for the treatment of local conditions. This ensures a high local concentration of the drug e.g. hydrocortisone acetate in the treatment of RA.

(c) Transcutaneous

(i) Iontophoresis- galvenic current is used for bringing about the penetration of drugs into the deeper tissues where they may act upon the tissues in the neighbouhood of the point of application.

(ii) Inunction- Certain drugs when rubbed into the skin can get absorbed and may produce systemic effects e.g. nitroglycerin ointment in angina pectoris.

(iii) Jet injection- the transcutaneous introduction of a drug by means of a high velocity jet produced through a microfine orifice. It does not require needle e.g. Insulin being tried in the form of jet injector.

(iv) Adhesive units- a transdermal therapeutic system in the form of an adhesive unit has been developed to deliver the drugs slowly, producing systemic effect e.g. scopolamine for prevention of motion sickness.

(d) Trans-mucosal route

(i) Sublingual route- when placed under the tongue the active agent get dissolved in mouth and absorbed through buccal mucosa directly into systemic circulation. It ensures rapid onset of action, quick termination of drug effect, and prevention of degradation in the stomach. e.g. nitroglycerine in angina pectoris.

(ii) Trans-nasal route- the drug is applied to nasal mucosa for quick absorption and action e.g. dDAVP, synthetic analogue of varopressin in administered by this route. No poisonous drug be administered by this route, as it may reach brain along with lymphatic channels.

(iii) Trans-rectal route- certain drugs can cross the rectal mucosa like other lipid membranes; thus, ionized and lipid soluble substances are readily absorbed from the rectum.

(e) New Drug delivery systems

(i) Ocusert- when placed directly under the eyelid, can deliver a steady flow of pilocarpine for 7 days.

(ii) Progestasert- an IUCD, produces controlled release of minute quantities of progesterone within the uterus for a year.

(iii) Prodrug- is an active chemical derivative that, after administration, undergoes biotransformation to the pharmacologically active drug.

Apart from these routes, compouterized, miniature, syringe pumps are now available for continous or intermittent administration of drugs. 'Targeted' delivery of anti-cancer drugs using monoclonal antibodies against cancer cell antigens is one of the newer innovations in drug delivery systems.

It is important to realize that a drug may exert different effects when given by different routes e.g. oral $MgSo_4$ is saline purgative; I.M. $MgSo_4$ is anticonvulsant; hypertonic $MgSo_4$ (as retention enema), reduces intracranial tension.

(9) Prescription Writing

The term "prescription" is associated with the order for a specific medication for a certain person at a particular time.

It is necessary to know the way of selection of the most suitable drug and dosage where in palatability, stability, rate of absorption, patient safety, therapeutic index and other important factors are considered.

Traditionally, a prescription follows a definite pattern in modern medicine in order to facilitate its interpretation. It is usually written on a special form. A prescription should possess the date first and then the name and address of the patient. The symbol Rx indicates Greek meaning Recipe i.e., take. Then the drugs required must be prescribed in the original brand name but not in generic name in block letters e.g., AMPICILLIN, ACETYL SALICILIC ACID, PARACETAMOL etc. This should be accompanied by type of preparation indicated (Tablet, Syrup etc). alongwith dosage and how many times to be administered i.e., times of administration. Finally the prescription should by signed by the physician.

A model prescription

(1) August 31, 2000.

(2) Satyanarayana K.

1-20-371/4,
Subrahmanian colony,
Kottivakkam
Chennai-91.

(3) Rx

(4) (i) Abhraka Bhasma 250 mg b.d.s.

(with honey)

(ii) Chyavana Prasa 5 gm b.d.s.

(5) Signature of the physician.

Here it is important to note that the prescriptions are now written by noting down chief complaint etc., history of illness, physician observations followed by diagnosis. This may be noted down for practical convenience.

Chapter-XV

Brief History of Dravya guna in Vedas and Samhitas

1. Brief History of Dravya guna

It is generally concluded that Dravya guna sastra was never considered as one among the eight branches of Ayurveda before Raja Nighantu. At the same time many do not understand that Ayurveda always emphasized the concept of 'pharmacotherapeutics' but not pharmacology and therapeutics seperately. The concept of 'Chikitsa chatushpada' (the quartet in treatment) substantiates this view. Basing upon this view Dravya (the drug) and chikitsa (the treatement) are denoted with same nomenclature and synonyms.

चिकित्सितं व्याधिहरं पथ्यं साधनमौषधम् ।
प्रायश्चितं प्रशमनं प्रकृतौस्थापनं हितम् ।।
विद्याद्भेषज नामानि....................।
(च.चि.१अ)

During the earliest times, the pharmacological and therapeutic utility of herbs was assumed on the basis of 'Doctrie of Signature' e.g.: usage of lac (Laksha) in haemorrhage (Raktapitta), Manjishta in blood born disorders (Rakta Vikaras), Haridra (turmeric) in Jaundice (Kamala), testicle- shaped seeds of Kapikachchu as aphrodisiac (Vajikarna) etc.

Dravyaguna and its development through ages can be classified into three periods basing upon the available historical evidences. Acharya P.V. Sharmaji divided the history into:

(1) Prachina kala - 4000 BC to 7AD i.e., upto post-Gupta period (ancient times)

(2) Madhyama kala - 8 to 15 AD (medeival period)

(3) Adhunika kāla - 16 AD onwards (modern times)

Vedic literature and Brihat Trayee texts (Charaka Samhita, Sushrita Samita & Vagbhatam) are placed under the ancient times. Two of the Laghu Trayee texts (Rigvinischaya & Sarngdhara Samhita) and other main Nighantus belong to the medeival period. Modern era begins with Bhava Prakasa & Raja Nighantu etc.

2. Dravyaguna in the Vedic Literature

Systematic utility of herbs will be found in the Rigveda-Oushadhi Sukta (10.97.1-23) and also in Atharvaveda (8.7.1-8 and 11.6.16-17). We also find references about the drug acting at the site of action i.e., different organs, joints etc., recieving the drug administered orally.

Plants were also used as Mani (amulet) to ward off the evil spirits. Vedic literature did mention that the drug acts because of its inherent power (Veerya).

There are different versions over the conclusion of vedic period. Some of them are:

Dr. Avinash Chardra	-	25,000 B.C.
Sri Bala Gangadhara Tilak	-	6.000 B.C.
Mc. Donald	-	1,500 B.C.
Max Muller	-	1,200 B.C.

In Satapath Brahmana Padarthas are divided into two groups viz., Amula (without root system) and Mulinyah (with root system)- "पशवोऽमूला:, ओषधयो मूलिन्य:"। (श.ब्रा. २-२-३-१०).

Sun and earth were considered to be the father and the mother for the plants [AVS-3/23/6]. Water is stated to be the basis for the development of plants [AVS-1/33/1]. It is also said that oushadhis (herbs) will grow due to rains and the animal kingdom survive by consuming these plants. This is accepted on the basis of modern concept of 'energy' chapter in Biochomistry plant utilizing energy from sun through photophosphirilation is the cause of survival of entire animal kingdom.

Many plants were used for 'Yajnas' (rituals) is the vedic period. Sruva, Chamasa, Idhma and Upamanthani are the four items of Yajna, which are prepared from Udumbara. They are also known as Chaturoudumbara (Bri,6-3-13). Other important plants are: Bilwa,

Khadira, Palasha, Rohitaka, Kashmarya, Rajjudala, Sugandhi tejana etc.

Vedic practice of medicine is enriched with single drug therapy. There are very few indications for each herb. Basing upon their therapeutic utility drugs are classified into four groups:

(1) Atharvani - drugs used for rituals.

(2) Angirasi - drugs which act as anti microbial.

(3) Daivi - drugs used for Rasayana purpose.

(4) Manushyaja - drugs used in the treatment of different conditions.

Fundamental Principles of Dravyaguna in the Vedic Period

(1) Rasa is considered to be Apya (water) in nature-

"आपां रसाः ओषधिभिः संचताम् ।" (अ.के.शा.४/५/२)

(2) Rasa, Veerya, Vipaka are described in detail in Atharva veda (AVS-6-96-1).

(3) The principal ingredient of a herb which is responsible for the phar-macological action is regarded as 'Veerya'.

"आपां तेजो ज्योतिरोजो बलं च वनस्पतीनामुतवीर्याणि" ।(अ.वे.शा. १य३०/३)

(4) Different types of 'Karma' i.e., biological and pharmacological activities are also mentioned in the vedas.

Some of them are:

1. Prameha (diuretic)
2. Grabha Prasāvana (oxytocin-like activity).
3. Grabhādhana (pro-fertilization activity).
4. Garbha dosha nivarana (drugs for ante-natal care).
5. Vajikarana (useful in infertility)
6. Vishaghna (anti-dote)
7. Sarpa visha nivarana (anti-snake venom)
8. Rakshoghna (antiseptic)
9. Kesa vardhana (hair growth promoting)
10. Kesa Brimhana (hair tonic)
11. Vasikarana (hypnotic)

12. Masaka Bhanjana (Mosquito repellent)
13. Krimi Nasaka (anti-microbial)
14. Kasa hara (anti-tussive)
15. Medha janana (brain tonic)
16. Kleeba karana (contraceptives?)
17. Soubhagya vardhana (aromatic)
18. Rasayana (antoxidants)
19. Nidra janana (sedatives)
20. Krityadushini
21. Balya (tonic)
22. Deepana (appetizers)
23. Rohana (growth promoting)
24. Sandhana (fracture healing etc.)
25. Sleshma sleshana (mucolytics?)

Classification of herbs in the vedic Period

During the vedic period, food and drugs are mainly divided into two categories viz., Oshadhi (smaller plants) and Vanaspati (bigger plants). The former group are used as food while the later are used as drugs. Further, each group is sub-divided into two more groups i.e., Virudha and Vānaspatya.

While classifying the herbs, various aspects have been considered. The morphological, pharmacological, therapeutic, aspects are mainly concentrated. We also come across signature and simile while classifying the herbs. Therefore their classification appers to be complete and scientific.

The following are the basis for classifications of medicinal plants in the vedic period:

(1) Classification on the basis of habit *(वानस्पतिक संज्ञानुसार वर्णीकरण:)*

Plants are classified into four caterogories on the basis of natural habit viz., (1) Vanaspati (2) Vānaspatya (3) Oushadhi (4) Veerudha

वनस्पतीवानस्पत्यानोषधीरूत वीरूधः। (अ.वे. ११-५-२४)

(2) Morphological classification *(अङ्गानुसार वर्गीकरण:)*

Plants are denoted on the basis of characteric features of stem, leaves, flowers, fruits etc.

(3) As per their stem *(काण्डानुसार वर्गीकरण)*

(a) Kandini (काण्डिनी)	trees which have trunk and branches e.g. Neem, Mango tree etc.
(b) Visakha (विशाखा)	trees which have leaves at the tip of the main stem e.g. coconut tree, palm tree etc.
(c) Eka shuga (एकशुंगा)	plants with cauline (smooth) stem or plants which germinate from single bud (AVS 8-7-4)
(d) Namasyanti (नमस्यन्ती)	bushy type trees i.e., trees with stems bent down due to weight of flowers and fruits e.g. Lemon [AVS.3-57-3]
(e) Arohini (आरोहिणी or रोहिणी)	climbers (AVS 8-7-1]
(i) Pratanvati (प्रतन्वती)	tendril climber (RV. 10-97-2).
(ii) Teekshna Sringya (तीक्ष्णशृग्य:)	thorny strangler (AVS 8-7-9)
(iii) Parāgatā (परागता)	which spreads to very long distance (R.V. 10-97-21)
(iv) Prasumati (प्रसूमती)	runners (?).
(v) Bhumi Santanvati (भूमिसंत्वती)	procumbents.
(vi) Seerah (सीरा:)	which moves from one place to the other (R.V. 10-97-9).

(4) As per leaf *(पत्रानुसार वर्गीकरण)*

(a) Parna Vasati (पर्णवसति:)-	leaves with medicinal value
(b) Suparnah (सुपर्णा:)-	plants with beautiful leaves.
(c) Sahsraparni or Parnini- (सहस्त्रर्पी, पर्णिनी)	which has innumerable leaves

(5) As per flower *(पुष्पानुसार वर्गीकरण)*

(a) Apushpa (अपुष्पा)	without flowers

(b) Pushpavati (पुष्पवती)	with flowers
(c) Stambini (स्तम्बिनी)	with big inflorasence of with bunches of flowers

(6) As per fruits *(फलानुसार वर्गीकरण)*

(a) Aphala (अफला)	without fruits
(b) Phalini (फलिनी)	with fruits
(c) Supippala (सुपिप्पल)	with beautiful fruits

(7) Classification on the basis of life span *(औषधनीवनानुसार वर्गीकरण)*

(1) Punarnava (पुनर्नवा)	which takes rebirth every year.
(2) Dhruva (ध्रुवा)	which live for centuries together
(3) Purvajata (पूर्वाजाता)	which live for thousands of yeras (Yuga)

(8) On the basis of biological activity *(गुणकर्मानुसार वर्गीकरण)*

(1) Masaka Jambhani (मशकजम्भनी)	musquito repellent
(2) Visha dushini (विषदूषणी)	antidote
(3) Sepha harshini (शेफहर्षिणी)	which causes penile erection
(4) Kesa Brihmani (केशबृंहणी)	hair tonic

(9) Therapeutic classification *(चिकित्सानुसार वर्गीकरण)*

(1) Viswa bheshaji (विश्वभेषजी)	universally used drug
(2) Yakshma nasini (यक्ष्मनाशनी)	used in fevers
(3) Durnama Chatana (दुर्नामचातन)	used in skin diseases
(4) Kilasa bheshaja (किलासभेषज)	used in leucoderma

(10) On the basis of taste *(रसानुसार वर्गीकरण)*

(1) Madhumad Agram (मधुमदग्रम्)	tip or terminal bud is sweet
(2) Madhuman Madhyam (मधुमन्मध्यम्)	the middle part or medulla of the stem is sweet.
(3) Madhuman Mulam (मधुमन्मूलम्)	the root is sweet.

(11) On the basis of colour *(वर्णानुसार वर्गीकरण)*

(1) Sukla (शुक्ला)	white coloured (Alba)
(2) Krishna (कृष्णा)	black coloured (nigrum)

(3) Rohini (रोहिणी)	red coloured (rubra)

(12) On the basis of contents *(तद्गतविशिष्टद्रव्यानुसार वर्गीकरण)*

(1) Apamgarbha (अपांगर्भ)	contain planty of water
(2) Payaswati (पयस्वती)	contain latex
(3) Medini (मेदिनी)	contain oily substances

(13) On the basis of specific activity *(प्रभावात्मक वर्गीकरण)*

(1) Divya (दिव्या)	herbs with extraordinary powers (RVS 10-97-4 & AVS 8-7-3)
(2) Amsumati (अंशुमती)	illuminating plants (AVS. 8-7-4)
(3) Prachetasa (प्रचेतस)	with hidden activity inside (AVS8-7-7)

(14) Economic classification *(व्यापारिक वर्गीकरण)*

(1) Apakrita (अपक्रीता)	herbs or drugs purchased from the foreign countries (AVS 8-7-11)
(2) Dhanam Sanishyanti (धनंसनिष्यन्ती)	costly drugs purchased from foreigners (RVS 10-97-8)

(15) Commonly available drugs *(सर्वसाधारण औषधि)*

(1) Bahvi (बह्वी)	abundantly available
(2) Viswah (विश्वा)	available all over the world
(3) Sahasranamni (सहस्रनाम्नी)	with several names in different places

(16) According to habitat *(उत्पत्तिस्थानानुसार वर्गीकरण)*

(1) Udakatmanah (उदकात्मान:)	aquatics
(2) Anakolvah (अनकोल्वा:)	hydrophytes (AVS 8-7-9)
(3) Go bhaja (गोभाज:)	xerophytes (RVS 10-97-5)
(4) Mulam Samudra (मूलं समुद्र:)	see weeds etc (AVS 8-7-2)
(5) Avapatanit Divah (अवपतन्ती दिव:)	brought from the heaven (RVS 10-97-17)

(17) On the basis of originator's name *(ज्ञातनामानुसार वर्गीकरण)*

(1) Brihaspati Prasuta (बृहस्पति प्रसूता)	created by Brihaspati

(2) Mamushyaja (मनुष्यजा)	originated by human beings or cultivated plants (?)
(3) Angirasi (आङ्गीरसि)	found by 'Angira' followers.
(4) Atharvani (अथर्वणी)	found by 'Atharva' followers

(18) Classification of poisonous plant *(विषौषधि वर्गीकरण)*

(1) Sthavara visha: (plant and mineral poisons)

(a) Madavati (मदवती)

(b) Girijata visha (गिरिजात विष)

(c) Kanda visha (कन्दा विष)

(2) Jangama visha: (poisons of animal origin)

(a) Sarpa visha (सर्पविष)	snake poison
(b) Vrischika visha (वृश्चिकविष)	scorpion poison
(c) Keet visha (कीटविष)	wasp poison etc

(19) Classification of diet *(आहारविषयक वर्गीकरण)*

(1) Andha (अन्ध)	people pray for it
(2) Vāja (वाज)	it nourishes the tissues (dhatus)
(3) Kshu (क्षु)	people pray for it because of good qualities
(4) Sina (सिनः)	which reduces appetite.

Basis of Nomenclature in the Vedic period

The name and etymology of the herbs provide some idea about the characters and properties. There are certain names which exist in the same way even today. Similarly some have disappeared while some have been introduced later.

(1) Udumbara, Aswatha etc., names are existing from vedic period.

(2) 'Atasa' (अतस) of Rigveda is modified as 'Atasi' (अतसी)

(3) Gulgulu (गुल्गुलु) and Kashmarya (काष्मर्य) are changed into Guggula (गुग्गुलु) and Kasmarya (काश्मर्य) respectively

(4) Names like Jangida (जङ्गिड), Khalkula (खलकुल) etc., have disappears or renamed.

(5) Dravanti, Jyotishmati, Trivrit, Viswa bheshaja etc., are the names used in Rigveda. But they may not represent the same drugs of vedic period. It is expected that the botamical source for those drugs might have changed at later period.

(6) Araṇi, which is the synonym for Agnimantha was used to denote another drug in vedic literature.

(7) Ghritachi (घृताची) become the synonym for Laksha (lac).

(8) Jeevanti is added to Vedic Materia Medica from the period of Atharva veda only.

(9) Karanja and Aralu are the names of two gaints in Rigveda and they have become names of trees later.

(10) Maha Bala and Mucha kunda are the names of a god/godess and of a great saint respectively.

Anatomy of plants in Vedas

A comparision is made between Purusha (human) and Vanaspati (plant). Some of them are:

	Purusha	Vanaspati
1.	Loma	Parna (leaf and hairs)
2.	Twak	Bahirutpatika (Eetoderm)
3.	Rakta	Niryasa (latex)
4.	Mamsa	Sakara (mesoderm)
5.	Snayu	Kinata (endoderm)
6.	Asthi	Abhyantara kashta (heart kashta)
7.	Majja	Majja (pith or medulla) (Sa.Br. 3-7-1-8)

3. Dravya Guna Aspects in the Samhitas

Ayurvedic treatises have mainly elaborated the fundamental concepts of Dravyaguna in the beginging and later discussed about their utility in different diseases. But these texts did not concentrate upon the properties individual drugs.

(1) Charaka Samhita

This text starts with 'Bheshaja chatushka', indicating the importance of Dravyguna. The following Dravyaguna aspects are discussed in this treatise:

(1) Sutra Sthana 1. chapter *(दीर्घंजीवितीयम्)*

(i) Concept of Samanya and Visesha

(ii) Nine causative factors of creation (Nava Karana Dravyas)

(iii) Two types of dravyas- Chetana & Achetana (living & non-living)

(iv) Dravya, Guna & Karma

(v) Samavaya

(vi) Rasa and its effects on doshas

(vii) Dravya classifications and their utility

(2) Sutra Sthana 2. chapter *(अपामार्गतण्डुलीयम्)*

Drugs used in Panchakarma are discussed.

(3) Sutra Sthana 3. chapter *(आरग्वधादीयम्)*

Different herbs and minerals used for external application are discussed.

(4) Sutra Sthana 4. chapter *(षड्विरेचनशतीय:)*

(i) 600 preparations used for purgation and emesis.

(ii) 50 vargas (group of drugs) containg 10 drugs each i.e., 500 drugs are discribed. Each group is mentioned with one indication e.g.: Hridya, Balya, Seeta prasamana, Krimighna etc.

(5) Sutra Sthana 6. chapter *(मात्राशितीयम्)*

Heavy and easily digestible food items and their quantities are discussed.

(6) Sutra Sthana 9. chatper *(खुड्डाकचतुष्पादम्)*

Qualities of ideal drug are mentioned

(7) Sutra Sthana 13. chapter *(स्नेहाध्याय:)*

4 types of fats and their utility is described.

(8) Sutra Sthana 22. chapter *(लङ्घनबृंहणीय:)*

Six types of drugs viz., Langhana, Brimhana, Rukshna, Snehana, Swedana & Sthamubhama drugs and their use in therpeutics are discussed.

(9) Sutra Sthana 25. chapter *(यज्जः पुरुषीयः)*

(i) Naturally available healthy and unhealthy foods & drugs.

(ii) Best drugs for a specific purpose (Agrya oushadhas)

(iii) Pathya & Apathya

(iv) Posology and its importance

(10) Sutra Sthana 26. chapter *(आत्रेयभद्रकाप्यीयः)*

(i) The entire chapter is very important as far as fundamental concepts of Dravyaguna are concerned.

(ii) It mainly deals with Rasa and its number. After discussing about Rasa, Veerya, Vipaka, Prabhava were discussed.

(iii) The Panchabhoutikatwa of Dravyas, is mentioned .

(iv) Incompatibility (विरूद्धद्रव्य) is also described.

(11) Sutra Sthana 27. chapter *(अन्नापानविध्यध्यायः)*

It mainly deals with dietary substances under 12 varges (7 concerned with Anna varga and 5 concerned with Pana varga)

(12) Vimana Sthana 3 chapter

In this chapter the side effects of Pippali, Lavana & Kshara on long term usage are mentioned.

(13) Çhikitsa Sthana 1& 2 chapters *(रसायन और वाजीकरण)*

These two chapters deal with the concepts of Rasayana and Vajeekarana. Many single drugs are indicated in these chapters.

(14) Kalpa Sthana 1 to 6 chapters

Entire part covers the Vamana (emetic) and Virechana (purgative) dravyas

Note: Above mentionings clarify that Charaka did give much importance to drugs and Dravyaguna aspects in relation to management of different conditions.

(2) Suśruta Samhita

It contains more number of drugs as well as more elaborate classification compared to Charaka Samhita.

(1) Sutra Sthana 1. chapter (*वेदेत्पत्तिमध्याय*)

Classification of durgs- Sthavara & Jangama (inanimate & animate)

(2) Sutra Sthana 20 chapter (*हिताहितीयाध्याय*)

(i) Hita & Ahita dravyas (good & bad dietary materials)

(ii) Viruddha dravyas (incompatible substances)

(3) Sutra Sthana 34 chapter (*युक्तसेवीयमध्याय*)

Qualities of drug (22-23 verses)

(4) Sutra Sthana 36 chapter (*भूमिप्रविभागीयमध्याय*)

(i) Soil & soil types

(ii) Panchabhuta configuration of drugs

(iii) Properties of best drug

(5) Sutra Sthana 37 chapter (*मिश्राकाध्याय:*)

Different drugs are described as per their therapeutic effects.

(6) Sutra Sthana 38 chapter (*द्रव्यसंग्रहणीयाध्याय:*)

It is a very important chapter for Dravyaguna since 37 Ganas are described. This classification is based upon the concept of different drugs having different indications. (But Charaka classified on the basis of different drugs with single indication in the given context).

(7) Sutra Sthana 39 chapter (*संशोधनसंशमनीयाध्याय:*)

Sodhana drugs - 4 vargas

Samana durgs - 3 vargas

(8) Sutra Sthana 40. chapter (*द्रव्यरसगुणवीर्यविपाकविज्ञानीयाध्याय:*)

The fundamentals of Dravyaguna i.e., Rasa, Veerya etc., except Guna are described in this chapter.

Another important feature is that the importance of each aspect is discussed (प्राधान्यताहेतु:)

(9) Sutra Sthana 41. chapter (*द्रव्यविशेषविज्ञानीयाध्याय:*)

(i) Panchabhuta aspect of drug

(ii) Seeta (cold) & Ushna (hot) concept in relation to dravyas

(10) Sutra Sthana 42. chapter (*रसविशेषविज्ञानीयाध्याय:*)

Rasa (taste) is discussed in detail

(11) Sutra Sthana 43 chapter (*वमनद्रव्यविकल्पविज्ञानीयाध्याय:*)

Drugs having emetic property are discussed

(12) Sutra Sthana 44. chapter (*विरेचनद्रव्यविकल्पविज्ञानीयाध्याय:*)

Drugs having purgative proterty are discussed

(13) Sutra Sthana 45. chapter (*द्रवद्रव्यविज्ञानीयाध्याय:*)

Different fluid diets in 10 vargaas

(14) Sutra Sthana 46. chapter (*अन्नापानविध्यध्याय:*)

Different solid foods in 13 vargas

**Guna (phyical property) is explained from 514 to 524 verses.

(15) Chikitsa Sthana 26th chapter for Vājkarana and 27th to 30th (4 chapter) for Rasayana Chikitsa.

(16) Uttara Sthana 63. chapter (*रसभेदविकल्प:*)

Rasa (teste) and its different combinations are discussed.

Note: Being a surgeon Sushrita gave importance to Surgical aspects in the beging of his treatise and later discussed about Dravyaguna aspect. While Charaka described Dravyaguna in the begining.

(3) Ashtanga Sangraha

(1) Sutra Sthana 1 chapter (*आयुष्कामीयम्*)

Rasa, Guṅa, Veerya, Vipaka are described

Drug ȧdministering times are also mentioned

(2) Sutra Sthana 6 chapter (*द्रवद्रव्यविज्ञानीयम्*)

(3) Sutra Sthana 7 chapter (*अन्नस्वरूपविज्ञानीयम्*)

(4) Sutra Sthana 9 chapter (*विरुद्धान्नविज्ञानीयम्*)

(5) Sutra Sthana 12. chapter (*द्विविधौषधविज्ञानीयम्*)

(6) Sutra Sthana 13. chapter (*अन्यसंग्रह:*)

(7) Sutra Sthana 14. chapter (*शोधनादिगणसंग्रह:*)

(8) Sutra Sthana 15 chapter (*महाकषायसंग्रह:*)

(9) Sutra Sthana 16. chapter *(विविधगणसंग्रह:)*

(10) Sutra Sthana 17. chapter *(द्रव्यादिविज्ञानीयमध्याय:)*

(11) Sutra Sthana 18. Chapter *(रसभेदीयमध्याय:)*

(4) Ashtanga Hridayam

(1) Sutra Sthana 1. chapter *(आयुष्कामीयमध्याय:)*

(i) Rasa, Guna, Veerya, Vipaka & Prabhave are described

(ii) Types of Desa (place)

(iii) Drug administering timings

(iv) Classification of drugs

(v) Qualities of a drug

(2) Sutra Sthana 5 chapter *(द्रवद्रव्यविज्ञानीयाध्याय:)*

(3) Sutra Sthana 6. chapter *(अन्नस्वरूपविज्ञानीयाध्याय:)*

(4) Sutra Sthana 7. chapter *(अन्नरक्षाध्याय:)*

(5) Sutra Sthana 9. chapter *(द्रव्यादिविज्ञानीयाध्याय:)*

Fundamental concepts of Dravyaguna are discused.

Panchabhuta aspects are also mentioned.

(6) Sutra Sthana 10. chapter *(रसभेदीयाध्याय:)*

Rasa, Ras types and their properties etc.

(7) Sutra Sthana 15. chapter *(शोधनादिगणसंग्रहोध्याय:)*

Note: Laghu Vagbhata appears to follow the concepts of Charaka mainly. He accepted Sushrita's classification of durgs to a great extent. He also added 2,3 new vargas.

Among As. Sangraha and As. Hridaya we find many common aspects. The matter covered by former text in the first 11 chatpers of Sutra Sthana is covered under first 7 chapters by the later text.

(5) Sarngdhara Samhita

Sarngdhara's work belongs to 13 AD. It gained considerable popularity and authority after Madhava Nidana. It is the second in the series of Laghu trayee.

First part (Prathama Khanda) of the text deals with the measurements and general principles on collection of raw materials etc., in the first chapter. The second chapter deals mainly with the times of drugs administration (Bhaishajya Prayoga kāla). Third chapter introduces the concept of pulse into the Ayurvedic system of medicine for the first time while the fourth chapter is one of the most important chapters of all Samhitas. It deals with various actions of the dravyas which is not found with any other earlier texts.

Second part (Madhyama Khanda) of this treatise deals with the pharmaceuticals and pharmacy procedures which are closely related to pharmacology and pharmacotherapeutics. Preparations like Swarasa, Kalka, Kwatha, Seeta Kashaya, Phanta, Mantha, Churna, Avaleha, Gutika, Āsava-Arishta, Ghrita, Taila etc., are described along with preparatory procedures and relavant examples. 11th chapter deals with the mineral drugs and their purification procedures. This is also a new contribution of Sarangdhara.

Third part (Uttara Khanda) mainly deals with Sodhana procedures (Pancha karmas) and other general procedures of E.N.T & ophthalmological diseases (viz., Aschyotana, Anjana, Kavala, Gandusha, Karnapurana, Siro vasthi etc.)

The first two parts of this Samhita are very useful for the field of Dravyaguna. The commentary of Adhamalla is added attraction to this text. For example, Ādhamalla quoted clearly for the first time that Vājikarana is meant for both males and females.

(6) Bhava Prakasa

It is the classical work of 'Bhava Mishra'. This work forms a connecting link between medeival period and modern period of Ayurveda, just like Vagbhatam which is the connecting link between ancient and medeival period of Ayurveda. Though the author followed other books like Madanapala Nighantu etc., Still maintained individual identity in describing fundamental concepts and also in introducing new diseases and drugs. Bhava Prakasha is the last in the series of 'Laghu Trayee'.

Bhavamishra's father is 'Latakana Mishra'. He might have lived at Varanasi or Kanyakubja. He is a strong believer in Shaiva religion.

Period of Bhava Mishra

He mentioned about 51 authors of several Ayurvedic texts viz., form Charaka to Vishnudharmottara. He mainly followed Sarngdhara (13 AD) in general concepts and management. He copied Madana pala Nighantu (1347 AD) for the Nighantu part. 17 AD books like Yoga Ratnakara, Yoga Tarangini and Lolamba Rajeeya have quoted Bhava Prakasa.

Among treatment aspects most important one is administration of Rasa Karpura, Chopchini etc., in Phiranga Roga. Phiranga Roga is first mentioned by him. Though Rasa Karpura is known earlier to Bhava mishra its utility in Upadamsa and Phiranga Roga was first described by Bhavamishra.

There fore he may be placed between 15-17 AD. But the manuscript obtained from Jammu Library belongs to 1665 AD. Thus, it must be safely placed at about 16 AD. He had also written a 'Bhāshya' in the name of "Guna Ratna Māla".

Chapters in Bhava Prakasha

The whole book is divided into three divisions namely Purva Khanda, Madhyama Khanda and Uttara Khanda.

(1) Purva Khanda– Ayurvedavatarana, Srishti Prakarana, Garbha Prakarana, Bāla Prakarana, Dina-Rutu charya Prakarana & Mishraka Prakarana.

(2) Madhyama Khanda– Diseases are discussed in four parts

(i)	Prathama bhaga (Part-I)	:	Jwara to Grahani
(ii)	Dwitiya bhaga (Part-II)	:	Arsas to Vata Rakta
(iii)	Tritiya bhaga (Part-III)	:	Sula to Bhagna
(iv)	Chaturtha bhaga (Part-IV)	:	Nādi Vrana to Bāla Rogas

***Note–** Total 71 chapters are present in Madhyama Khanda.

(3) Uttara Khanda– Rasayana and Vajikarana are delineated.

Contribution of Bhava mishra to Dravyaguna :

(1) Integration of Hindu and Muslim culture will be visible from Madana pala's period. The same trend is seen with Bhava mishra.

Hence name like: Pārasika yavāna, Ahiphena, Bhanga, Jaya pāla, Kharbuja, Pinda Kharjoora, Amrita phala etc.

(2) Some new drugs have been introduced by Bhava mishra. They are: (a) Pārasika vacha (b) Dweepantara vacha (c) Ākāra karabha (d) Pudina (e) Dāru haridra (f)(Mārkandika (g) Souveera etc.

(3) Apart from the following there are few more worth considering drugs viz., (i) Chandra sura, (ii) Kulanjana (iii) Āmragandhi Haridra (iv) Aranya Haridra (v) Chukra (vi) Latā Kasturi (vii) Gandha Kokila (viii) Chillaka, (ix) Charmakaraluka (x) Āmravarta (xi) Gandha Mālati (xii) Kukumda beeja (xiii) Chinaka (xiv) Chichinda (xv) Makkhanna (xvi) Garjara (xvii) Āluka (xviii) Khasa taila (xix) Sarja Rasa taila.

(4) Some of the drugs with specific importance for their description and identity are as following:

(1) Pushkaramula as Kushta variety or Substitute.

(2) Swarna Ksheeri root as 'Choka'

(3) Two types of Karpura viz., Pakwa & Apakwa.

(4) Three types of Kasturi vix., Kāmarupi (Assam), Naipali (Nepal), and Kashmiri (Kashmir).

(5) Three types of Kumkuma namely, Kashmiri (Best variety), Bahlika (Iran) & Pārasika (Persion).

(6) Two types of Tagara i.e., Tagara & Pinda Tagara.

(7) Ashmantaka as the synonym of Kanchanara.

(8) Three types of Karanja i.e., Nakta Māla, Puti Karanja and Karanji

(9) Madana Pala's Kukkuradru is described as Kudundara.

(10) Chavika phalam is considered as Gaja Pippali.

(11) Vriddha Kāraka is two types viz., Chagalantri & Virddha dāraka.

(12) Detailed description of Ashta vargas is available.

(13) Newly Chātur beejas (four seeds) are described.

(14) Five types of Swarna and three types of Rajata are delineated.

(15) Yasada is mentioned for the first time.

(16) Though a list of substitutes were mentioned for various drugs, it is advised not to substitute the main ingredient of any com pound preparation*.

(17) He appears to follow Raja Nighantu for the classification of plant kingdom. The divisions are: Vanaspati, Vānaspatya, Kshupa, Valli & Oushadhi.

(18) Different parts used are described along with suitable examples.

(19) Definitions of Deepana, Pachana etc., Karmas are provided similar to Sarngdhara.

(20) The drvya constitnents are claimed to be five viz., Rasa, Guna, Virya, Vipaka and Sakti (Prabhava).

The Nighantu Part consists of 23 vargas Totally. They are:

1. Haritakyadi	9. Sāka varga	17. Ghrita varga
2. Karpuradi	10. Mamsa varga	18. Mutra varga
3. Guduchyadi	11. Kritanna varga	19. Taila varga
4. Pushpa varga	12. Vāri varga	20. Sandhana varga
5. Vatāda	13. Dugdha varga	21. Madhu varga
6. Amradi	14. Dadhi varga	22. Ikshu varga
7. Dhātwadi	15. Takra varga	23. Anekartha Nama varga
8. Dhanya varga	16. Navaneeta varga	

Commentaries on Bhava Prakasa

(1) No Sanskrit commentary is available.

(2) Jayadeva wrote incomplete commentary in Pāndu Lipi.

(3) Rādha krishna wrote 'Sarvanighantu Sarwaswa teeka' in Hindi.

(4) Oldest edition was published by Jeevananda, Calcutta in 1985.

(5) Nirnaya Sagar, Mumbai edition by Dattaram Choube as editor 1855.

(6) Venkateswara Press, Mumbai edition by Saligram Vaidya in 1906.

After wards many authors have edited and Published Bhava Prakasa.

---

* योगे यदप्रधानं स्यात्तस्य प्रतिनिधिर्मत:
यत्तु प्रधानं तस्यापि सदृशं नैव गृह्यते ॥ (भा.प्र. १/६/१६७)

4. Number of Drugs mentioned in the ancient literature

Conclusion on the total number of drugs deliniated in the ancient Indian medical texts is highly contraversial. Different authors provided different numbers. According to Acharya Priya Vrata Sharma the number of drugs deliniated in Rigveda, Yajurveda and Atharva veda are about 67,81 and 289 respectively. This increase in the number of medicinal plants will indicate the development in the utility of herbs during vedic period.

In the preface, on his work 'Gloosary of Vegetable drugs in Brihat Trayee'. Thakur Balwant Singh dissussed regarding the number of medicinal plants in the Samhitas : "As regards the total number of drug plants mentioned in the three Samhitas, it appears, on a rough estimate, that, it lies some where between six and seven hundred or it may be about 600 if the unidentified food grains, divine drugs and vegetable poisons are excluded including, of course, the food-cum-drug plants and some of the drastic poisons accepted for use after some treatment.

The number of the Sanskrit names (excluding their derivatives) are about 1900 out of which, on a rough conuting, about 670 are common to all the three texts and about 240, 370 and 240 have been exclusively mentioned only in C.S., S.S., and A.H. respectively. Thus the total number of the Sanskrit names are about 1270, 1100 and 1150 in S.S., C.S. and A.H. respectively. Their numerical superiority in S.S. indicates that a much larger number of plants were known and used by Susruta. While that in A.H. over C.S. may be explained by the fact that vagbhata borrowed freely from both to make his treatise more comprehensive and practical, although with the same object in view he dropped most of the divine drugs plants and the vegetable poisons from his perview.

The natural follow-up step after this analysis should be to assess the actual size of the drug stock in each of the Samhitas and to determine the pace of its enrichment or depletion as time advanced. There are insurmountable difficulties in the achievement of this object. Although the chronological priorities or the order of their appearance are more or less established, the present day editions of the two parent Samhitas are not what they were at their first appearance".

The author feel it really unfortunate to document that not even hand ful of P.G. or Ph.D. thesis have been submitted so far on reidentification or number of vegetable drugs from the major Samhita books. Some of the studies are:

1. Sathe N.B., Charaka Samhita Ki Anirnita Aushadiya.
   Jamnagar: IPGTR, Dept. of D.G., 1960 (M.D. Thesis)
2. Sharma A.N., Sushrita Samhita ke Nirneeta Evam Anirneeta Dravya.
   Jamnagar: IPGTR, Dept. of D.G., 1963 (M.D. Thesis)
3. Singh R.; Atharva Vanaushadhi Vivechana.
   Varanasi: IMS, BHU, Dept. of D.G. (1980) Ph.d. Thesis)
4. Singh Savitri; Rigveda mein Vanaushadhiyon Ka Vivechana.
   Varanasi: IMS, BHU, Dept. of D.G. Ph.D. Thesis.

At present Govt. of India officially reported an estimate of 8000 as the total number of medicinal plants in India (Editorial, AMRUTA. Bangalore, December 1998). From published literature, the FRLHTdatabase gives a lower estimate of 7195 species of medicinal plants. The following is the information on no of medicinal plants in different systems of medicine:

System	**Ayurveda**	**Folk**	**Homoeo**	**Modern**	**Siddha**	**Tibetan**	**Unani**
Ayurveda	<u>1773</u>	731	164	55	743	271	653
Folk	731	<u>4720</u>	147	56	636	201	486
Homoeo	164	147	<u>296</u>	60	142	70	155
Modern	55	56	60	<u>105</u>	41	17	50
Siddha	743	636	142	41	<u>1122</u>	227	486
Tibetan	271	201	70	17	277	<u>280</u>	224
Unani	653	486	155	50	486	224	<u>751</u>

The family and genera analysis of 7195 medicinal plants shows that 387 families and 2220 genera are included. Some of the major families are: Asteraceae (424), Euphorbiaceae (219), Lamiaceae (218), Fabaceae (217), Rubiaceae (210), Poaceae (169). Papilionoceae (167), Acanthaceae (143), Rosaceae (130) and Apiaceae (118).

Since the work on inventorisation of the medicinal plants of India is incomplete, there is naturally a gap in our understanding of the distribution and distribution pattern of the species and therefore, a gap in our knowledge of the 'conservation status' of the species also exists. Global trend show that 12.5% of all plant life is already facing the threat of extinction. With the present level of unconcern, we do not know if medicinal plants conservation or their extinction will prevail.

We have already learnt from the ancient literature that many excellent medicinal plants like Soma, Brahma Suarchala etc., have become extinct today. The same may happen to drugs like Kushta, Sathi, Daru Haridra also. It is the high time to reidentify all the botanical sources of classical Ayurvedic herbs and conserve and preserve them for the future generations.

✸

Chapter - XVI
Knowledge about various Nighantus and their authors Dravya guna books by modern scholars

1. Dravya Guna Lexicons in Medieval Times

Foreign invasion and foreign rule have affected every walk of life in India during the medeival period. So Ayurvedic literature is no exception to this. With a change in the socio-economic conditions the traditional practice of Ayurveda is badly affected. Many problems shooted up especially in the identity of herbs and in understanding the meanings of the original treatises.

Therefore, Nighantus (lexicons or dictionaries) dealing with Indian Materia Medica have their origin between 8-10 AD. These Nighantus are simile to 'Nirukta' on vedas. As we know. Nirukta will point out the concealed or secret meanings of Vedas-निगूढं अर्थं गमयन्ति ज्ञापयन्ति इति निगम: ।- (यास्क). Similarly, 'Nighantu throws light on to the secret meanings of the terms denoting different synonyms of the vegetable kingdom"-एकार्थवाचिनाम् पर्यायशब्दानां सङ्घो यत्र प्रायेण उपदिश्यते तत्र निघण्टुशब्द: प्रसिद्ध:।'' (वाचस्पत्यम्) ।

On identifying the importance, Raja Narahari quotes in his work-

निघण्टुना विना वैद्यो, विद्वान्याकरणं विना ।
आयुधं च विना योद्धा स्त्रयो हासस्य भाजनम् ।। (रा.नि)

i.e., the physician entering into practice without any knowledge on Nighantus is simile to a Pandit without knowledge on grammer and a warrier without weapon.

It may be noted that the literature which goes under the term 'Kosha' is not the same as Nighantus. Keith differentiated between 'Kosha' and 'Nighantu'. Even the purpose which intiated the development of Nighantus was quite different from that of the Koshas. 'The former was written to facilitate interpretation of vedic texts, while the later was a simple dictionary to help writers and not based on any particular text.

It is very difficult to conclude about the period when the system of writing Ayurvedic Nighantus came into vogue. However, it can be realized that the earlier nighantus were concerned mostly with the description and synonyms of medicinal plants.

It the chronology, these Nighantus have introduced some new herbs to Indian Materia Medica. During the process they also created confusion by using same synonym for different plants. However, it would be interesting to study the different medicinal plants from the vedic period to the period of Ayurvedic Nighantus. This might throw a good deal of light on the general chronology of different texts, and may also help in the study of the development of knowledge of medicinal plants in ancient India.

One of the greatest contributions of Ayurvedic Nighantus is that their authors have collected and documented the then existing information on medicinal plants. Though it is very difficult to fix the chronology of these Nighantus, many writers and scholars place Dhanwantari Nighantu (10AD) as the oldest of the available Nighantus.

The writing of nighantus in the classical fashion ends with Raja Nighantu in 7AD. Therefore 10-17AD is considered to be a golden era for Nighantu writers in India. The last recognized Nighantu is saligrama-Nighantu (19AD).

Among the 'Koshas' a significant work of Shivadatta Mishra (1625-1700AD) is more related to Dravyaguna Vijnana. His book 'Shiva Kosha' describes about the identity of many plants.

In more recent period, some works like 'Nighantu Ratnakara' of Vishnu Vasandera Godabole; 'Nighantu Adarsh' of Bapalal Vaidya etc., are also seen. Certain lexicons are also written in vernacular languages e.g. Nighantu Ratnakar of Datar, Mahabal, Patil etc.

It is also not possible to finalize the total number of lexicons on Indian Materia Medica some of the important Nighantus are picked up and explained in this chapter. They are:

1. Ashtanga Nighantu
2. Paryaya Ratnamāla
3. Dhanwantari Nighantu
4. Sodhala Nighantu

5. Siddha Mantra
6. Hridaya Deepaka Nighantu
7. Mādhava Dravya Guna
8. Dravya guna Sangraha
9. Madana Pala Nighantu
10. Raja Nighantu
11. Kaiyadeva Nighantu
12. Shiva Kosha
13. Dravya guna Sataka
14. Abhidhana Ratnamala
15. Raja Vallabha Nighantu
16. Nighantu Ratnakara
17. Sāligrama Nighantu
18. Madanādi Nighantu
19. Nighantu Ādarsh.

It appears from the dates that are approximately fixed by various authors, that the majority of lexicons have come into existance between 11-16 AD.

In more recent period, some works appeared in vernacular languages, collected from the then existing ocean of Sanskrit literature on the subject. The Nighantu Ratnakara of Datar, Mahabal, Patil etc., can be mentioned as one good example for vernacular lexicon.

It is not even possible to obtain correct knowledge on the existing manuscripts in different oriental libraries of the world and particularly of this century. It was, therefore, found very difficult to select a manuscript for publication and find its availability in different libraries. A rough estimate of about 95 Nighantu manuscripts are reported so far from various libraries. The total number of lexicons unpublished with critical enditing will be about 100 or so.

Before concluding it is important to realise that in the earlier days lexicons were written to denote various synonyms of a single drug. At the later period, especially, after the invasion of westerners, the medical lexicons too took some change as was the case with literary lexicons and are arranged alphabetically.

The literature of Dravyaguna is therefore available in two forms:

(1) Texts which describe only synonyms of drugs: e.g. Ashtanga Nighantu, Paryaya Ratnamala, Hridaya Deepaka Nighantu etc.

(2) Texts which explain synonyms along with properties & action etc: e.g. Dhanwantari Nighantu, Sodhala Nighantu etc.

The individual Nighantus are described in detail including the authors identity, time, subject contents etc.

2. Certain Important Nighantus and their Introduction

(1) Ashtanga Nighantu

The manuscripts of "Ashtanga Nighantu' or 'Ashtanga Hridaya Nighantu' are available in Tanjore library. Basing upon that Acharya P.V. Sharmaji published one lexicon (Kuppuswamy Sastry Research Institute, Madras, Series No. 4, 1973). This book deals with the drugs mentioned in Ashtanga Hridaya along with different synonyms.

A.S. Paranjape etal., in their introduction to Laghu Nighantu mention about Ashtanga Nighantu of Vagbhata (M.S. No. 13256/GOMM/CCS).

But the original author of this text is believed to be different from the other two vagbhatas (authors of As.Hr.& As.Sau.) significant critera to decide this fact is that some of the drugs mentioned in this text are not prosent in Ashtanga Sangraha and Ashtanga Hridaya. Similarly, authors like Jejjata (9AD), Madhavakara (9AD), Chakrapani (11AD) etc., have quoted about this lexicon. There fore Ashtanga Nighantu must be placed between 7th-9th AD.

**** Suśruta Nighantu**

Though it is not well documented, Acharya P.V. Sharmaji quoted about Suśruta Nighantu which is the lexicon part of the original Suśruta Samhita. It is believed that all the Brihat Samhitas were having a lexicon part which may be missing today.

The references about Suśruta Nighantu and Ashtanga Nighantu provide some clues in favour of Sharmaji's theory. Further study may be needed in this direction.

(2) Paryaya Ratnamāla

It is written by Madhava (Madhavakara) son of Indukara, who hails from a place called Silahrada. On review of literature we come across three Madhavas mainly viz.,

(1) Author of Rigvinischaya – son of Chandra kara

(2) Author of Paryaya ratnamala – son of Indukara.

(3) Author of Dravya Guna – son of Chakrapani.

From the above view it is clear that Indukara's son is the author of Paryaya ratnamala. But Tarapada Chowdary consider that the author of Rigvinischaya and Paryayaratnamala are same.

This book is first deleniated by Sarvananda Vanda Ghatiya (1159 AD) who is the commentator on Amarakosha. It is also quoted by Medini Kosha (13 AD), Ray Mukut (1430AD) and Bhanoji Dixit (1650AD).

Rigvinischaya in not reported before Vrinda (9AD). Chakrapani (11AD) mentioned twice about Paryaya ratnamala and Ksheera Swamy (11AD) quoted it several times. In the final verses he imitated the style of poet Magha (7-8AD). Therefore Paryaya ratnamala is placed between 8-9AD.

This text mainly deals with Synonyms like Ashtanga Nighantu. A part from them measurements, technical words are also provided. On the basis of the contents this text appears to be earlier to Dhanwantari Nighantu. For example, Ahiphena, Bhanga and Yasada are described in Dhanvantari Nighantu and Rasa Ratna Samuchchaya. These aspects are missing with Paryayaratnamala.

Vijaya name is synonymously used for both Haritaki and Tarkari. Vartaka term is replaced with Vatigan basing upon a Parsi word Vārdigān.

This text deals with mercury, sulphur, mica etc., indicating the development of Rasa Sastra during contemparary period.

Treatment of hydrocele (Bradhna roga chikitsa) is mentioned only in Paryayaratnamala and Vrinda Madhavam. But it is missing in Madhava Nidana.

This Nighantu has a unique approach i.e., 13-216 slokas for synonyms, 217-578 are half slokas, 580-1424 are Pada, (पद), 1425-1472 are names of Padartha or drugs. From 1474-1654 three types of sabdas were used viz.,

(1) the drugs with one meaning (1474-1504)

(2) the drugs with two meanings (15050-1586) &

(3) the durgs with many meanings (1587-1754)

It is first published in 1946 from Patna university.

(3) Dhanwantari Nighantu

Of all the extant Nighantus, this is believed to be the oldest. But really it is not so. Dhanwantari-the author is not the lord Dhanwantari but seems to be another person. It is apparent from his prayer on lord Dhanwantari- "नमामि धन्वन्तरिमादिदेवं........" (I bow to God Dhanwantari).

The original name of the book appears to be 'Dravyavali Samuchchaya'. It is still a mystery how this name 'Dhanwantari Nighantu' emerged.

Various manuscripts availabe at Pune mention the author's name as Mahendra Bhogik. The author of this text is inspired by treatises of Charaka, Sushrita etc., and compiled the quotation either partially or completely from the earlier texts. The author has made use of colloquial, Sanskrit as well as foreign languages in this texts-'अनेकदेशान्तरभाषितेषु सर्वेष्वथ प्राकृतसंस्कृतेषु ॥'

He further adds-'after knowing both local and Sanskrit names of the plants one should see them, ask their names to others, should touch the plants to ascertain the texture etc., and thus should try to know about many plants.

Totally there are 7 groups under which the plants are described. Total drugs or drug groups (excluding Misraka Varga) are claimed to be 373 but the over all number of individual drugs will be 527. For example 'Triphala Gana' contains three individual herbs and 'Pancha Lavana' contains five types of salts.

Though being the first author of a lexicon, he narrated the drugs on the basis of Rasa, Veerya, Vipaka etc., First the synonyms scattered here and there are compiled and then the properties of the drug are discussed. Many others have imitated his style and method at later periods.

P.V. Sharmaji put this work between 10-13 AD, Yasada is described in it therefore this work can not be earlier to 13AD. Moreover, it mentions about Ahiphena, Jayapala, Agnijara, Vijaya etc., which were brought to India from foreign countries during Muslim rule. It also mentions the purification methods of mercury which may be borrowed from Rasa Sastra texts written in 13AD. The author quoted regarding Hemadri and Arunadatta. So he can not be earlier to 13AD. Ksheera Swamy (11AD) and Hemachandra (commentator) on Abhidhana Chudamani (12AD) mentioned this work in their writings. Thence, it is placed between 11-13AD.

Evidences prove that the author borrowed this work from *Dravyavali*. Another possibility is that there might have been another work known as *Dhanwantari Nighantu* from which the existing text emerged as a mixture of Dravyavali & Dhanwantari Nighantu.

Merits of this text are:

(1) Both Charaka & Suśruta have mentioned one drug under many Ganas/Vargas. But, this text described one drug under one Gana only.

(2) While grouping the drugs under different Ganas, Dhanvantari Nighantu followed a new and unique procedure which was not there earlier.

(3) The drugs are named on the basis of the first drug under that varga. Then each Varga is divided into different Ganas basing up on pharmacological properties.

(4) Synonyms and properties are described in an order for each and every drug.

(5) The author described some extra drugs also in the end of each Varga. They are actually not mentioned in the original Vargas.

(6) Though the author is inspired by Charaka and Suśruta he maintained his speciality. For example Dadima is mentioned under Phala varga in the treatises. But in this text, Dadima is not mentioned under Amradiphala varga. Infact it is mentioned in the Satapushpadi varga. Like wise Banana is described in Karaveeradi varga.

The seven Vargas narrated in this text are:

1. GuduchyadiVarga– plants combating different diseases e.g.: Guduchi, Sathi, Shaliparni, Jeevaka etc.

2. Satapushpadi Varga– herbs used as stomachic digestive etc. e.g.: Satapushpa, Misrcya, Ela, Nagakesara etc.

3. Chandanadi Varga– plants with volatile oils/flavonoids and minerals. e.g.: Chandana, Manalusila, Tutha etc.

4. Karaveeradi Varga– herbs used in skin, krimi, Visha & haemorrhage. e.g.: Karaveera, Rasona, Sinduvara, Akshu.

5. Amradi Varga– plants used for their furits, flower, creepers and barks. (some aromatic drugs are also present) e.g.: Amra, Bhavya, Kadamba, Arjuna, Jati etc.

6. Swarnadi Varga– both herbal, mineral and animal sources which are used for different diseases are described under this e.g.: Gold, tin, Mercury, Masura, Godhuma etc.

7. Misrakadi Varga– drugs with miscellaneous properties e.g.: Oushadhi Gana & Visha Gana.

Total number of Drugs in Dhanwantari Nighantu:-

S.N.	Name of the Varga	No. of Ganas	No. of dravyas	Drugs mentioned at chapter ending	Total Drugs
1.	Guduchyadi	11	89	1	90
2.	Satapushpadi	2	42	1	43
3.	Chandanadi	3	64	6	70
4.	Karaveeradi	4	56	4	60
5.	Amradi	3	61	4	65
6.	Suvarnadi	10	94	36	130
7.	Misrakadi	2	69	-	69
	Total	35	475	52	527

(4) Sodhala Nighantu

This work is a valuable contribution of Gujarat state to Ayurvedic materia medica. Author Sodhala is a physician, scholar, grammarian and astrologer too. He took lot of pains in compiling this text by refering several contemporary works.

This Nighantu is otherwise known as 'Guna Sangraha' or 'Nama Sangraha'.

In the introductory verses Sodhala express his view that students of Ayurveda in his time are facing great difficulty as the list of drugs, propar classification, nomenclature etc., are not available. Therefore he composed this work after consulting earlier works of Agnivesa etc. He claims that this text will solve controversies among various texts and would describe the properties of drugs with their Rasa, Veerya, Vipaka etc., in not too detailed or too concise style so that the same may be easily understood.

Between Astanga Sangraha and Ashtanga Hridaya, he preferred the later treatise because of its concised style. He quoted much from As. Hridaya, although he borrowed sufficiently from Charaka and Suśruta as well. Similarly while writing Gada Nigraha he followed Rigvinischaya of Madhava for pathophysiology and followed Siddha Yoga of Vrinda for management.

This text has intimate relation with Dhanwantari Nighantu. There are 27 groups or drugs totally. The first 7 are common with Dhanwantari Nighantu. The difference is that 7th group is *Misrakadi Varga* in Dhanwantari Nighantu while it is named as *Lakshmanadi Varga* in this text. As the style adopted by Dhanwantari Nighantu became absolete after some time, Sodhala made an attempt to revive the same. At the same time he left some unnecessary details given in Dhanwantari Nighantu. He described the properties of the drugs in a concise manner so as to enable the students to grasp the subject easily e.g.: वासः क्षयकासघ्नो रक्तपित्त कफापः ।

It appears that he utilized Dalhana's commentary on Suśruta Samhita e.g.: his description of Madhu (Honey). Therefore Sodhala must be placed later to Dhanwantari Nighantu (10AD) and earlier to Dalhana (12AD). To fix the lower limit Bhava mishra's descriptions are also essential. Bhavamishra (16AD) had taken enough material from Sodhala Nighantu such as description of Haritaki, Chavika,Gaja Pippali, Karpura, Parasika Yavani, Lata Kasturi, Bala Chatushtaya etc. The magical action of *Chetaki* (a variety of Haritaki) is first described in this book and latter borrowed by Bhava mishra.

चेतकीपादपच्छायामपसर्पन्ति येनराः ।
भिद्यन्ते तत्क्षणादेव पशुपक्षिमृगादयः ।। (शो.नि.)

Sarangdhara (13AD) and Madanapala (14AD) have imitated Sodhala in their writings. Narahari (15AD) also accepted many things from Sodhala Nighantu. Kesava (13AD) and Bopadeva (14 AD) have utilized Sodhala's work. Several passages are commonly found in Sodhala Nighantu and Madhava Dravya Guna (12-13AD). The description of Ahiphena is found in Madhava Dravyaguna while it is missing in Sodhala's work prove that Madhava's work is posterior to Sodhala's. Therefore this text may be placed between 11-13AD.

The following facts are worth remembering:

(1) Yasada is not mentioned among Dhatus. (Yasada is not found in the texts before 14AD).

(2) Jayapala is not mentioned in this text while, Sarangdhara (13AD) used it.

(3) Bhanga, Ahiphena, Akara karabha, Rumi mastagi etc., described in Gada Nigraha are missing in this text.

(4) Mercury and its purification is mentioned. It indicates that this text is developed after 10AD.

(5) Kankushta and Swarna Ksheeri are the terms used synonymously in Ashtanga Nighantu (10AD). Dalhana (12AD) consider it as the Niryasa of Swarnaksheeri while later texts mentioned both the drugs seperately. Sodhala too, mentioned Kankushta and Swarnaksheeri seperately.

The entire text is classified into 27 vargas:

1.	Guduchyadi Varga–	Katu, Tikta, Kashaya dravyas, Jivaniyas, Sodhana drugs.
2.	Satapushpadi Varga–	Spices etc, having volatile oils and carmirnative action.
3.	Chandanadi Varga–	aromatic drugs, gum-resine, minerals, gems etc.
4.	Karaveeradi Varga–	Upa vishas, Sakas (leafy vegetable), acquatic plants.

5. Amradi varga– fruits, big trees, flowers and stems.
6. Swarnadi Varaga– metals and mercury
7. Lakshmanadi Varga– contains many peculior plants and drugs not described in other Nighantus.
8. Paniyadi Varga
9. Paniya Varga
10. Ksheera varga
11. Dadhi Varga
12. Takra Varga
13. Navaneeta Varga
14. Ghrita Varga
15. Taila Varga
16. Madhu Varga
17. Ikshu Varga
18. Madya varga
19. Mutra Varga
20. Suka dhanya Varga
21. Jurna Varga
22. Trinadhanya Varga
23. Simbi dhanya Varga
24. Kritanna Varga
25. Anupana Varga
26. Mamsa Varga
27. Misraka Varga- definitions of techni cal terms, personal hygene

(5) Siddha Mantra

Its author is Vaidyacharya Kesava. At the end of the text he informed that he is the son of Madhava. Bopadeva also quoted that Madhava belongs to Veda pada or Deva pada in Maharashtra.

Kesava's scholarship and profissiency in practice are indicated by the titles or epithets Vadyanatha, Vaidya vandya, Vaidyacharya etc. However this text is a forgotten work on Indian Materia Medica now. "This work enables one to know the properties of drugs easily and in no time miraculous results are achieved quickly simile to the Mantras of Siddhas". Hence the title Siddha Mantra. The author further emphasize that the drug which is not understood here, can not be known elsewhere.

Kesava was the king physician of Singhana (1210-1247 AD). Singhana is known as Simharaja belonging to the Yadava dynasty. Therefore this text belongs to 12 AD.

The speciality of this work is that the drugs are arranged according to their effect on Doshas first followed by their Rasa, Veerya, Vipaka etc. The drugs are classified into eight groups. They are:

(1) Vataghna Varga
(2) Pittaghna Varga
(3) Kaphaghna Varga
(4) Vata Pittaghna Varga
(5) Kapha-Vataghna Varga
(6) Kapha-Pittaghna Varga
(7) Doshaghna Varga
(8) Doshala Varga

He described about 57 types of sub-groups of drugs according to variation of effect on doshas and their combinations.

A commentary entitled as 'Prakasa' has been written by his son Bopadeva. The basic concepts of Dravya Guna are discussed in the first nine verses (Nava sloks) on the same pattern of Panchalakshana Nidana of Rigvinischaya.

(6) Hridaya Deepaka Nighantu

Its author Bopadeva (Vopa deva) is a grammarian and author of certain religious books. Hence he is a land mark in the medieval period. He had a rich heritage of medical tradition from his father Kesava (13 AD) who was the royal physician. Dhaneswara is said to be the teacher of Bopadeva. He resided at a place called Veda pura which is situated on the bank of river Varada in Maharashtra. This was the capital of king Simha raja.

He is believed to be at least two and half centuries earlier to Bhavamishra i.e., 12-13 AD. Thus he became a valuable link between the ancient and modern era of Ayurvedic literature.

Hemadri (1260-1271) is contemporary to Bopadeva. Hemadri was the Prime/chief minister of king Mahadeva of Yadava dynasty. Bopa deva is said to be the physician/Pandit of king Mahadeva. Hence he is fixed in 13 AD. Some reference quote that Hemadri had written commentaries on Bopadeva's works-Hari leela and Mukta phala.

Altogether Bopadeva wrote 26 books. They are: 10 books on Sanskrit grammer, 9 books on Ayurveda, 1 book on Jyotisha, 3 books on literature and 3 books on Bhagavadgita. Out of these works, a book on medicine entitled as 'Sata Sloki' with Chandrakala commentary was edited by Vayaskar N.S. Moss of Kottayam (Kerala) and published in 1962. However his work on materia medica and Prakasa commentary on his father's work (Siddhamantra) are less popular.

This work was actually intended to explain the drugs mentioned in Ashtang a Hridaya. Hence the name Hridaya deepaka nighantu.

The subject matter of this text is divided into eight Vargas viz.,

(1) Chatushpada Varga-	Yashtimadhu to Swarnam.
(2) Tripada Varga-	Āragwadha to Kamalam.
(3) Dwipada Varga-	Madana phala to Vetasa.
(4) Eka pada Varga-	Swarna Ksheeri to Rishabhaka.
(5) Dwi Nāma Varga-	Tinisa to Surana.
(6) Eka Nāma Varga-	Sankhini to Hilamochika
(7) Nanartha Varga-	Koshataki to Haritaki
(8) Mishraka Varga-	food materials etc.

The author followed the material style of Paryayaratnamala rather than alphabetical order/style. Under Mishraka Varga, items other than drugs i.e., diet, Pancha Karma, other therapeutic measures have been described.

There is some peculiarity in arrangement of the matter. Sometimes, the chapter ends abruptly with the half verse and the subsequent chapter starts with the remaining half of the verse. e.g.: Eka pada varga ends with "मेदा परा महामेदा विषाण्यृषभको वृषः" a helf verse and the next chapter begins with the other half-"तिनिशः स्यन्दनो दूर्वा शाद्वलः बीजकोऽसनः।"

There is much similarity in the descriptions of Amara Kosha and Hridaya dipaka Nighantu.

Certain common aspects are:

(1) कर्कन्धुर्बदरी कोलिः ।	(3) यासो यवासो दुःस्पर्शाः ।
(2) गायत्री बालतनयः खदिरः ।	(4) हरेणू रेणूका कौन्ती । etc.

(7) Madhava Dravya Guna

Its author Madhava must be different from the author of Rigvinischaya and Paryayaratnamala. A part from this text, a work known as Dravyaguna Sangraha of Madhava was quoted by some commentators leading to an inferecnce about existance of another work on Indian Materia Medica.

A manuscript of Madhava's Dravyaguna (Sl. No. 5895; Accn. No. B 3773) is located in the Collection of the Bharata Kala Bhavan of B.H.U., Varanasi. This book is often quoted as 'Bhava Swabhava Vada' in the manuscripts.

Basing up on Sushrita Samhita the subject matter is arranged under two broad heads- (1) Drava dravya (liquids) and (2) Anna pana vidhi (diet). Though Madhava did not use these words directly, he adopted the same arrangement. There are totally 29 vargas in this text. They are:

1. Vividhoushadha Varga
2. Lavana Varga
3. Ikshu Varga
4. Madhu Varga
5. Ksheera Varga
6. Dadhi Varga
7. Takra Varga
8. Navaneeta Varga
9. Ghrita Varga
10. Taila Varga
11. Sneha Varga
12. Madya Varga
13. Kanjika Varga
14. Mutra Varga
15. Toya Varga
16. Sali Varga
17. Kudhanya Varga
18. Simbidhanya Varga
19. Mamsa Varga
20. Matsya Varga
21. Phala Varga
22. Saka Varga
23. Sreshta Varga
24. Rasa Varga
25. Manda Varga
26. Anna Varga
27. Pana-Bhakshya Varga
28. Anupana Vidhi
29. Prakeerna Varga (deals with Swastha Vritta).

First chapter starts with Haritaki which is Sara (purgative) in nature. He also described other purgatives like Trivrit, Katuki, Trayamana in continuation. Later Grahi (Astringent) drugs like Pata, Kutaja, Indrayava, Musta, Bilva etc., are described. Aromatic substances are divided into Pittaghna, Vātaghna & Kaphaghna such as Chandana, Kumkuma and Karpura respectively. Drugs effective in upper respiratary trrat and fevers were described in the end. After vegetable drugs minerals and animal products have been described. A part from Suśruta Samhita the author has closely followed As. San. and As. Hri. Among his sources hte author mentions Charaka, Suśruta, Parasara, Vagbhata, Bhattara-Harichandra, Bhela, Vaideha, Hareeta etc.

A part from the ancient sources, certain latest works like Sodhala Nighantu etc., were also consulted by author. Like Charakapani he had given importance to dietetic substances in a concized manner.

Some scholars observe that this work is transcribed in 1452 AD and the original work is anterior to this . Swami Laxmi Ram (20 AD) in his note on an Siddha Bheshaja Manimala & Siva datta Mishra (17 AD) quoted this work. Adhamalla (15-16 AD), Siviadas sen (15 AD) and Bopa deva (13-14 AD) have mentioned about this text in their works. Neither Dalhana (12 AD) nor Chakarpani quoted this text in their commentaries. But Sarvananda (12 AD) quoted a verse from this book in his commentary on Amarakosha.

There are several passages common in Dravyaguna Sangraha of Chakrapani and Madhava's Dravyaguna (vide: verses 12 to 20 in Dhanya varga of former text and 1-7 in the later text). Sivadas Sen is of the openion that the author of Dravyaguna and Rigvinischaya are same. Some verses tally with Sodhala Nighantu also.

The following subject matter is of some special importance in this text:

(1) Mentioning of Jayapala indicates it as a medeival period text in India.
(2) Vijaya is described
(3) Ahiphene is also mentioned which is found in Dhanwantari Nighantu (10-13 AD) and onwards.
(4) Yasada is not mentioned. That means it is earlier to 14 AD.

Considering the available evidences Madhava will be placed in the later part of 13 AD.

(8) Dravya Guna Sangraha

It is a Dravyaguna text written by Chakrapani datta in 11 AD. He is the author of 'Ayurveda Dipika' commentary on Charak Samnhita and 'Chakradatta'. This book mainly deals with the herbs used in diet. Fundamentals like Rasa, Guna, Veerya, Vipaka are described in the begining of the first chapter.

The contents are divided into 15 Vargas. They are:

1. Dhanya Varga
2. Mamsa Varga
3. Saka Varga
4. Lavanadi Varga
5. Phala Varga
6. Paniya Varga
7. Kshoudra Varga
8. Taila Varga
9. Ikshvadi Varga
10. Madyadi Varga
11. Kritanna Varga
12. Bhakshya Varga
13. Ahara Vidhi
14. Anupana Vidhi
15. Misraka Varga.

The author claims that this text is the essence of many books he referred.

तन्त्रणां सारमाकृष्य द्रव्याणां गुणसंग्रहः ।
भिषजामुपकाराय रचितश्चक्रपाणिना ।। (द्र.गु.सं.)

(9) Madana Pala Nighantu

This text was written by king Madana pala of 'Tika' dynesty. His capital city was 'Kashta Nagara'. This book is also known as 'Madana Vinoda'. According to the mentionings at the end of the text, it is assessed that this book is written during 1374 AD.

The author explained about the necersity in writing this work that "some nighantus are very less descriptile while some are too elaborate, some are very difficult to understand and voluminous. Hence this text is being written to expand the concised aspects and to edit the elaborated descriptions, by mentioning the well known nomenclature and by clear description of their properties for the sake of wise people".

केचित् सन्ति निघण्टवोऽतिलघवः केचिन्महान्तः परे
केचिद्दुर्गमनामकाः कतिपयो भावाः स्वाभावोच्छ्रिताः ।।
तस्मान्नातिलघुर्न चातिविपुलः ख्यातादिनामा सतां
प्रीत्यै द्रव्यगुणान्वितोऽयमधुना ग्रन्थो मया बध्यते ।। (म.पा.नि.१/५)

He mentioned about Bhanga, Ahiphena, Jayapala, Parasika Yavani, Chouhara, Sulemani Kharjura, Amrita phala, Grinjana, Madhu karkati etc.

Yasada is found in the 1954 edition edited by Vaidya Ram Prasad Sharma, published from Mumbai. But Acharya P.V. Sharmaji is of the openion that Yasada is not mentioned in Madana pala Nighantu.

There are about 13 vargas totally in this text:

1. Abhayadi Varga–	with 165 drugs e.g.: Haritaki, Bakuchi, Ahiphena etc.
2. Sunthyadi Varga–	with 39 drugs e.g.: Sunthi, Yavani, Tankan etc.
3. Karpuradi Varga–	with 84 drugs e.g.: Karpura, Chandana, Guggulu etc.
4. Suvarna Varga–	with 44 mineral & metallic drugs etc.
5. Vatadi Varga–	with 50 drugs e.g.: Vata, Aswatha, Salmali, Agustya etc.
6. Phala Varga– (Drakshadi Varga)	with 56 drugs e.g.: Draksha, Jambu, Naranga, Pugiphala etc.
7. Saka Varga–	with 56 drugs e.g.: Kushmanda, Vastuka, Lasuna etc.
8. Panadi Varga– (Drava Varga)	Jala, Ksheera, Taila, Mutra etc.
9. Ikshukadi Varga– (Madhura Varga)	Ikshu, Madhuka, Madu etc.
10. Dhanyaguna Varga– (Dhanya Varga)	Cearls, pulses etc
11. Dhanya Kritannadi – Varga (Kritanna Varga)	Yavagu, Peya, Vilepi etc.
12. Mamsa Varga–	different types of non-vegetarian foods.
13. Mishraka Varga–	Anupana, Dinacharya, Rutu charya etc.

The total number of substances or dravyas described by Madanapala are about 494 (450 vegetable and 44 metallic other drugs).

(10) Rāja Nighantu

This book is known with the names-'Abhidana Chudamani' and 'Nighantu Raja'. The author claims that this book is compiled after consulting works like Dhanwantari Nighantu, Madanapala Nighantu,

Halayudha Nighantu, Viswaprakasa Nighantu, Amarakosa, Bhojaraja Kosa. Another important aspect is this work deals with names of the plants in various languages. Thus some named it as 'Dravyabhidana Gana Sangraha'. But the author himselfs prefered the name 'Raja Nighantu meaning that this is the king among various Nighantus.

तस्मादयं जयति सर्वनिघण्टुराजः ।......

.......प्रारंभि भेषजहिताय निघण्टुराजः । (रा.नि.)

There are two persons known as the authors of this work.

(1) Narasimha Pandita- Cat.No. 231 BORI 926/1887-91

Cat.No. 13254 GOMM

Cat.No. 11289 SMT

Cat.No. 935 OMU 3398

(2) Narahari-Cat.No. 205 MOIB 1587

Cat.No. 1641 SMU

Cat.No. CCS.

Many consider that both the author are one and same. Cat.No. 231 BORI also quotes Narasimha as Narahari Pandita (Saka 1719). Therefore Narahari son of Iswara Suri is considered as the author of this work. He was the chief administrator/king of the Kashmir dynasties. (Some scholars express doubt about king Narahari as the son of Suri who is a religious head).

Narahari mentioned Madana pala Nighantu (1374 AD). So his date may be assigned as 14 AD or beging of 15 AD. He is after Amara Simha and Prof. H.H.Wilson puts him in 12-13 AD. It is also opined that he belongs to Deccan as many names indicate the terms used in Maharashtra and Karnataka.

For the first time Narahari gave first place to Dravyaguna among Ashtangas of Ayurveda. द्रव्याभिदानगदनिश्चय कायसौख्यं, शल्यादिभूतविषनिग्रह-बालवैद्यम् । (रा.नि. २०/४२)

This is the first leixcon which recognized the importance of nomenclature of plants.

नामानि क्वचिदिह रूढितः स्वभावात् देशोक्तया क्वचन च लाञ्छनोपमाभ्याम् ।
वीर्येण क्वचिदितराह्वयादिदेशात् द्रव्याणां ध्रुवमिति सप्तधोदितानि ।। (रा.नि.)

He introduced many new plants. Being a learned physician and grammarian the material is well discussed and arranged. Therefore we can certify that "of all the Nighantus available at present, this is the best one."

This text contains 23 vargas. But only 10 vargas (3 to 12 vargas) are allotted for vegetable drugs i.e.; 780 herbs, excluding 74 drugs of Suvarnadi varga. The remaining 13 vargas deal with other general aspects and diet etc. The total vargas are:

(1) Anupadi (2) Bhumyadi (Dharanyadi) (3) Guduchyadi (4) Satahvadi (5) Parpatadi (6) Pippalyadi (7) Mulakadi (8) Salmalyadi (9) Prabhadradi (10) Karaveeradi (11) Amradi (12) Chandanadi (13) Suvarnadi (14) Paniyadi (15) Ksheeradi (16) Shalyadi (17) Mamsa (18) Manushyadi (19) Simhadi (20) Rogadi (21) Satlwadi (22) Misrakadi (23) Ekarthadi.

Some writers place this text even later to Bhavaprakasa basing upon the following points.

(1) Peeta Karaveera is described in this text but missing in Bhavaprakasa.

(2) Karpura tail, Taila Pipilika, Krishna beeja, Surakshara etc., described in Raja Nighantu are not found in Bhavaprakasa.

(3) Kulanjan is described in Raja Nighantu but it was called as Mahabhari Vacha in Bhavaprakasa.

(4) Raja Nighantu mentioned about Jhandu which is not there in Bhavaprakasa.

Therefore Ra.Ni. is placed in and around 17 AD.

The vargas possessing vegetable drugs are as following:

1. Guduchyadi or Valli Varga - creepers or climbers are present. It deals with Guduchi to Palasi-52 drugs.

2. Satahvadi varga - small shrubs are present. e.g.: Satahva, Chakramarda, Apamarga, Kasa marda etc-80 drugs.

3. Parpatadi varga	- herbs are present e.g.: Parpati, Jeevaka, Rishabhaka, Brahmi, Kulutha etc -60 durgs
4. Pippalyadi varga	- products of economic value are de scribed in it as Panyaoushaddhas e.g.: Hingu, Sunthi, Ela, Maricha etc. -95 drugs.
5. Mulakadi or Saka varga	- vegetables are present e.g.: roots, tu bers leaves and fruits- 104 drugs.
6. Shalmalyadi varga	- trees and grasses growing in forest areas are present. It deals with Shalmali to Hijjala -72 drugs.
7. Prabhadradi or Vriksha varga	- mostly wild trees are present. e.g.: Agnimantha, Kutaja, Karanja, Bhurja etc. -65 durgs.
8. Karaveeradi or Uttamsa varga	- flowering plants are present. e.g.: Jasmine, lotus, Artemisia etc -86 drugs.
9. Āmradi Varga	- mostly fruits are described -109 drugs.
10. Chandanadi Varga	- This is a class of aromatic plants -57 drugs.

He divided the plants basically into four groups: (i) Vanaspathi (ii) Vānaspathi (iii) Kshupa or Valli and (iv) Oushadhi.

Some of the important drugs are:

Lingini, Somavalli, Amrita Srava, Dhumra Patra, Rudanti, Hasthi Sundi, Dugdha pheni, Jhandu, Kulanjan, Kaaraskara etc.

(11) Kaiyadeva Nighantu

This book is otherwise known as 'Pathya pathya Vibodhini'. Its author Kaiyadeva is the son of 'Saranga' and grandson of Pandita Padmanabha. He is the author of another text-'Nama Ratnakara, which deals with synonyms of various herbs. It is assumed therefore that Kaiyadeva might have written this lexicon to mention the properties (Guna-Karmas) of the herbs described in his earlier text.

P.K. Gode consider his period as earlier to 1450 AD. Though Ahiphena, Bhanga and Yasada were mentioned in the Chikitsa Granthas during 12 AD, Nighantu incorporated them during 13 AD. Kaiyadeva Nighantu do not possess Ahiphena. Bhanga is also reported in Dhanya Varga. Seetalika, Soma roga are only described during 12 AD texts. These two are described under Vihara Varga in Kaiyadeva Nighantu. Hence this book is definitely placed after 12 AD. It resembles Madana pala Nighantu in description style. Peeta Karaveera which is missing with Madanapala's book is present in Kaiyadeva nighantu. However Madanapala did mention about Sweta & Rakta varieties of Karaveera. From these references it is desirable to place this text around 15 AD. Therefore many consider it as belonging to 1425-1450 AD. The author might have belonged to Gujarat as he described Jhule, Vellantara, Tilaparni etc.

This text is divided into 9 vargas. They are:

1. Oushadhi Varga
2. Dhatu Varga
3. Dhanya Varga
4. Drava Varga
5. Pakwanna Varga
6. Mamsa Varga
7. Vihara Varga
8. Mishraka Varga
9. Nanartha Varga.

Acharya Surendra Mohan edited and published the first volume (Oshadhi Varga) through Meharchand Lakshman das from Lahore in 1928. The editor quotes that the manuscript found in Mumbai is the best and complete. However, Acharya P.V. Sharma opines that no manuscript is possessing 9th varga i.e.: Nanartha Varga.

Under Oushadhi varga Madhu Karkati, Pinda kharjura, Kanta-karanja, Babbula, Sinduri, Markandi etc., are described. Grinjana terms is used as synonym for both carrot and onion. Maha nimba is considered to be Bakayana. Amla vetasa is mentioned as Sakhamla. Revandachini's branch-like material was used as Vrikshamla.

(12) Shiva Kosha

Its author Shivadatta Mishra belongs to a traditional Ayurvedic family and his father is famous Vaidya Chaturbhuja Mishra.

This text is composed of 540 verses. The Oushadha dravyas and their synonyms are described alphabetically in Sanskrit. The author claimed his work as 'Nanartha Oushadha Kosha'. It is compiled on the basis of many lexicons of earlier times. This book is written in 1677 AD.

He also wrote another book called 'Sanjna Samuchchaya' (1719 AD) which deals with Nidana, Chikitsa and Dravyaguna. He also wrote a commentary on his own text Sivadatta Kosha with the name Siva Prakasa.

This text was edited and published by Harshe R.G., of Deccan college, Pune in 1952.

P.K. Gode concluded Sivadatta's period as 1625-1700 AD.

(13) Dravya Guna Sataka

Its author Trimalla bhatta also written another book called 'Yoga Tarangini'. This book is also known as 'Dravya Guna Sata Sloki'. It mainly deals with diet substances. Initially the effect of tastes (Rasa) on doshas is discussed and there after subject matter is discussed in 15 vargas (Starting with Jala varga and ending with Suvarnadi varga). After including the concluding verse there are 102 verses in this text.

Lead and Zinc are missing under the Suvarnadi varga. His style resembles that of Madana pala. Carrot is given a new name 'Garjara' instead of 'Grinjana'. In Kritanna varga also several new items were included: e.g.: पुष्पवती (कुलौडी), कचवती (कचौडी), जलवलिवलय (जलेबी) etc.

(14) Abhidhana Ratnamala

There is no indication about the author except some information in a manuscript found at Madras (Ms. No. D 13257 of Govt. Oriental Mss Library, Madras) which mention that the work is composed by a person who is the elder brother of Chatura Rachita (Chatura Rakshita).

As the famous commentator Mallinatha (14 AD) quoted about this work, it may be placed in 12-13 AD. This text is otherwise known as 'Shadrasa Nighantu'. It is less known in North India.

The subject matter is arranged in six chapters on the basis of taste (Rasa). The classification is mainly based upon Charaka & Suśruta

Samhitas. At the chapter begining a list of drugs which are going to be discussed are provided followed by one by on description with synonyms. As Rasa is the criteria of classification, vegetable, animal and mineral drugs are included in the respective taste groups. They are as following:

1. Madhura Skandha		-	102 drugs
2. Amla	"	-	32 "
3. Lavana	"	-	1 "
4. Tikta	"	-	128 "
5. Katu	"	-	70 "
6. Kashaya	"	-	115 "
Total		=	448 drugs

(15) Raja Vallabha Nighantu

It was originally written by Rajavallabha Vaidya and later redacted by Narayana Dasa. This text is classified into six chapters (6 Paricchedas). Importance is given to the drugs used in Dina charya (daily regimen).

Though the authors time is doubtful he used some verses of Bhavamishra & Madana pala. Hence placed between 17-18 AD. The redactor Narayana Das belongs to 1760.

1. Prathama Parichcheda	-	about Dinacharya (daily regimen)
2. Dwitiya "	-	about the Dravya varga.
3. Tritiya "	-	about diet etc.
4. Chaturtha "	-	about learning process & teaching.
5. Panchama "	-	about age groups, Brahma charya
6. Shashtah "	-	Nanoushadhi Varga.

(16) Nighantu Ratnakara

This text is written by Vishnu Vasandeva Godabole in 1867 AD. In this the Sanskrit verses have translation in Marathi language also.

The subject matter is discussed under two parts viz., Prathama khanda & Dwitiya khanda. The first part (Guna Dosha Prakarana) deals with Dravyaguna aspects followed by Shareera, Ashta sthana Pariksha,

Mana-Paribhasha, Rasa Sastra, Arka Prakasa, Ajeerna Manjari etc. The second part deals with Nidana and Chikitsa.

Some of the important drugs mentioned in this text are: Ākara Karabha, Kākodumbara, Kulanjan, Kankushta, Agnijara, Tuvaraka, Tamra Patra, Karpura taila, Pudina, Makhana, Raktanga (Madayantika), Rasa karpura, Rudanti, Seetaphala, Nava Sadara etc.

(17) Saligrama Nighantu

This text is being considered as the last in the series of classical nighantus. It was written by Lala Saligrama Vaidya of Muradabad (U.P.) . It was completed in 1896 AD. The author mentioned about many new drugs brought to India by the foreigners in modern times.

This text is divided into two parts viz., Purvartha (part-I) and Uttarartha (part-II). First part contains 23 Vargas:

(1) Karpuradi (2) Haritakyadi (3) Guduchyadi (4) Pushpa (5) Phala (6) Vatadi (7) Dhatupadhatu (8) Visha (9) Dhanya (10) Saka (11) Vari (12) Dugdha (13) Dadhi (14) Takra (15) Navanita (16) Ghrita (17) Mutra (18) Taila (19) Arka (20) Madhu (21) Ikshu (22) Sandhana (23) Sankhya Vargas.

Second part possess only two vargas viz., Anupadi varga and Misraka varga. At the end of the text an annexure is provided.

He is the author of another book "Saligrama oushadha Sabda Sagara" and written commentaries on several books.

(18) Madanadi Nighantu

This book is a glossary in Sanskrit and is written by Chandranandana. It is other wise known as 'Guna Nighantu'.This author and the author of Padartha Chandrika commentary on Ashtanga Hridaya appear to be one and the same.

The work is based upon several groups of drugs i.e., Ganas described in Ashtanga Hridaya Sutra Sthana 15 chapt. As the text starts with Madanadi Gana it is named as Madanadi Nighantu.

Chandranandana is the son of Ravinandana and is often cited as an authority in lexicography by Ksheera Swamy. His time is fixed between 10-11 AD on the basis of available evidences.

Though it is claimed to possess 33 Ganas only 32 are available in the present text. The Paris manuscript alone seems to teach 33 Ganas.

(19) Mahoushadha Nighantu

It is written by Aryadasa Kumara Singha of Ceylone and published with Hindi commentary in 1971 from Varanasi.

The subject matter is compiled after consulting several other nighantus and treatises. It consists of 7 vargas. Coffee, Tea etc. are also mentioned in this work.

(20) Abhinava Nighantu

It is written by Pandit Dattaram Choube of Mathura. It mainly describes single drugs with their morphological features and pharmacological properties.

(21) Nighantu Sesha

This text was written by Jaina Acharya Hemachandra in 12 AD. It deals with synonyms mainly. There are six khandas (6 chapters) in this text: (1) Vriksha ḳanda (2) Gulma ḳanda (3) Lata ḳanda (4) Saka ḳanda (5) Trina ḳanda (6) Dhanya ḳanda.

Some of the important drugs are: Rudraksha, Putranjeeva, Chanakya Mulaka, Yavanala etc.

(22) Vanaushadhi Darsika

Author of this book Thakur Balavant Singh claimed it as a guide to sub-Himalayan herbs. It is compiled in 1950s.

After his post-graduation in Botany he worked as lecturer in Ayurvedic unit of B.H.U. and had done commendable work in the identification of herbs.

This text consists of about 269 drugs with botanical descriptions mainly.

He is the author of many books. "Glossary of vegetable drugs in Brihat Trayee" is his another great work.

(23) Vaidyavatamsa

It is very small nighantu with 7 vargas. The author Lolamba raju belongs to 11 AD. The text mainly deals with dietary materials and consists of only 57 verses totally. Aswabala is mentioned under leafy vegetables in this text.

(24) Ayurveda Vijnanam

The author of this text Kaviraj Vinodalal Sen (19 AD) belongs to West Bengal. It consists of four parts viz., (1) Sutra Sthana (2) Sareera Sthana (3) Dravya Sthana (4) Nidana-chikitsa Sthana

Under Dravya Sthana several drugs with their synonyms, properties, uses, dosage are mentioned along with pictures. Drugs are classified on the basis of their pharmacological action e.g.: Vrishya Varga, Vataghna Varga etc.

New drugs like Dhusa Raja (Rumi Mastagi), Sudha muli (Salammisri), Katu veera, Shyam Parni (tea), Sardula kanda (Vana Palandu), Seeta Beeja (Isafgol) etc. are mentioned.

The substitutes for Ashta varga are mentioned in the following way:

(1) Jeevaka	-	Guduchi
(2) Rishabhaka	-	Vamsa lochana
(3) Meda	-	Aswagandha
(4) Maha meda	-	Sariva
(5) Kakoli (6) Ksheera Kakoli	}	Shatavari
(7) Ridhi	-	Bala
(8) Vriddhi	-	Maha bala

(25) Siddh Bheshaja Mani Mala

It is written by Krishna Rama Bhatta in 1886. The subject matter is discussed in 5 Gucchas (5 chapters). The author mentioned about many of his experiences along with classical compound preparations. Many practical experiences of physicians in and around Jaipur are also documented.

He himself claimed that he performed mercury purification several times.

In the second chapter totally 18 vargas are described. Under Haritakyadi varga drugs like Mamira, Kasani etc. are described.

(26) Nighantu Adarsh

Its author Vaidya Bapalal is born at Sanasoli village of Gujrat in 1896. His knowledge on drug identification and contraversial drugs is exquisite. Most of his works are in Gujarati while some are translated into Hindi.

This text is available in two volumes at present which deals with synonyms, etymology, botanical descriptions, properties & therapeutic uses. This is one of the complete texts on Dravyaguna.

(27) Dravya Guna Vijnanam

Yadavji Trikamji Acharya is the author of this work which is published in two parts. Sri. Yadavji Trikamji born in 1881 at Porbundar.

He is a man with high scholarship. He edited and published Charaka Samhita, Suśruta Samhita & Madhavanidana from Nirnaya Sagar Press, Mumbai.

He also edited: Rasa Prakasa Sudhakara, Gada Nigraha, Raja Martanda, Nadi Pariksha, Vaidya Manorama, Dhara Paddhati, Rasa Kamadhenu, Kshema Kutuhalam etc.

His other works are: Siddha Yoga Sangraha, Rasamrita and Ayurveda Vyadhi Vijnanam.

The first part of Dravya Guna Vijnana consists of fundamental concepts on Dravya, Guna, Rasa, Vipaka and Veerya as five chapters. Under this, the openions of Dr. Balakrishna Amarji Pathak (a modern physician) are also published.

The second part is meant for the single drugs which are described with names, properties and uses etc.

(28) Dravya Guna Vijnanam

Acharya Priya Vrata Sharmaji published his work in 5 volumes form Varanasi (Chaukhambha Press)

Vol. I - fundamental principles of Dravyugna

Vol. II - herbal drugs

Vol. III - animal & mineral drugs

Vol. IV - pictures

Vol. V - literature of Ayu. herbs etc.

P.V. Sharmaji published and edited several books.

(29) Sandigdha Nirnaya

This is written by Sri Bhagiratha Swamy (Ayurveda Mahamahopadhyay) in 1936 from Calcutta. It deals with the controversial aspects on several drugs.

Siddhoushadha Manimala, Atma Sarwaswa and Ayurveda Vijnana are his other books.

(30) Vanoushadhi Darpanam

Its author is Kaviraj Virajacharan Gupta. It is published in two parts i.e., first part in 1908 and second part in 1909.

(31) Vanaspati Sastra

Jayakrishna Indraji Thakur written and published in 1910. He learnt a good deal of subject on medicinal herbs through Vaidya Bapalal. K.R. Kirtikar who is the author of Indian Medicinal plants consulted him several times to know about contraversial drugs. This indicates about his knowledge on contraversial drugs.

3. Modern Books on Medicinal Plants

(1) Pharmacographia Indica

It was written by William Dymogk, C.J.H. Wardon & David Hooper in 1890. It is considered to be the first book on Indian medicinal plants which is published along with the reports of Scientific/experimental studies. Even toxicity studies are also reported.

(2) Indian Medicinal Plants

K.R. Kirtikar and B.D. Basu published it from Delhi in 1918. Being a botanist Kirtikar described the morphological and taxonomical aspects. Most importantly the picture drawings of many medicinal plants are made available for the first time through this work.

Kirtikar expired in 1917 and then Basu completed this work.

This book is published in four parts of description and four parts of plates consisting of pictures.

(3) Indian Materia Medica

Dr. K.M. Nadkarni is the author of this work. After an extensive study it is published in 1908 in two parts. First part deals with fundamental concepts of Ayurveda, measurements, posology, times of administration etc., along with 2671 herbs. The second part deals with the animal products and mineral drugs.

(4) Dictionary of Economic Products of India

George Watt published this work in 1908. This work consists of economic products arranged in the alphabetical order in English. Many of the medicinal herbs their identity and utility are discussed in this work.

(5) Indigenous Drugs of India

Col. R.N. Chopra had written this in 1954. He is a modern doctor who studied Ayurvedic herbs and conducted research on them. He published the results of his experimental studies in this work.

He is the author of Glossary on Medicinal plants also.

Few more important books are the following:

i. Wealth of India (11 volumes) – Chopra et al., CSIR.

ii. Indian Medicinal Plants (2 volumes) – G.V. Satyavati et al, ICMR.

iii. Treatise of Indian Medicinal Plants (5 volums) – CSIR.

iv. Compendium of Indian Medicinal Plants (6 volums) – CSIR

v. The Indian Medicinal Plants (5 volums) – Orient Longman.

vi. Materia Medica of Hindusthan – Ainsle (1813)

vii. Flora India – Roxburgh (1874)

viii. Bombay Drugs – Sakharam Arjun (1879)

ix. Materia Medica of the Hindus – V.C. Dutt (1922 2nd edition)

REFERENCE BOOKS

1. Amara Kosha with "**Rāmāśrami" commentary**
   Varanasi: 1983.
2. Ambikadatta Shastri; **Rasa Ratna Samuchchaya**
   Varanasi: 1976.
3. Ambikadatta Shastri; **Bhaiṣhajya Ratnāvaḷi**
   Varanasi: 1987.
4. Atridev Gupta; **Ashtānga Sangraha**
   Mumbai: 1951.
5. Atridev Gupta; **Ayurvēd Kā Brihat Itihās**
   Varanasi: 1982.
6. Balwant Singh Thakur & Chunekar K.C.
   Glossory of Vegetable Drugs in Brihat Trayee
   Varanasi: 1990.
7. Bapalal Vaidya; **Some Controversial Drugs in IndIan Medicine**
   Varanasi: Chaukhambha Orientalia, 1982.
8. Chunekar K.C.; **Bhāva Prakāśa Sighantu**
   Varaṇasi: 1984.
9. Clarenece Wilbur Taber; Tabler's **Cyclopedic Medical Dictionary**
   Philadelphia: 1960.
10. Dāmodar Joshi; **Rasa Sastra**
    Trivandrum: 1986.
11. Dharmananda; **Rasatarangini**
    Delhi: 1979.
12. Dhawan B.N. et al.; Use of Pharmaceutical Techniques for Study of Natural Products. Lucknow: 1992.
13. Dhyani s.c.; **Dravya guna siddhānta**
    Varanasi: 1986.
14. Dhyani s.c.; **Rasa Panchak** (Ayurvedic Principles of Drug Action)
    Varanasi: 1982.
15. Dwarakanath c.; **"Digestion and Metabolism in Ayurveda"**
    Calcutta: 1967.
16. Dwarakanath c.; **Fundamental Principles of Ayurveda.**
    vol. I to vol. III. Mysore: 1952.

17. Bhagavan Dash; **Concenpt of Agni in Ayurveda**
Varanasi
18. Eric W. Marbin; **Husa's Pharmaceutical Dispensing**
Easton Pensylvania: 1959.
19. Goodman L.S. & Gillman A.; **The Pharmacological Basis of Therapeutics**
New York: 1996.
20. Govardhana Sharma Changani, **Aṣaṭāñga Samgraha (Sutra)**
Varanasi: 1986.
21. Gune; **Oushadhi Gunadharma Sāstra (5 Vols.)** Pune
22. Hanumantha Rao M.; **Tri-ḅhāsha Dictionary**
Rajahmundry: 1987.
23. Hanumantha Rao N.; **Panchabhuta Theory**
Vijayawada: 1996.
24. Hari Shastri P.; **Ashtānga Hridaya**
Varanasi: Chaukhambha Orientalia. 1982.
25. Khemraj Sri Kishan Das; **SāligrĀma nighantu**
26. Kulkarni A.D.; **Rasa Ratna Samuchchaya**
New Delhi: 1982.
27. Mohammad Ali; **Text Book of Pharmacology**
Delhi: 1994.
28. Mohanlal G.; **Guna parijnānam**
Jamnagar: 1961.
29. Narayana Vittal Purandhare; **Rājani Ģhaṇtu Sahita Dhanwantari Nighaṇtu,** Pune: 1896.
30. Neal M.J.; **"Medical Pharmacology at a glance"**
London: 1989.
31. Nisteswar K.; **Dravya Guna Maulika Siddhāntamulu**
Vijayawada: 1986.
32. Parashu Rama Shastri; **Śārangḍhara Samhita.**
Mumbai: 1920
33. Pawan Kumra R. Godatwar; **Ayurvedic Check-List (CCIM syllabus and Text Books)**.Varanasi: 2000
34. Phadke; **Draya Guna Sāstram.**
Mumbai: 1989.
35. Ramgopal Shashtri; **Vedon Mein Ayurveda**
Delhi: 1956.

36. Rajeswara, Datta Shastri; **Bhaishajya Ratnavali**
Varanasi: 1979.
37. Ram Prasad; **Madana Pāla Nighantu**
Mumbai: 1954.
38. Rama Raksha Pathak; **Padārtha Vijnāna.**
Nagpur: 1978.
39. Ranajit Rai Desai; **Āyurvēdīya Padārtha Vijnāna.**
Nagpur: 1974.
40. Sastry J.L.N.; **Introduction to Oncology in Ayurveda**
Hyderabad: 1999.
41. Sastry V.L.N.; **Koumārabhritya Sāramu**
Hyderabad: 1989.
42. Sastry V.V.S.; **Tridosha Theory**
Kottaikkal: 1981.
43. Satoshkar & Bhandarkar; **Pharmacology and Pharmacotherapeutics**
Mumbai: 1996.
44. Satyadeva Dube; **Dravyaguna Sutram**
Varanasi
45. Sarandini A. Dahanukar & Urmila M. Tatte; **Ayurveda Revisited**
Bombay: 1998.
46. Satyavati G.V. etal.; **Medicinal Plants of Inida. Vol. I& II)**
New Delhi: 1978 & 1987.
47. Sharma P.V.; **Ayurveda Ka Vaijnanika Itihas**
Varanasi: 1981.
48. Savnur H.V.; **Ayurvedic Materia Medica**
Delhi: 1950 & 1988.
49. Sharma P.V.; **Chakra Datta**
Varanasi: Chaukhambha Orientalia. 1995.
50. Sharma P.V.; **Dōsha Kāraṇa Tattwa Mīmāmsa**
Varanasi: 1986.
51. Sharma P.V.; **Dravyaguna Vijnanam. (Vol. I)**
Varanasi: 1984.
52. Satya Pāla; **Kashyapa Samhita**
Varanasi: 1953.

53. Sharma P.V.; **History of Indian Medicine**
New Delhi: 1995.
54. Sharma P.V.; **Introduction to Dravya Guna**
Varanasi: 1984.
55. Sharma P.V. & Guru Prasad Sharma; **Kaiyadeva Nighantu**
Varanasi: 1979.
56. Sharma P.V.; **Mādhava Dravya Guna**
Varanasi: 1993.
57. Sharma P.V.; **Siddha Mantra & Hridaya Dīpikā**
Varanasi: 1977.
58. Sharma P.V.; **Soḍhala Nighantu**
Varanasi: 1972.
59. Udupa K.N.; **Advances in Research in Indian Medicine**
Varanasi: 1970.
60. Venkatacharya P.B.A.; **"Kaya Chikitsa Siddhantamulu"**
Hyderabad: 1988.
61. Viswanatha Dwivedi; **Āyurvēdīya Oushdhiyon Ka Vargikarna**
Jamnager: 1966.
62. Editor; **Rasa Vaiseshika** (with Nārasimha Bhashya).
Trivandrum: 1976.
63. Viswanatha Dwivedi; **Oushadha Vijnana Sastra**
Panta: 1987.
64. Tripathi S.N. etal., **Concept of Jātharāgni and Ḍhātwagni in Ayurveda.**
New Delhi: 1987.
65. Yadavji Trikamji; **Dravyaguna Vijnana Vol. I**
Nagpur: 1986.
66. Yadavji Trikamji; **Charaka Samhita**
Mumbai: 1924.
67. Yadaji Trikamji; **Sushrita Samhita**
Varanasi: 1980.
68. Venkateswara Sastry Mukkamala; **Bhava Prakasa**
Vijayawada: 1959.
69. Yeturi Srinivasa Charyulu; **Yoga Ratnākaramu**
Nellore: 1939.

70. Wallis T.E.; **Text Book of Pharmaco Gnosy**
Delhi: 1985.

71. Dwarakanath C.; **The Development of Indian Medicine Sarngadharaś Contribution**
New Delhi: 1991.

72. Ashutosh Kar; **Medicinal Chemistry**
New Delhi: 1996.

73. Parimoo P.; **A Text Book of Medicinal Chemistry**
New Delhi: 1995.

74. Dinesh Chandra Sharma; **Vedon Mein Dravyaguna Sāstra**
Jamnagar: 1989.

75. Chaudhri R.D.; **"Herbal Drugs Industry"**
New Delhi: 1996.

Index

A

Abhava dravya
Achetana dravy
Achintya 81
Abhidāna Ratnamala 423
Abhinava Nighantu 426
Adbhuta karma 182
Āgneya dravya 10,21
Agni bhuta 7
Āgama 182
Ahamkāra 7
Āhāra dravya 28
Classification 43,44
Ākasa bhuta 7
Ākasa dravya 10,21
Anasana 19
Andaja 23
Anupana 357-361
Ap bhuta 7
Āpya dravya 10,22
Āptopadesa 169
Ārambha samarthya 16
Ashta Prakriti 8
Āsrayatwa 16
Ashta vidha virya vada 162
Ashtanga nighantu 405
Ātma 10
Ātma guna 78,79
Avastha paka 131-133
Āyurveda Vijnanam 427
Avyakta 7,9
Āyurveda 1

B

Bhuta 5
Bhumi 296
Bhutadi 7
Bhouma dravya 22,26
Bheshaja Prayoga-Marga 381,385
Bombay Drugs 430

C

Charakokta varga 41,42
Chaturvimsati tattwas 8
Chetana 19
— Antah 19
— Bahirantah 19
Chikitsa chatushpada 11
Circadian Rhythms 370-372,379
Compendium of Indian-Medicinal Plants 430

D

Darsana 181
Daivapratighata 181
Dhatupadehat 153
Dhanwantari Nighantu 407-409
Dictionary of Economic products of India 430
Dravya 1,4
— Medicinal properties of 10

Dravya Importance of 12
— gata Panchapadarthas 1
— Guna–Karma 1
— guna Sangraha 416-417
Dravyaguna sataka 423
Dravyaguna vijnanam
— P.V. Sharma 428
— Yadavji Tri Kamji 428
Dravya virya vada 161-162
Drisyabhuta 6
Drug combinations 339-340
Dwi-vidha Vipaka vada 144-145
Dwi-vidha Virya vada 162-163
Dwyanuka 6

E

Endothermic 2
Ekadasa Indriyas 7
Ekadesa Sadhyatwa 17
Exothermic 2

F

Flora India 430
(Flora of British India)
Formulation of compound-
drugs 338-339,345

G

Gulma 25
Guna 1,2
— etymology of 45
— characters of 45-46
— classification of 47-48
— Importance of 85-87
— Pharmocological
— activity of 79-81
Guna References of 88
— virya vada 162-163
Gurvadi gunas 48-66

H

History of Dravyoguna 381-399
–brief history of DG 381-382,388
–DG in vedic literature 382-389,395
–DG in Samhita
–granthos 389-499
Hridaya deepaka
nighantu 413-416,421

I

Ideal drug 337-338
Incompatibility 343-349,355
Indian Materia Medica 430-431
Indian Medicinal Plants
— Kirtikar & Basu 429
— Satyavati G. 430
Indigenous Drugs of India 430
Index 436-441

J

Jala Bhuta 7
Jangama dravya 22
Jarayuja 23

K

Kaiyadeva nighantu 421-422,429
Karma 1,3
Karma Karana 169
Karma virya vada 163-164
Kramapekshitatwa 16

L

Lata 25

M

Madanadi nighantu 425
Madanapala nighantu 417-418
Madhava Dravyaguna 414-416
Mahabhuta 6
Mahat 7
Mahoushadhi nighantu 426
Materia Medica of Hindus 430
Materia Medica of Hindusthan 430
Matra 349-357

N

Neutron 7
Nighantus of medieval times 402-405
Nighantu Ādarsh 428-429
Nighantu Ratnakara 424
Nirindriya 19
Nishta paka 133-135
Nityatwa 14
Number of drugs inancient literature 399-401,407

O

Oudbhida 22,24
Oushadha dravya 28
Oushadha Prayogakala 363-379
  modern view 370-373
Oushadhi 25

P

Pancha bhutas 7,8
Pancha bhuta theory 5
Panchendriya grahyatwa 15
Pancha padarthas 1
Pancha tanmatras 7,8
Pancha vidha vipaka vada 142-143
Paradi gunas 66-76
Paribhashika virya vada 162-163
Parthiva 22,26
Parthiva dravya 10,22
Parts used 340-343
Paryaya ratnamala 405-407
Pharmacographia Indica 429
Physical properties in drug action 81-85
Posology 349-357
Prakriti sama samaveta 178
Pratighata Samarthya 18
Prescription writing 379-380
Prabhava–2; 172-182
— etymology of 172
— characters of 172-177
— functions of 177-178
— superiority of 181-182
Purusha 10

Q

Quality (Guna) 1,2

R

Rajah 7
Raja nighantu 418-421,428
Raja vallabha nighantu 424
Rasa–2; 89-129
— etymology 89
— definition 90
— characters 91
— number of 91-94

Rasa-2; modern view 94-96
— panchabhowtikatwa 96-98
— chemistry of 98-101
— effects of season 103-104
— method of testing 105-108
— transformation 108-111
properties & functions 111-112
— local actions 112-114
— systemic actions 114-117
— degree of activity 117-118
— combination &
— permutations 118-120
— exceptions to general
laws 120-121
— effect on dosha 121-122
— usage in Āhāra 123
— usage in vyādhi 122
— (usage in oushadha)
— Madhura (sweet) 123
— Amla (sour) 124
— Lavana (saltish) 125
— Katu (pungent) 125
— Tikta (bitter) 126
— kashaya (astringent) 126-127
— superiority of 127-128
— References 129
Rasa-Anurasa 102-103
Rasabhibhava 169
Rasopalabdhi 104-105
Routs of drug administration 373-385
Reference Books 431-435,442

S

Sakti Virya vada 161-162
Saligrama nighantu 425-426,432
Sandigdha nirnaya 429-430
Sapta padarthas 1
Sastra pramanya 16,153
Sattwa 7
Sendriya 19
Shadvidhi vipaka vada 141-142
Shiva kosha 422-423
Shodasa vikriti 8
Siddha bheshaja manimala 427
Siddha Mantra 412-413
Sodhala nighantu 409-412,418
Sravana 182
Sukshma bhuta 6
Suśruta nighantu 405
Sushrutokta vargas 38-40
Swajatyavasthanatwa 15
Swastha Urjaskara 11
Swedaja 23
Skandha 27-30
— (Madhura–Amla–Lavana–Katu–Tikta–Kashaya)

T

Taijasa 7
Tamas 7
Taratama yoganupalabdhi 17
The Indian Medicinal Plants 429
Times of drug administration 362-373
— modern view 370-373

Treatise of Indian
Medicinal Plants 429
Trividha Ahamkara 7
Trividha Vipaka vada 143-144
Tulya Rasa guna visesha 182

U

Udbhijja 23

V

Vagbhatokta varga 38-40,41
Vaidyavatamsa 426
Vaikarika 7
Vaiseshika guna 76-78
Valance 7
Vanaspati 24
Vanaspatya 25
Vanaspati sastra 429
Vanoushadhi darshika 426,429
Vaya viya dravya 10,21
Vehicle (Anupana) 357-361
Vichitrapratyayara
bdhatwa 178-181
Vikalpa samarthya 17
Vikriti Vishama samaveta 178
Vipaka–2; 130-153
— etymology 130
— characters 130
— analysis & determination 130-135
— modern view 135-139
— site of drug metabolism 139-140
— types of 140-145
— qualities of 146-147
— properties & function 147-149
— assessing vipaka 149-150
— experimental models of 150-151
— difference between
— Rasa & Vipaka 151-152
— superiority of 152-153
— references 153
Vipakapekshatwa 153
Viruddha 25
Viruddhatwa 344-350
Visha pratighata 181
Virya–2; 154-171
— etymology 154
— characters 154-155
— modern findings 155-159
— analysis of virya
— concept 159-160
— number of viryas 160-163
— functions of 104-164
Upalabdhi of virya 166-167
-general principles
& exceptions 167-168
— superiority of 168-169
— references 170-171
Virya pradhanikatwa 169
Vyavasthitatwa 14

W

Wealth of India 430

X

Xenobiotics 137